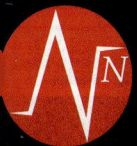

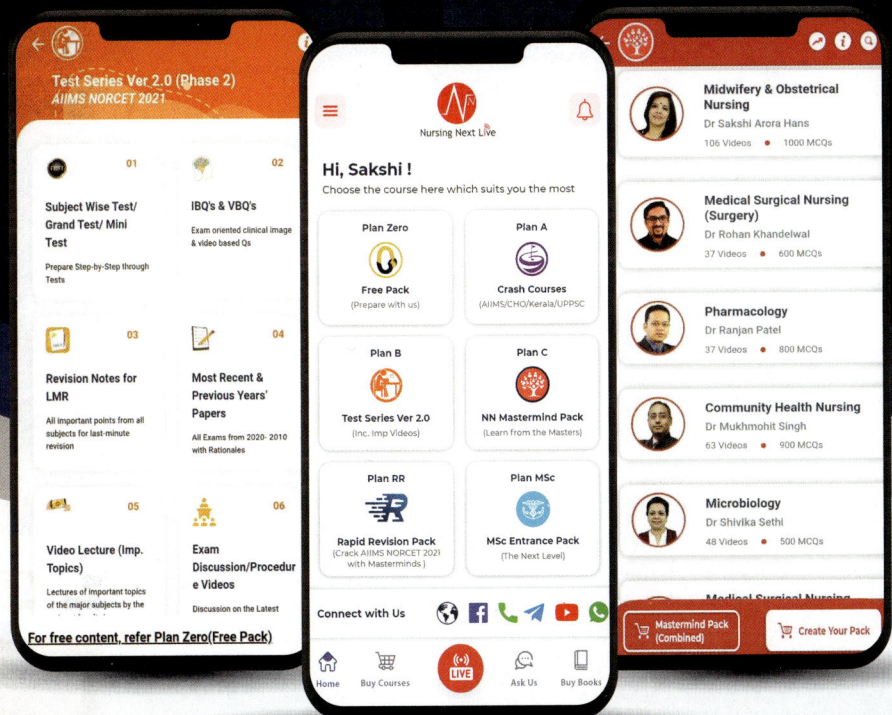
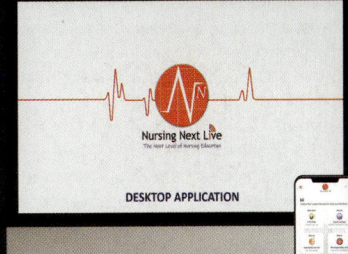
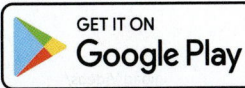
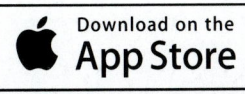

ABOUT US

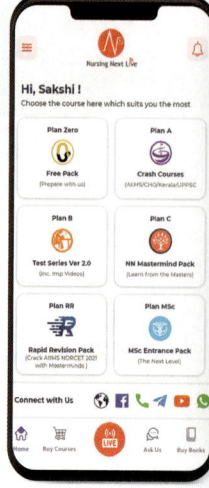

Nursing Next Live has been conceptualized based on the observation that there is a huge gap between the educational services available to the medical graduates and the nursing students. As these two are the strong pillars in providing holistic care to the patients, it is extremely vital that nurses should get equal exposure to access learning. To overcome this issue, we have come forward with the commitment of providing quality education to the nurses in India at their doorstep through Nursing Next Live. And therefore, we say **"We are bringing Learning to the People Instead of People Going for Learning".**

It is India's first and the biggest digital learning platform in the field of Nursing Education. The Nursing Next Live is an interactive self-assessment app, which helps you to build knowledge of nursing specialities any time and anywhere. In a span of one year we have magnified the nursing sector by upscaling it with the strategically designed Quality Content by the Top Medical Faculties of India. We at Nursing Next Live envisage that all students from Kashmir to Kanyakumari should get quality education. We pledge to give the best learning experience to all our students, under one single roof, and that is **"All-in-one and One-in-All platform".**

The Core Values and Principles of Nursing Next Live is:

• First Digital Learning platform for All Nursing Competitive & Undergraduates Exams with Futuristic Approach
• We are bringing Learning to People, Instead of People going for learning!
• Concept Based Teaching by TOP Medical & Nursing Educators (The Masterminds)
• "Quality Content" & "Smart-Study" Approach
• One in All, All in One! Nothing Beyond
• 360 Degree Approach for your complete Preparation
• Most Up to date & updated Content
• Best Guidance & Support at every step
• Best Interface with Unique & Advance Features
• Everything at one Platform ...Buy CBS Nursing Books at Special Discounts/Cashbacks

Nursing Next Live is the fastest-growing Edutech organization in the field of Nursing! With **70k+** downloads, **1200+** total number of selections, **150+** AIIMS NORCET 2020 Selections, and many backend achievements it is the Highest Ranked App on the Play Store. The idea was possible to bring into reality because it was backed by the team of best professionals who did not see time; had One vision and One Goal in Mind of providing the students Nothing but The Best! Their trust towards the vision for the brand and their efforts to continuously make it a success helped Nursing Next to reach to this position.

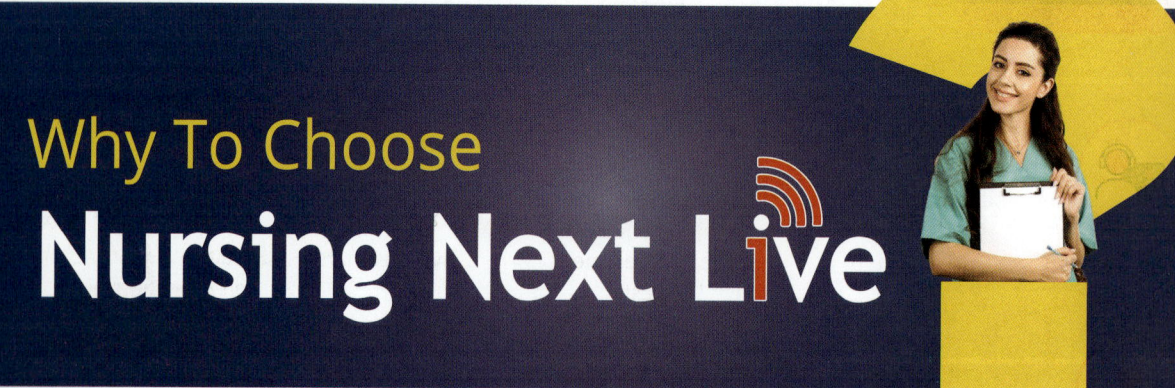

Why To Choose
Nursing Next Live

⊚ India's 1st Digital Learning Platform for all nursing competitive, nursing undergraduate and nursing postgraduate exams (One-in-All, All-in-One)
⊚ User friendly interface with unique & advanced features
⊚ Most Up-to-date & Quality Content based on New INC Syllabus
⊚ Conceptual learning with an integrated and futuristic approach
⊚ Smart Study under the guidance of India's Top Educators who are the masterminds of their subjects
⊚ Enhance your learning from Basic To Advance level with a 360-degree approach
⊚ Regular Live Doubt Sessions and Live Tests based on real-time exam pattern
⊚ TOP Selections in AIIMS NORCET, AIIMS MSc, BFUHS, CHO, SGPGI, JIPMER, RRB, DSSSB etc (From Rank 1 to 1000)
⊚ Study Planner that helps you to organize your study
⊚ Faculty-Student Meet (Forthcoming) that provides you an opportunity to meet with faculty and get clarify your doubts
⊚ Printed Booklet: You will get the printed notes of the video lectures that will save your time in notes making and organize your time in a better way
⊚ Customize Study which helps you to create your own pack depending on your needs and wants
⊚ Daily dose of information keeps you updated everyday with new information
⊚ One-in-all all-in-one: You will get exam oriented plan in the app for whatever exams you are targeting. Simulation Videos

THE COMPLETE PACKAGE

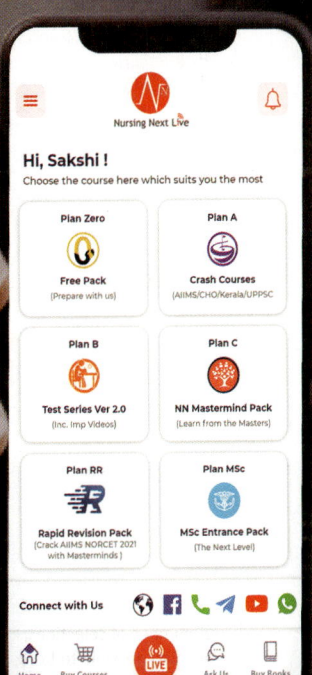

50,000+
MCQs with their Rationale

2000+
Hours of Recorded video lectures
(Covering All Subjects/All Topics/
Imp Topics Chanting Videos/Exam
Discussions/LMR/IBQ & VBQs
Discussions)

150+
Previous years' question papers
covering all National & State
Level Exams (2021-2010)

Monthly/Weekly/Daily
Live Doubt Sessions &
Faculty-Students' Meet (Forthcoming)

1500+
E-Notes/Flash cards of all the
subjects for Last-minute Revision

1000+
Image-based Questions with their
Rationale

200+
Video-based Questions with their
Rationale

Monthly
Special Mega Assessment Tests,
National Scholarship Test with up to
100% Scholarship & Reward points

200+
CBS Nursing Books available for
purchase

200+
Newly Created Subject-wise cum Topic-wise Test, Mini Test & Grand Tests
based on all important National Exams like AIIMS, PGIMER, JIPMER, DSSSB,
RRB & ESIC, also State level exams like Kerala PSC

Special Features

Live Classes

Live Doubt
Sessions

Mega Assessment
Tests

Live Webinars

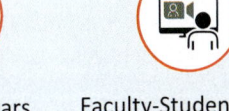
Faculty-Student Meet
on Zoom Sessions

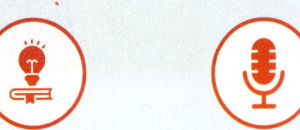
Study Plans

Success Stories

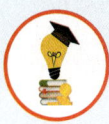
Daily Dose of
Knowledge

Blogs

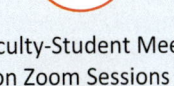
National Scholarship Test
with upto 100% scholarship

Any Doubt
Ask Us

Exam
Notifications

Buy CBS Nursing Books

Bookmark
Your Imp Topics

Download Videos/
Notes

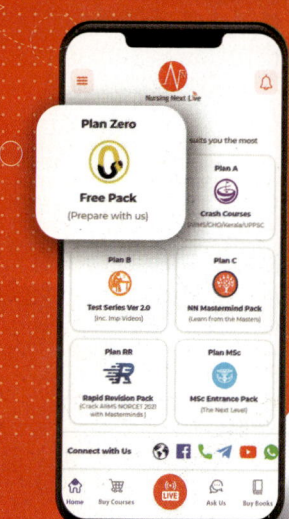

"जांचो, परखो, फिर खरीदो!"

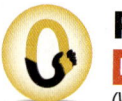

Plan ZERO

FREE PACK

(Validity Unlimited)

Nursing Next Live focuses on providing you the with the best and beyond, nothing less. In Plan ZERO we provide you the glimpse of the content from the various pack that gives you the rights to explore the contents in the App and help in taking the right decisions before selecting the pack.

WHY TO EXPLORE

- Glimpse of the content from the various packs
- TRY-TRUST-OPT. It provides you the rights to first analyze and then go for the best pack
- Enriched content

BEST FOR

- Those who want to explore before selecting the right pack
- Students who have an urge to gain the last momentum by giving a final touch to their preparation.

What all you will get

- **2000+** MCQs with Rationale covering All Subjects, Important Topics
- **150+** E-Notes covering All Subjects, Selective important Topics
- **100+** Hours of Lectures covering All Subjects (Topic-wise/Imp Topics/Chanting/Exam Discussions)
- **100+** IBQs & VBQs of All Subjects
- **15** Most Recent/Previous Years Papers with Rationale
- **5+** Grand Test & Bonus Test based on Real Time Exam Pattern
- **5+** National Scholarship test with negaitive marking, National Level Ranking & Cash Rewards
- Daily Dose of Knowledge— Word of the Day, Fact of the Day, Practice Pearls, Question of the Day
- Unsolved & Solved Question Papers of BSc 1st to 4th Year in a consolidated manner covering all Important Universities (Forthcoming)
- Monthly National Scholarship Test with Special Discount for Top Rankers
- How to Prepare for Exams (in the form of Study Planner/Videos)
- Complete Access to Target High Extra Edge Section – which includes additional MCQs & Golden Points in Video Form

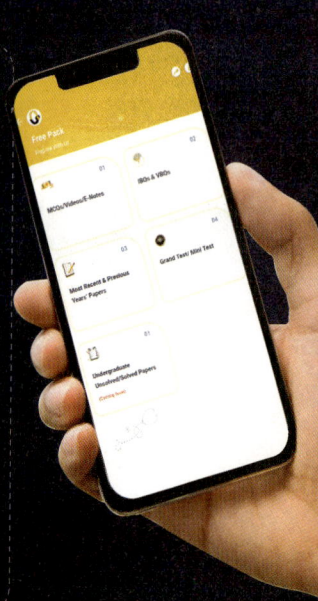

Selections in

Various Competitive Nursing Exams

What our glorified achievers say about Nursing Next Live

लक्ष्य तय है, तो PLAN A सही है!"

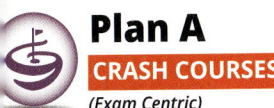

Plan A
CRASH COURSES
(Exam Centric)

you have a set target and working to achieve it then Plan A is the perfect plan for you. We have come up th this plan to help you prepare for a particular exam that includes exam-centric AIIMS NORCET 2020, PGI, CHO & Target Kerala PSC Crash Courses to help you get a hold of every topic in-depth. You get access in-detailed content of Real-Time Pattern of exams and their latest syllabus. Put your hands on the best!

WHY TO SUBSCRIBE
Exam specific, it targets the specific exam therefore its pattern syllabus is as per the targeted exam
Get Acquainted with exam pattern that helps you improve your skills
Helps in the last minute revision

BEST FOR
- Those who are preparing for specific exams and want to improve their knowledge by practicing
- Those who are working professionals and want to prepare for exams along with their jobs

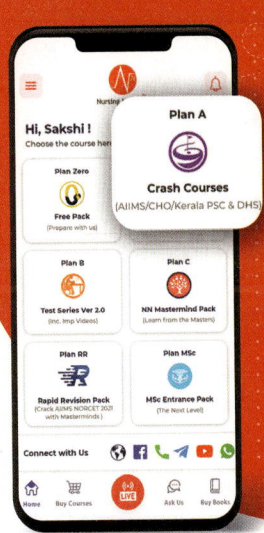

What all you will get

Plan A1
CHO Crash Course

- **35+** Subject-wise Tests & Grand Tests (including Bonus Tests & Previous Years Papers)
- **1500+** Questions with rationale
- **70+** E-notes for last-minute revision covering all he important topics as per the syllabus of CHO
- **30+** (Duration of 30+ Hours) Pre-recorded Videos given by top faculties in Hinglish covering every important topic from exam point of view

MRP ₹689/- | Validity 2 Months

Plan A2
AIIMS NORCET 2020 Crash Course

- **60+** Live Tests Subject-wise based on AIIMS Delhi pattern
- **1500+** Qs with Rationale including MCQs, IBQs, VBQs, Clinical skills, Priority setting, and case study
- **15+** Mock Test, Revision Test, and Grand Tests based on Real-time pattern of AIIMS Delhi with Negative Marking and National Level Ranking
- All Subject-wise Tests & Grand Tests are with Detailed Rationale
- **140+** Last-Minute Revision Notes based on Frequently asked Topics of previous Years
- **12+** Videos on Chanting Session by Top Educators/Subject Experts
- **35+** Multiple videos on special tricks for non-nursing subjects, tips on memory retention, strategies to attempt exams, etc.
- Success Guaranteed as we have had 150+ Selections (Rank 3 to 5k) in AIIMS NORCET 2020.

MRP ₹1499/- | Validity 2 Months

Plan A3
Target Kerala PSC Crash Course

- **60+** Subject-wise/Grand Tests with Rationale
- **320+** E-Notes in the form of Subject-wisesynopsis
- **50+** Hours of Videos in English (Important Topics Pre-loaded video + Chanting videos)
- In association with our Best-Selling Title- Target High Staff Nurse Entrance Exam

MRP ₹945/- | Validity 2 Months

Plan A4
UPPSC Staff Nurse Crash Course

- **40+** subject-wise tests which cover the complete syllabus from basics to advance
- **7** Grand Tests Based on real time exam pattern
- **3** Extra Edge Tests covering Important Positions, Important Nursing Procedures, Drug Calculation, suture techniques & COVID special)
- Previous Year Paper Discussion video helps you how to approach the correct answer
- **25+** Quick Revision videos in one-liner form that covers all the important points from the weightage subject
- **1** **"SUCCESS MANTRA"** video to guide you the right approach for preparation

MRP ₹1499/- | Validity 3 Months

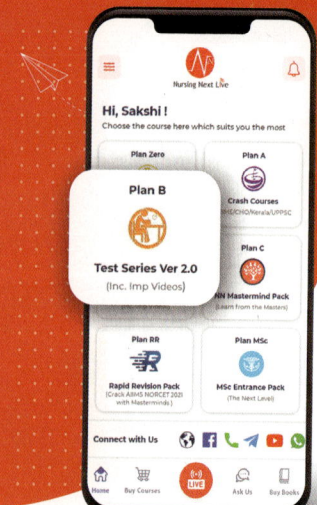

" आज का अभ्यास, आपके कल की सफलता! "

Plan B

Test Series Ver 2.0

(360° Approach)

Test series 2.0, as the name says to excel in any test, you need to base your learnings on two principles 1st practice, practice, practice, and then 2nd is a 360-degree approach. Variety of subject-wise and topic-wise test IBQs, and VBQs that follow the latest exam fashion to help you level up your preparatory work. To give complete touch to the preparation, we have covered all important national & state level last 15 years papers wit important topics/ exam discussion videos.

WHY TO SUBSCRIBE

- Comprehensive test pack with 360 degree approach for those who are targeting any staff nurse examination of National or State level
- Keep track of your progress through test analysis report
- Last-minute revision notes of important topics from all the subjects
- Detailed explanation helps you to enhance your knowledge

BEST FOR

- The students who want to delve into the topic and opt for extensive preparation for any staff nurse entrance exam.
- Who never want to stop learning and always look forward to upgrading their pre-acquired knowledge.
- Working students who don't want to compromise with their preparation and success.

What all you will get

Pre Loaded Content (Phase 1 + Phase 2)

- **190+** Newly Created Subject-wise, Mini Test and Grand Test focusing all important National Exams AIIMS, PGIMER, JIPMER, DSSSB, RRB and ESIC
- **15K+** Qs (MCQs, IBQs, VBQs) with Rationale and updated reference from standard textbooks. All the Tests are designed by the Subject Experts and Topper Students
- **400+** Hours Recorded Video Lectures of Nursing/Non-Nursing Subjects by some of India's best nursing faculties/subject experts. Lectures are in English/Hindi language focusing on concept-based learning.
- **5** Exam Discussion Videos of 2019 Exam papers (Duration 20 Hours)
- **150+** Hours of Recorded Video on Subject-wise Exam Discussion of previous years papers (2017-18) of all nursing exams delivered by subject experts
- **5** Skill Procedure videos demonstrating Nursing Skills in real-time
- **100+** Previous Year Exam Papers of all Nursing Exams from 2020-10 with Rationale (Attempt/View PDF Mode)
- **1500+** Flashcards/E-notes on all the important topics of all the subjects for last minute revision (In 6 months)
- **800+** Image-based Questions with Rationale
- **200+** Video-based Qs with Rationale
- **Complete Access to Plan A-Crash Courses**

New Content (Phase 3) Q Bank Pack

- **8000+** Qs in Q Bank form of all the topics from all the subjects
- **700+** E-Notes covering all subjects/all topics

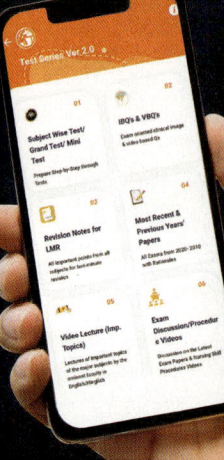

| MRP ₹3497/- | Validity 4 Months |
| MRP ₹6998/- | Validity 6 Months |

TESTIMONIALS

What our subscribers say about "TEST SERIES PLAN"

तैयारी आगे की!"

Plan MSc
MSc Digest

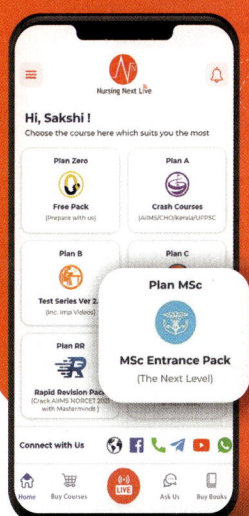

e cant be louder about It, Nursing Next Live is the only growing platform offering MSc preparations to e aspirants. As we say, that your success is our success, so we always look forward to providing the best d beyond study content with a futuristic approach. MSc Digest contains every vital information about e subjects in one place so that it gets easy for all to access the content on one platform.

WHY TO SUBSCRIBE

Make your preparation easy with your job
Enriched content helps you to prepare, revise and assess
Content is prepared by the top Medical & Nursing experts
Guidance and support

EST FOR

Who are always hungry to gain more knowledge from anywhere when they get a chance.
Who believe in focusing on one topic at a time
Who want to go further and upgrade their study content to the next level.

What all you will get

- Subject-wise synopsis covering image base illustrations and interesting Mnemonics to provide an extra edge preparation
- **3500+** MCQs covering the important topics of all subjects
- **800+** IBQs covering all subjects/topics
- **10+** Milestone papers covering more than 1000 MCQs to imbibe the environment of a real examination
- **3** Tests covering 150 IBQs
- **3** Tests covering 75 VBQs
- **10** Previous year papers (2020-2017) covering questions based on important topics/sub-topics from all subjects
- Exam capsules in the form of flashcards & tables
- **400+** LMR flashcards covering all subjects
- Hard copy of notes will be provided

MRP ₹1999/- **Validity 90 Days**

TESTIMONIALS

What our glorified achievers of MSc Entrance Exam say about Nursing Next Live

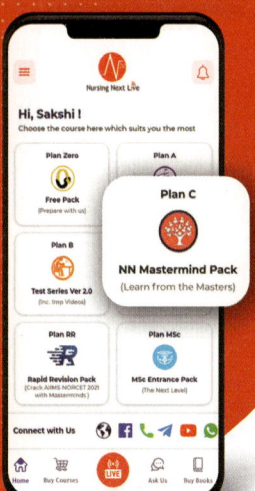

"ज्ञान हो बढ़ाना, तो PLAN C ही लेना!"

Plan C/C Plus
MASTERMIND Pack *(One-in-All, All-in-One)*

Nursing Next's One in all, all in one Mastermind pack for complete preparation! Plan C plus is a f package that contains all that you need for your 100% preparation for all the Nursing competiti exams. The content of this package is curated and drafted by the Top-Educators of Nursing Next Liv who are the masterminds of their subjects. NN Mastermind Pack is a gradual phase-wise learni journey with the option of Individual and combined pack and a validity of 12 months!

WHY TO SUBSCRIBE
- Detailed lectures as per the INC syllabus
- Helps you in building the strong foundation
- The MASTERMINDS : India's top medical & nursing faculty is here to guide you
- Sufficient content to cater your undergraduate and entrance exams needs
- Handwritten notes of the lectures that help you to revise the topic
- Question Bank with the topics that help you to assess your understanding in that particular topic

BEST FOR
- Students who are at a good progression level and want to build up their foundation more.
- Those who look forward to studying from the best and beyond educators.
- The students who want to upgrade their knowledge or the one aiming for Staff Nurse Entrance Exam, and also for the Undergraduates.

SPECIAL FEATURES
- Nursing Next's "Mastermind Pack", is a One-Stop solution for all your exam preparation needs for Staff Nurse Entrance Exams & Nursing Undergraduate Exams!
- It is our One-in-All, All-in-One pack for the nursing students of the Digital era!
- NN Mastermind Pack is exactly that 'learning tool' for all the nursing aspirants. It is carefully planned, and strategically designed, under the expertise of TOP Medical/Nursing Educators, just to make learni more authentic and easier for our students.
- Covering All Subjects, All Topics concepts from Basics to Advanced level pattern with the help of Videos/Question Banks & Handwritten Notes
- The Masterminds (TOP EDUCATORS) of NN Live have focused on ALL the upcoming Nursing Exams by giving two convenient options under 'Individual Subject Pack', & 'Combined (NN Mastermind Pack)'
- NN Mastermind Pack is a "road to success" for those who are preparing for any or all staff nurse entrance exams.

What all you will get

Plan C (Including Plan RR)
- **1200+ hours** of Video Lectures on All Subject/All Topics
- **11,000+** Questions with Rationale covering All Subject/All Topics
- IBQ/VBQ Video Discussions of All Subjects
- **Monthly Live Doubt Sessions/Live Classes**
- **80+Hours** of Rapid Revision Videos for **AIIMS NORCET**
- **2021** by Mastermind faculty
- **Handwritten Notes** of videos in PDF format integrated in the App
- Focusing on Quality study over quantity study, using the smart-study approach
- Monthly **Mega Assessment** Tests with National LevelRanking
- All upcoming exam's Important Topics & Exam/Discussions will be covered
- Complete **360-degree approach** for preparation
- Unlimited Watch Time, FREE Download Video option, National Level Ranks, Bookmark the content, Pause & Resume video option
- Best Guidance & Support at every stage
- Monthly Live Doubt Sessions/Live Classes/Live Webinars by Mastermind Faculty

Validity: 12 Months

MRP ₹12974/-

Plan C Plus (Including Plan A+B+C+RR)
- Plan A of NN Live (Complete access to Crash Courses—CHO/AIIMS NORCET 2020/KERALA PSC/UPPSC
  +
- Plan B of NN Live (Complete access to Test Series Pack Focusing AIIMS NORCET 2021 & Other Staff Nurse Exams)
  +
- Plan C of NN Live (Complete access to Plan C by the Mastermind Faculty
  +
- Plan RR of NN Live (Complete access to Rapid Revision Pack)

Validity: 6 Months
MRP ₹9995/-

Validity: 12 + 2 Bonus Months
MRP ₹15999/-

Validity: 24 Months
MRP ₹31998/-

Undergraduate Packs (Prof.-wise)

1st Year Students
✓ Anatomy
✓ Physiology
✓ Biochemistry & Nutrition
✓ Microbiology
✓ Fundamentals of Nursing

2nd Year Students
✓ Pharmacology
✓ MSN – Medicine
✓ MSN – Surgery
✓ Community Health Nursing
✓ Sociology
✓ CET

3rd & 4th Year Students
✓ Pediatric Nursing
✓ Midwifery & Obstetrical Nursing
✓ MSN – Medicine
✓ MSN – Surgery
✓ Mental Health Nursing
✓ Community Health Nursing
✓ Nursing Research & Statistics
✓ Nursing Management & Administration

Other Mastermind Pla

Mastermind Plan C
For 3rd & 4th Year Students those who are targeting for Sta Nurse Exams

Mastermind Plan C Plus
For Pass out Students those who are targeting for AIIMS NORCET Staff Nurse Exams

The Masterminds

Learn from the Top Educators of India

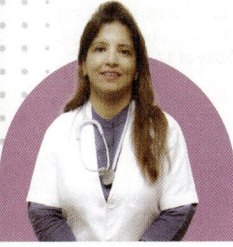

Dr Sakshi Arora Hans

Midwifery & Obstetrical Nursing

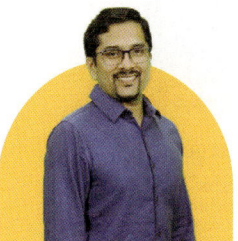

Dr Rohan Khandelwal

MSN - Surgery

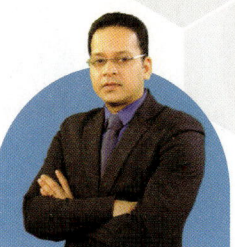

Dr Ranjan Patel

Pharmacology

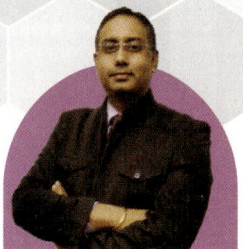

Dr Mukhmohit Singh

Community Health Nursing

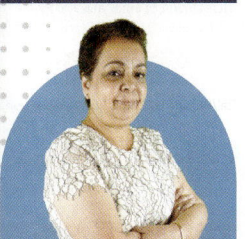

Dr Shivika Sethi

Microbiology

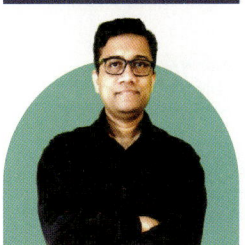

Dr Ashish Kumar

Physiology

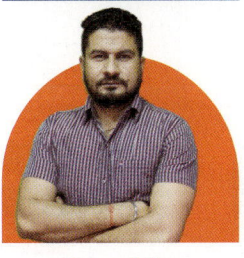

Dr Aman Setiya

MSN - Medicine

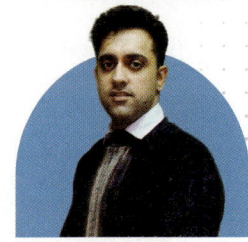

Dr Anand Bhatia

Pediatric Nursing

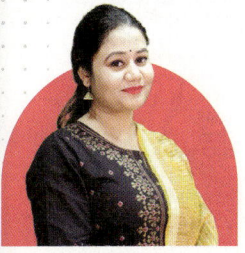

Ms Sabina Ali

Fundamentals of Nursing

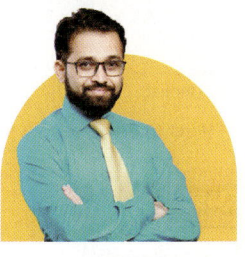

Dr Shrikant Verma

Anatomy

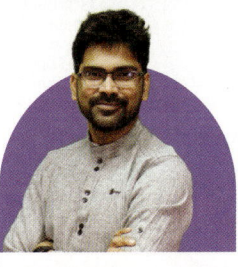

Dr Karthikeyan Pethusamy

Biochemistry & Nutrition

Ms Chetana

Mental Health Nursing

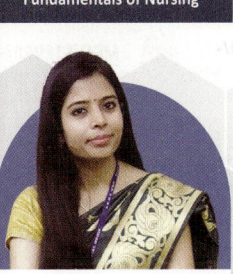

Saumya Srivastava

Nursing Management & Nursing Education

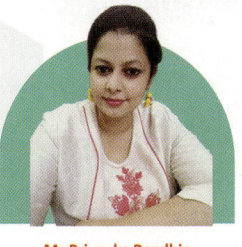

Ms Priyanka Randhir

Sociology & Computers

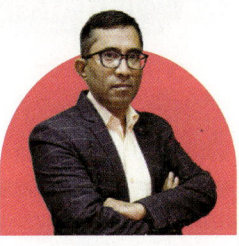

Mr Nitish Dubey

General Arithmetic

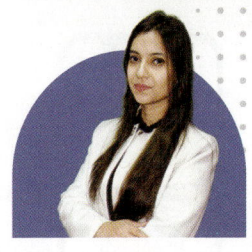

Ms Saloni Sharma

Aptitude & Reasoning

Individual

Midwifery & Obstetrical Nursing
By Dr Sakshi Arora Hans

What all you will get

- **100** hours of Videos on All topics
- IBQs & VBQs Discussion Videos
- **15** hours of Rapid Revision Videos covering Important Topics for AIIMS NORCET 2021
- **1000** Topic-wise MCQs with Rationale
- Live Doubt Sessions/Live Classes
- **88** Hand written Notes in PDF format

Validity: 6 months

MRP ₹1994/-

MSN - Surgery
By Dr Rohan Khandelwal

What all you will get

- **50** hours of Videos of All topics
- IBQs & VBQs Video Discussions
- **3** hours of Rapid Revision Videos covering Important Topics for AIIMS NORCET 2021
- **800** Topic-wise Qs with Rationale
- Live Doubt Sessions/Live Classes
- **51** Hand written Notes in PDF format integrated in App

Validity: 6 months

MRP ₹1499/-

Pharmacology
By Dr Ranjan Patel

What all you will get

- **50** hours of Videos of All topics
- IBQs & VBQs Video Discussions
- **10** hours of Rapid Revision Videos covering Important Topics for AIIMS NORCET 2021
- **800** Topic-wise Qs with Rationale
- Live Doubt Sessions/Live Classes
- **71** Hand written Notes in PDF format integrated in App
- **100** Probable Questions of Pharmacology for AIIMS NORCET 2021

Validity: 6 months

MRP ₹1499/-

Community Health Nursing
By Dr Mukhmohit Singh

What all you will get

- **90** hours of Videos of All topics
- IBQs & VBQs Video Discussions
- **7** hours of Rapid Revision Videos covering Important Topics for AIIMS NORCET 2021
- **900** Topic-wise Qs with Rationale
- Live Doubt Sessions/Live Classes
- **87** Hand written Notes in PDF format integrated in App
- **300** Probable Questions of CHN for AIIMS NORCET 2021

Validity: 6 months

MRP ₹1995/-

Microbiology
By Dr Shivika J Sethi

What all you will get

- **54** hours of Videos of All topics
- IBQs & VBQs Video Discussions
- **8** hours of Rapid Revision Videos covering Important Topics for AIIMS NORCET 2021
- **800** Topic-wise Qs with Rationale
- Live Doubt Sessions/Live Classes
- **75** Hand written Notes in PDF format integrated in App
- **100** Probable Questions of Microbiology for AIIMS NORCET 2021

Validity: 6 months

MRP ₹1499/-

MSN - Medicine
By Dr Aman Setiya

What all you will get

- **90** hours of Videos of All topics
- IBQs & VBQs Video Discussions
- **5** hours of Rapid Revision Videos covering Important Topics for AIIMS NORCET 2021
- **900** Topic-wise Qs with Rationale
- Live Doubt Sessions/Live Classes
- **90** Hand written Notes in PDF format integrated in App
- **400** Probable Questions of MSN - Medicine for AIIMS NORCET 2021

Validity: 6 months

MRP ₹1499/-

" जितनी जरूरत उतना पढ़ो!"

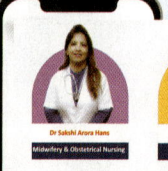
Dr Sakshi Arora Hans
Midwifery & Obstetrical Nursing

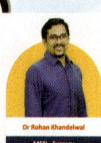
Dr Rohan Khandelwal
MSN - Surgery

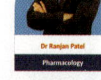
Dr Ranjan Patel
Pharmacology

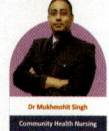
Dr Mukhmohit Singh
Community Health Nursing

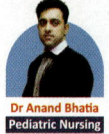
Dr Anand Bhatia
Pediatric Nursing

Now you have
The Freedom to Choose

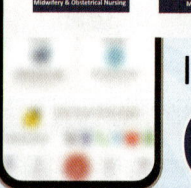

Introducing

CREATE YOUR PACK

Pack

Pediatric Nursing
By Dr Anand Bhatia

What all you will get

- **80** hours of Videos of All topics
- IBQs & VBQs Video Discussions
- **8** hours of Rapid Revision Videos covering Important Topics for AIIMS NORCET 2021
- **900** Topic-wise Qs with Rationale
- Live Doubt Sessions/Live Classes
- **81** Hand written Notes in PDF format integrated in App
- **300** Probable Questions of Pediatric Nursing for AIIMS NORCET 2021

Validity: 6 months | MRP ₹1994/-

Anatomy
By Dr Shrikant Verma

What all you will get

- **60** hours of Videos of All topics
- IBQs & VBQs Video Discussions
- **6** hours of Rapid Revision Videos covering Important Topics for AIIMS NORCET 2021
- **605** Topic-wise Qs with Rationale
- Live Doubt Sessions/Live Classes
- **86** Hand written Notes in PDF format integrated in App
- **100** Probable Questions of Anatomy for AIIMS NORCET 2021

Validity: 6 months | MRP ₹1299/-

Biochemistry & Nutrition
By Dr Karthikeyan Pethusamy

What all you will get

- **50** hours of Videos of All topics
- IBQs & VBQs Video Discussions
- **3** hours of Rapid Revision Videos covering Important Topics for AIIMS NORCET 2021
- **500** Topic-wise Qs with Rationale
- Live Doubt Sessions/Live Classes
- **45** Hand written Notes in PDF format integrated in App
- **100** Probable Questions of Biochemistry & Nutrition for AIIMS NORCET 2021

Validity: 6 months | MRP ₹1299/-

Physiology
By Dr Ashish Kumar

What all you will get

- **60** hours of Videos of All topics
- IBQs & VBQs Video Discussions
- **8** hours of Rapid Revision Videos covering Important Topics for AIIMS NORCET 2021
- **600** Topic-wise Qs with Rationale
- Live Doubt Sessions/Live Classes
- **55** Hand written Notes in PDF format integrated in App

Validity: 6 months | MRP ₹1299/-

Fundamentals of Nursing
By Ms Sabina Ali

What all you will get

- **200** hours of Videos of All topics
- IBQs & VBQs Video Discussions
- **14** hours of Rapid Revision Videos covering Important Topics for AIIMS NORCET 2021
- **900** Topic-wise Qs with Rationale
- Live Doubt Sessions/Live Classes
- **200** Hand written Notes in PDF format integrated in App
- **300** Probable Questions of FON for AIIMS NORCET 2021

Validity: 6 months | MRP ₹1994/-

Mental Health Nursing
By Dr Dharmendra Singh & Ms Chetana

What all you will get

- **90** hours of Videos of All topics
- IBQs & VBQs Video Discussions
- **6** hours of Rapid Revision Videos covering Important Topics for AIIMS NORCET 2021
- **900** Topic-wise Qs with Rationale
- Live Doubt Sessions/Live Classes
- **300** Probable Questions of MHN for AIIMS NORCET 2021

Validity: 6 months | MRP ₹1994/-

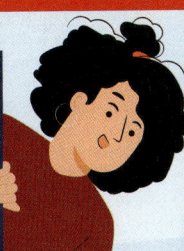

Select any **5 Subjects**
by **The Masterminds** and Create Your Own Pack

MRP ₹8450/- | Validity: 9 Months

Wondering, HOW? Call us at our helpline number +91-9999117411

Undergraduate Packs
By THE MASTERMINDS

Undergraduate Pack - 1st Year

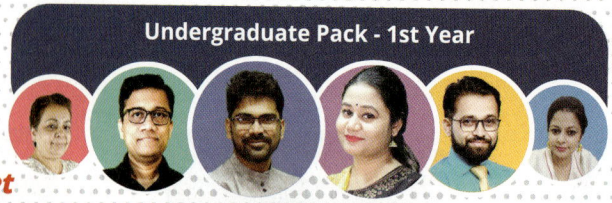

What all you will get

Main Subjects	Video Duration	No. of Questions
Anatomy	60+ Hours	600+ Qs
Physiology	60+ Hours	600+ Qs
Biochemistry & Nutrition	50+ Hours	500+ Qs
Microbiology	50+ Hours	500+ Qs
Fundamentals of Nursing	200+ Hours	400+ Qs

Bonus Subjects:- Computers & Psychology

MRP ₹7997/-

Validity: 18 months

Undergraduate Pack - 2nd Year

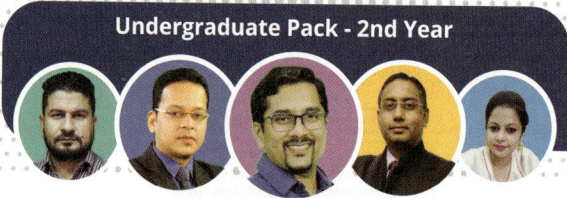

What all you will get

Main Subjects	Video Duration	No. of Questions
Pharmacology	50+ Hours	800+ Qs
MSN - Medicine	90+ Hours	900+ Qs
MSN - Surgery	50+ Hours	600+ Qs
Community Health Nursing	90+ Hours	900+ Qs
Sociology	40+ Hours	250+ Qs

MRP ₹7997/-

Validity: 18 months

Undergraduate Pack - 3rd & 4th Year

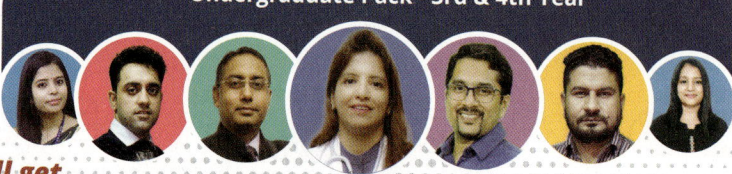

What all you will get

Main Subjects	Video Duration	No. of Questions
Pediatric Nursing	80+ Hours	900+ Qs
Midwifery & Obstetrical Nursing	100+ Hours	1000+ Qs
MSN - Medicine	90+ Hours	900+ Qs
MSN - Surgery	50+ Hours	600+ Qs
Mental Health Nursing	90+ Hours	900+ Qs
Community Health Nursing	90+ Hours	900+ Qs
Nursing Research & Statistics	35+ Hours	400+ Qs

Bonus Subjects:- Nursing Managment & Nursing Education

MRP ₹12992/-

Validity: 24 months

Special Features

- Handwritten Notes of Videos in PDF Format
- IBQs/VBQs Discussion Videos of above mentioned Subjects
- Monthly Mega Assessment Tests
- Monthly Live Doubt Session/Live Classes/Live Webinar by MM Faculty
- Best Guidance & Support
- Get your query directly resolved by MM faculty

"कम समय में जीत पक्की!"

Plan RR

Rapid Revision Pack

(Ready, Steady & Rapid)

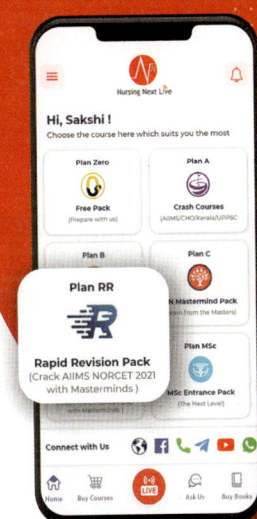

We are here to make you a Mastermind for all your Nursing exams, and for that, we believe the last-minute revision works like a wonder. Rapid Revision Pack, as the name says is to make you all ready and rapid for all your Nursing Competetive exams. Learn from basics to advance level and get a hold of every topic. Gain the last-minute momentum with this pack and open the gateway to excellence for yourself.

WHY TO SUBSCRIBE

- Rapid and intense course of study
- Covers important topics in concise yet complete form
- Most probable Qs which have large rate of incidence in exam
- If your foundation is good, then this is good pack to revise before the exam

BEST FOR

- Those who believe in doing extensive preparation for their Nursing competitive exams.
- The students who want to clear all of their last moment doubts.
- Working professionals who never want to compromise with their learnings for the competitive exams.

What all you will get

Plan RR

- **80-100 Hours of Rapid Revision Videos** covering Most Imp Topics for NORCET 2021 (Major Subjects including Nursing Management & Nursing Education)
- **2000+** Probable Qs with Rationale (MCQs + NCLEX Pattern)
- IBQ & VBQ Video Discussions by Master Mind Faculties (Relevant Subjects)
- **10 Special Mega Assessment Test** based on AIIMS NORCET Pattern
- Various Imp Tips/Trick & How to Prepare for NORCET 2021 Videos
- **15+** Imp Videos on COVID 19/Test & Discussion covering MCQ & NCLEX Pattern Qs
- COVID-19 Capsule (MCQs & Videos)
- Rapid Revision eBook in PDF format

MRP ₹2777/- | Validity: 2.5 Months

Plan RR+Mini TSP

Complete Content of RR Pack + Mini TSP:

- **15k** Questions with Rationale
- **1000+** IBQs/VBQs with Rationale Subject-wise/System-wise approach
- **190+** Tests (Subject-wise/Grand Test)
- **1500** E-notes/Clinical Gems
- **400+** Hours of videos Lectures/Subject-wise Exam discussion/Skill Procedure Videos

MRP ₹7520/- | Validity: 3+1 Months

TESTIMONIALS

What our Subscribers say about our Rapid Revision Pack

SELF-EVALUATION IS THE KEY!
"It has proved the best plan if you look forward to self evaluate before your exams. Great initiative."

Sushma Rani

LESS TIME CONSUMING AND MORE LEARNING!
"Through the Rapid revision pack and test series 2.0, I learned from excellent educators in a time-saving way"

Usha Rani

EXPERIENCE REAL-TIME EXAM VIBE!
"Rapid Revision Pack has helped me clear my doubts by providing real-time exam experience preparation. I gained an overall improvement in my studies."

Akansha Sharma

INNOVATIONS DETERMINES EFFECTIVENESS!
"Excellent pack if you want to do a quick revision effectively. The lectures are in a very comprehensive manner which makes it one of the best initiatives by NNL. "

B. Snegha Varshini

NN LIVE BECAME MY PARTNER-IN-LEARNING!
"Mastermind C Plus Pack became an amazing opportunity for me as I got everything from MCQs to High Standard Questions. Got the RR plan as a bonus too. Also, the faculty is always there to boost you up!"

Rahul Sain

IMPROVING RESULTS AND CHANGING STUDY PERSPECTIVES!
"Even the micro-content helped me to study in a macro way. With NNL, it has become very simple for me to understand the topics in a very comprehensive way. The Live sessions just work as an advantage. Thank you Nursing Next Live!"

Yashpal Vishvakarma

GLORIFIED ACHIEVERS

With over 150+ AIIMS NORCET 2020/100+ CHO &

AIIMS NORCET 2020

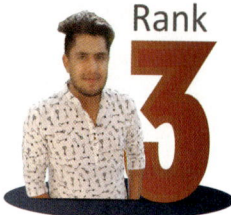

Rank **3**

Rahul Dahiya
Roll No. 9016060

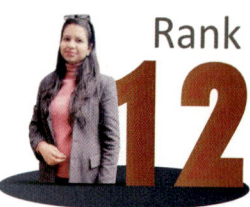

Rank **12**

Nisha Singla
Roll No. 9101820

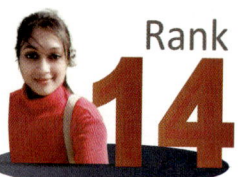

Rank **14**

Arushi Mittal
Roll No. 9079646

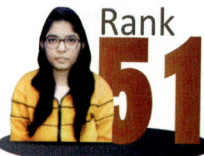

Rank **51**

Komal Dhull
Roll No. 9024458

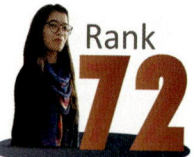

Rank **72**

Shivani Bourai
Roll No. 9092877

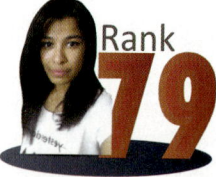

Rank **79**

Nivedita Saini
Roll No. 9004587

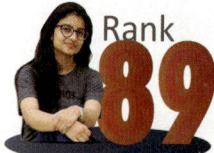

Rank **89**

Rupali Garg
Roll No. 9054544

And many more

CHO 2020

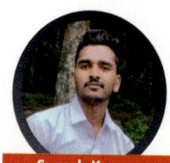

Suresh Kumsr
Rank- 1
Roll No. 12090
MP

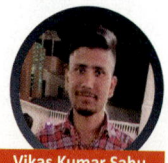

Vikas Kumar Sahu
Rank- 14
Roll No. 10011
MP

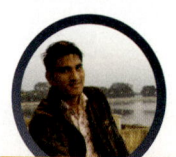

Harish Kumar Lodha
Rank- 18
Roll No. 7930
MP

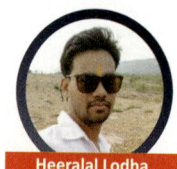

Heeralal Lodha
Rank- 33
Roll No. 10009
MP

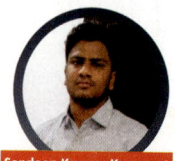

Sandeep Krumar Kumawat
Rank- 44
Roll No. 12585
MP

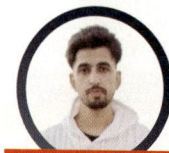

Mahadev Aanjan
Rank- 50
Roll No. 10130
MP

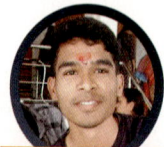

Nilesh
Rank- 81
Roll No. 10572
MP

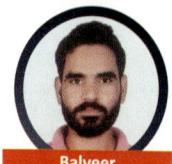

Balveer
Roll No. 619175
RAJASTHAN

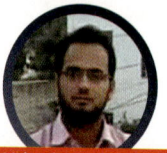

Mahendra Singh Gurjar
Roll No. 626167
RAJASTHAN

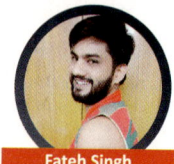

Fateh Singh
Roll No. 108169
RAJASTHAN

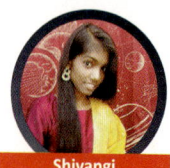

Shivangi
Roll No. 406105
RAJASTHAN

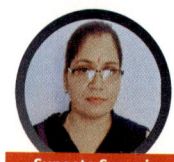

Suneeta Swami
Roll No. 619378
RAJASTHAN

And many more

OF NURSING NEXT LIVE

1200+ STUDENTS who cleared Various National/State Level Nursing Exams

BFUHS 2021

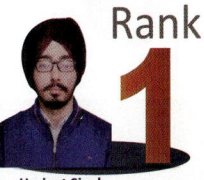
Rank **1**
Harjeet Singh
Roll No- 472478

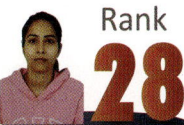
Rank **28**
Kuljit Kaur
Roll No. 473956

Rank **32**
Karan Sharma
Roll No. 469134

Rank **38**
Smriti Rana
Roll No. 463342

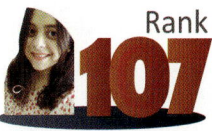
Rank **107**
Harpreet Kaur
Roll No. 474125

And many more

AIIMS MSc ENTRANCE EXAM 2021

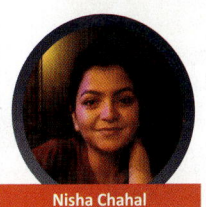
Nisha Chahal
AIIMS AIR-18

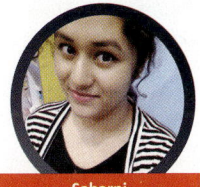
Sabarni
AIIMS AIR-21

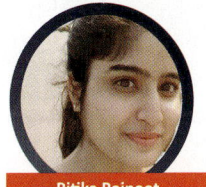
Ritika Rajpoot
AIIMS AIR-23

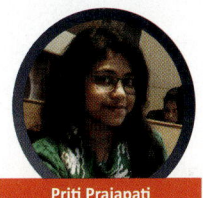
Priti Prajapati
AIIMS AIR-39

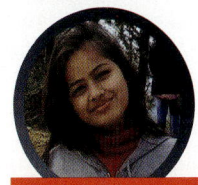
Shivangi Patwal
AIIMS AIR-64

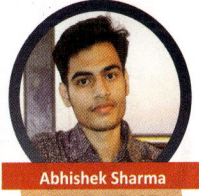
Abhishek Sharma
AIIMS AIR-97

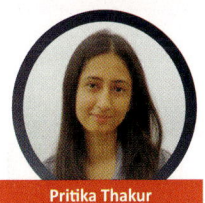
Pritika Thakur
AIIMS AIR-119

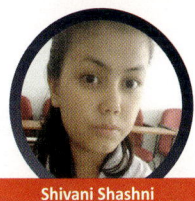
Shivani Shashni
AIIMS AIR-173

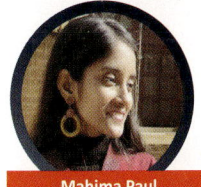
Mahima Paul
AIIMS AIR-175

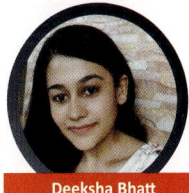
Deeksha Bhatt
AIIMS AIR-281

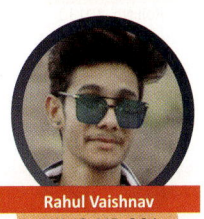
Rahul Vaishnav
AIIMS AIR-301

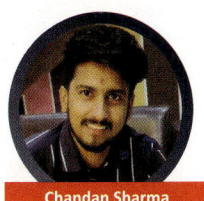
Chandan Sharma
AIIMS AIR-310

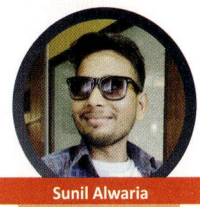
Sunil Alwaria
AIIMS AIR-677

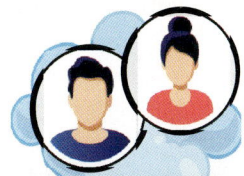
You Will Be The Next...

Scan the QR code to visit to our
YouTube Channel to hear their success stories.

ONE PLACE FOR ALL! AN INVITATION FOR ALL THE NURSING FACULTY MEMBERS TO COME.

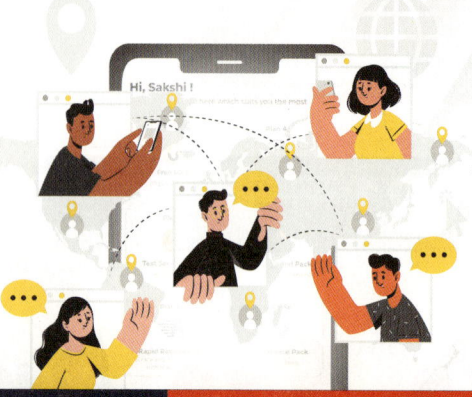

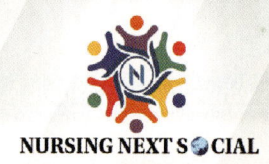

NURSING NEXT SOCIAL

Carrying on the legacy of being the best networking platform for the Nursing Segment!

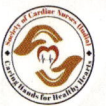 

NOW DISTANCE WILL NOT BE A BARRIER

Knowledge is like money: to be of value, it must circulate, and in circulating it, it can increase in quantity!

Nursing Next Live always focuses on providing you with the best and beyond and nothing less than that. We aim to bring all the Nursing Faculties from across the nation closer and together on a single platform.
No social distancing can stop the circulation of learnings from the teachers to students now. With Nursing Next Social, all the faculties from every corner of the country can join at one platform without any barriers.
Nursing Next Social at your service!
ONE PLATFORM TO BECOME THE MENTORS AND MENTEE!

Rewards For You

• Get Acknowledgement & Appreciation Certificates • Get Sponsorships for Educational Programs • Get Credit hours for attending Webinars • Get Free Access to Nursing Next Live Content & CBS Nursing Books   • Get Latest Updates related to your subject • Get a chance to become Reviewer, Contributors in Nursing Next Live, Target High & in CBS Nursing Titles

BE THE MENTOR OR MENTEE

SHOWCASE YOUR ACHIEVEMENTS ➡ SHARE YOUR KNOWLEDGE ➡ ENHANCE YOUR KNOWLEDGE

Purposes
• Attend Webinars/ E- Workshops
• Connect with other Faculty Members
• Share Your Knowledge. Be the Mentor or Mentee
• Get Complimentary Books
• Latest Updates on State/National/International Conferences & Webinars

Special Features
• Create your profile
• Add your accomplishments to level up your portfolio
• Earn Reward Points & Redeem through various options
• Set your Professional GOALS with timelines
• Regular Updates on Upcoming Conferences, CNEs & webinars
• Become Mentor or Mentee
• Get a chance to become Reviewer, Contributor or Author
• Get Certificates with credit hours issued by renowned nursing societies

PRE-REGISTER FOR **NURSING NEXT SOCIAL**
& Get 60 Days Free Subscription of **Nursing Next Live App**

ARE YOU A NURSING FACULTY ?
BE THE PART OF NURSING NEXT LIVE SOCIAL!

Scan the QR Code & Fill the form to Pre-register

Or Use the below link to fill the form
http://nursingnextlive.com/NNSocial/

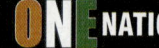 NATION **ONE** NURSING COMMUNITY

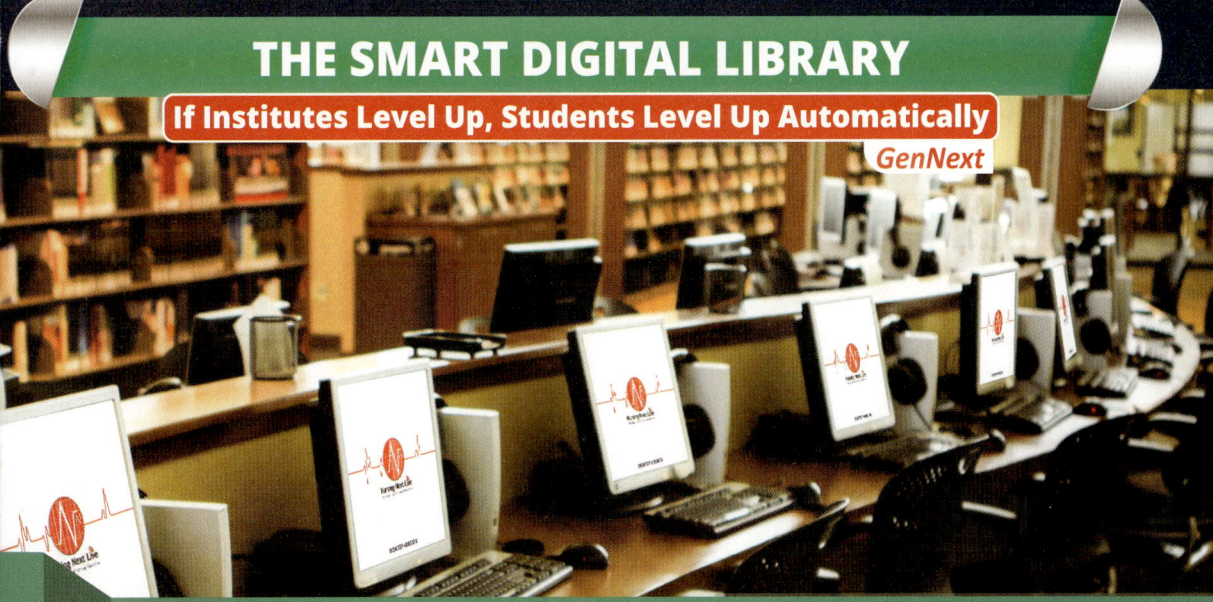

THE SMART DIGITAL LIBRARY

If Institutes Level Up, Students Level Up Automatically
GenNext

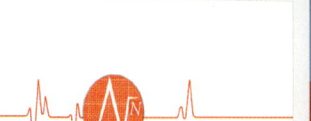

DESKTOP VERSION

GET ACCESS TO A VARIETY OF CONTENT
Unlike the traditional library methods, we are here to provide you with the impeccable online learning resource where you avail yourself of diversified content to study from. Learn with a futuristic approach and make yourself ready for the in-trend competitions.

TAKE-ON FUTURISTIC STUDY PATTERN
The digital libraries store a wide range of content as per the trends in a virtual environment to give a complete in-vogue experience to the learners.

INCREASE YOUR INSTITUTION'S BRAND VALUE
Be the best Digit-ally to all the learners and increase your brand value. Enhance your traditional library methods by giving it high-tech touch and give your students and the institute the best learning e-learning resource.

COST & TIME-EFFECTIVE
Utilize your money where it needs to be utilized! Digital libraries cover a small space but give boundless information and content to study from. Moreover, if we look forward to our environment, it helps eliminate the paperwork and the time-consuming manual checking of papers.

NO OPENING OR CLOSING HOURS
To offer a sublime 24*7 study experience to your students the digital library works like a wonder. The students can get access and read the library content in digital format anytime and anywhere using their preferred devices. Many readers these days prefer digital libraries over conventional libraries to access the content at their own pace and convenience.

What all you will get

- Complete access to all the Content of all Courses (Crash Courses, Test Series Ver 2.0, Mastermind Pack) with Unlimited Watch Time & the option of re-attempting test.
- All Topics of All Subjects (as per INC syllabus) are covered in form of Video Lectures, MCQs with Rationales, E-Notes, Hand Written Notes (PDF form will be integrated in the app by Feb '21) & Subjective Qs along with IBQs, VBQs, Most Recent & Previous Year Papers, and Live Doubt Sessions per month with Faculties.
- New Content will be added every month. Therefore, the Quantity of your Content will increase gradually throughout your subscription period.

- Regular Online Training Sessions for Best Guidance & Support on "How to Prepare for Nursing Competitive Exams" from the Top experts.
- Get a Dashboard to monitor your Students Progress Chart and Total Usage. *(Forthcoming)*
- Smart Digital Library is available in 2 versions 1) Tablet Version 2) Desktop Application Version.
- Avail Best Discounts & Special Offers on Smart Digital Library. The Institutional Subscription starts with a minimum of 20 subscriptions

For Business Proposal-related enquiries, contact:

Bhupesh Arora
(Project Director)
+91-9555590180
bhupesharora@nursingnextlive.in

	Plan Zero	Crash Course	Test Series	Rapid Revision	Mastermind Plan C	Mastermind Plan C Plus
Videos						
1. All Subjects /Topics Videos	—	—	—	—	—	✓
2. Video Lectures of Imp Topics	✓	—	✓	✓	✓	✓
3. Exam Discussion Videos	—	—	—	—	—	✓
4. Procedure Videos	—	—	—	—	—	✓
5. Rapid Revision Videos	—	—	✓	✓	✓	✓
6. IBQ/VBQ/Clinical Qs Discussion	—	—	—	✓	—	✓
7. Live Doubt Sessions	—	—	—	—	—	✓
8. Student-faculty Meet	—	—	—	—	✓	✓
9. Zoom Sessions/Webinar	—	—	—	—	✓	✓
10. Youtube Videos	✓	—	✓	✓	✓	✓
Tests						
11. Special Mega Assessment Tests	—	—	✓	✓	✓	✓
12. Grand Tests	✓	✓	✓	—	—	✓
13. Subject-wise Tests	✓	✓	✓	—	—	✓
14. Mini Tests	✓	✓	✓	✓	—	✓
15. IBQs/VBQs	—	✓	✓	—	—	✓
16. Most Recent Papers	—	✓	✓	—	—	✓
17. Previous Years Papers	—	✓	✓	—	—	✓
18. Kerala Psc Crash Course	—	✓	✓	—	—	✓
19. CHO Exams Crash Course	—	✓	✓	—	—	✓
20. AIIMS NORCET 2020 Crash Course	—	✓	✓	✓	✓	✓
21. UPPSC Crash Course	—	✓	—	—	—	✓
22. Most Probable Qs	—	✓	✓	✓	✓	✓
23. National Scholarship Test	✓	✓	✓	✓	✓	✓
24. Subject-wise Qs of All Topics	—	—	—	—	—	✓
Notes						
25. Handwritten Notes Integrated With Lectures	✓	—	—	—	—	✓
26. Last-minute Revision Notes	✓	✓	✓	✓	✓	✓
27. Notes Integrated With Rapid Revision Videos	—	—	—	✓	✓	✓
28. Printed Booklets(*Forthcoming*)	—	—	—	—	—	✓
Features						
29. Desktop Version	—	✓	—	✓	✓	✓
30. Any Doubt Ask Us	—	✓	✓	✓	✓	✓
31. Report A Query	—	✓	✓	✓	✓	✓
32. National Level Ranking	—	✓	✓	✓	✓	✓
33. Blogs	—	✓	✓	✓	✓	✓
34. Daily Dose Of Knowledge	—	✓	✓	✓	✓	✓
35. Forums Get Latest Info	—	✓	✓	✓	✓	✓
36. Resume Learning	—	✓	✓	✓	✓	✓
37. Buy Books	—	—	—	—	✓	✓
Supports						
38. Guidance & Counseling	—	—	—	✓	✓	✓
39. Faculty Telegram Channel	—	—	—	✓	✓	✓
40. Faculty Facebook Page	—	—	—	✓	✓	✓

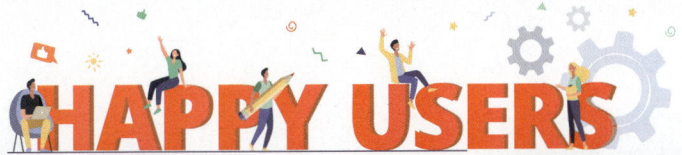

HAPPY USERS

Anisha Manna
★★★★★

DIVERSIFIED SPECIAL FEATURES TO BRACE YOU UP!

"The app is highly recommended for all nursing aspirants. The app has numerous special features with thorough information and is the best Nursing preparation option during these Pandemic times. Used for just 1 year and cleared my M.Sc. with excellent results."

Abhishek Kushwaha
★★★★★

RESULTED TO BE THE BEST NURSING PREPARATION APP!

"Hands down, it is the best Nursing app I have come across. All the tests, study content, CHO Crash Course will not let your expectations down but will prove to be really impressive. If you are a Nursing student/aspirant, then don't think just go for it."

Swatilekha Das
★★★★★

BECOME AN ACHIEVER FROM JUST AN USER WITH NURSING NEXT LIVE

"It has proved to be the best platform for me. If any student is looking for the perfect platform for Nursing Preparations, this is it. To become an achiever from just a dreamer, install this app and study from the plans now."

Nursing Guide Hindi
★★★★★

BEST PLAN FOR THE 1ST YEAR NURSING STUDENT

"The question bank, video lectures are amazing. Extremely helpful for any Nursing Aspirant. It is more preferable if you are in 1st year of Nursing. Do use this app if you want to make your knowledge vaster and achieve all your Nursing goals."

Harshit Upadhyay
★★★★★

IT HAS PROVED TO BE THE BEST NURSING PREPARATION ALLY!

"All the faculties especially Dr Sakshi, Dr Mukhmohit, Dr Rohan, Ms Sabina, all are excellent. The only drawback is that Dr Dharmendra needs to be a bit quick to make the notes and data. Else, it is an excellent prepping platform."

Naga Venkat
★★★★★

GET THE REAL-TIME TEST EXPERIENCE BY USING THE NNLIVE APP

"It is an excellent platform for learning and practicing for Nursing Competitive Exams. It consists of topic-wise explanations and helps us hold command of all. After attempting the real-time tests, I was able to progress gradually."

Sarangi Patel
★★★★★

THE ONE-STOP SOLUTION AS IT SAYS!

"I am grateful to the Nursing Next Live team for making great efforts towards providing us with the best and beyond preparation experience. The video lectures, e-notes, MCQs, and so on will suffice all your preparation needs and take it to the next level."

Deepak Kumar
★★★★★

10/10 RECOMMENDATION FOR THE NN LIVE APP!

"This app is best for all Nursing students as it has the best quality content to study and learn from."

Shafat Maqbool
★★★★★

CLEAR ALL YOUR DOUBTS-101!

"The video lectures, study content is highly informative and the topics are understood effectively. Clear all your doubts with NNL in no time"

Video Testimonials

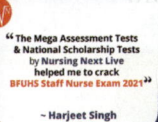

"The Mega Assessment Tests & National Scholarship Tests by Nursing Next Live helped me to crack BFUHS Staff Nurse Exam 2021"
~ Harjeet Singh
Rank -1

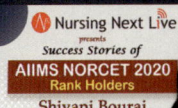
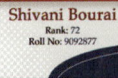
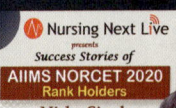

Nursing Next Live presents
Success Stories of
AIIMS NORCET 2020 Rank Holders
Shivani Bourai
Rank: 72
Roll No: 9092877

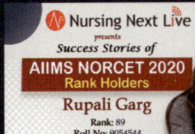
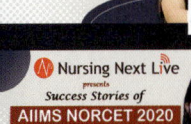
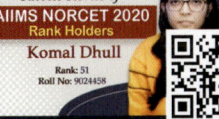

Nursing Next Live presents
Success Stories of
AIIMS NORCET 2020 Rank Holders
Rupali Garg
Rank: 89
Roll No: 9054544

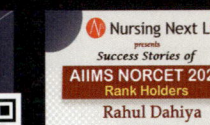
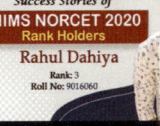

Nursing Next Live presents
Success Stories of
AIIMS NORCET 2020 Rank Holders
Rahul Dahiya
Rank: 3
Roll No: 9016060

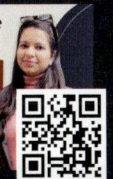

Nursing Next Live presents
Success Stories of
AIIMS NORCET 2020 Rank Holders
Nivedita Saini
Rank: 79
Roll No: 9004587

Nursing Next Live presents
Success Stories of
AIIMS NORCET 2020 Rank Holders
Nisha Singla
Rank: 12
Roll No: 9101820

Nursing Next Live presents
Success Stories of
AIIMS NORCET 2020 Rank Holders
Komal Dhull
Rank: 51
Roll No: 9024458

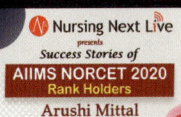
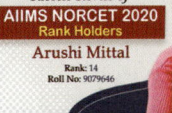
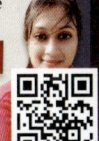

Nursing Next Live presents
Success Stories of
AIIMS NORCET 2020 Rank Holders
Arushi Mittal
Rank: 14
Roll No: 9079646

Scan the QR Codes to watch the videos on our YouTube Channel.

We Are Here 24X7

24×7 Guidance & Support

We provide personalized guidance and counseling to all our Subscribers, to ensure that their preparation is in the right direction, that is, toward success. That's why we have an active support service, handled especially by our:`

Nursing Counselors/Academic Counselors – To suggest you what to refer as per your need and want
Relationship Managers – To guide you throughout your learning journey and help you on every step
Guidance & Counselor – To teach you what to study and how to study
Scientific Team – To clear your Scientific Doubts within 24-48 Hours

How to connect with us?
Any Doubt, Ask Us : (In App Support 24x7)
Helpline and WhatsApp No : 9999117411 (Mon-Sat 9:00 am to 8:00 pm, Sunday 9:00 am to 2:00 pm)
Email : feedback@nursingnextlive.in
Web : www.nursingnextlive.com

Follow Us
(Scan the QR Code to Visit to Our Social Media Pages)

FACEBOOK
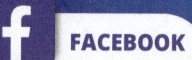
- Latest Updates & Discount Offers
- Read students feedbacks & Testimonials
- Fun & Learn Activities- Participate and win exciting prizes & free subscription

INSTAGRAM

- Latest updates of upcoming events
- Participate in giveaways, contests, and quizzes
- See what's latest

YOUTUBE

- Watch Success Stories, Tips & Tricks for easy preparation, from the top rank holders
- Videos of all Subjects/Important Topics by the mastermind faculty
- Various Last-minute revisions, motivational, and chanting videos
- Live Doubt Sessions every month for paid subscribers

LINKEDIN

- Behind-the-scenes of Nursing Next Live
- Significant days of the staff members
- Get insights into the insides of NNLive

TELEGRAM
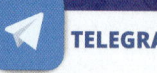
- Exclusive content for both paid and free subscribers
- Get Daily MCQs/IBQs, E-Notes, Video Teasers
- Latest updates, Daily dosage of learning, Quiz, Special discounts & Offers

Introducing TARGET HIGH DIGITAL
Now Read & Practice Together

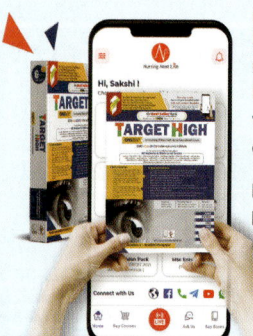

India's No. 1 and the most trusted book with exclusive & complete coverage of all National & State Level Exams is now going digital with no restrictions & additional content.

Explore The Next Level Of Best Preparation, Now!

Buy Best-Selling CBS Nursing Books

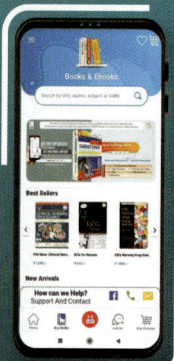

Read, Review & Buy

Now, buying CBS Nursing Books is extra convenient with Nursing Next LiveApp!

Get a Glimpse of **Sample Pages and TOC** before you proceed to buy the books.

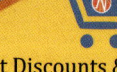

Best Discounts & Special Offers on all the Books.

 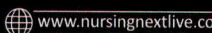

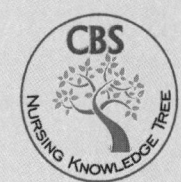

Textbook of
Nursing Education
for BSc Nursing

(As per the Syllabus of Indian Nursing Council for BSc)

Editor

RATNA PRAKASH MSc (MSN), PhD

Principal
Pal College of Nursing & Medical Sciences
Haldwani, Uttarakhand, India
Former Dean
Manipal College of Nursing
Manipal, India

Contributors

- **Alka Kalambi**
- **Anil Parashar**
- **Assuma Beevi TM**
- **Gitumoni Kanwar**
- **Jagadheeswaran P**

- **Mamtaz Begum**
- **Nagendra Prakash**
- **Nancy Fernandes Pereira**
- **Piti Koul**

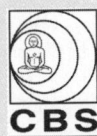

CBS
Dedicated to Education

CBS Publishers & Distributors Pvt Ltd

- New Delhi • Bengaluru • Chennai • Kochi • Kolkata • Lucknow
- Mumbai • Hyderabad • Nagpur • Patna • Pune • Vijayawada

Textbook of
Nursing Education
for BSc Nursing

ISBN 978-93-86827-34-0
Copyright © Publishers

Reprint: 2021

First Edition: 2018

Published by **Satish Kumar Jain** and produced by **Varun Jain** for

CBS Publishers & Distributors Pvt Ltd

4819/XI Prahlad Street, 24 Ansari Road, Daryaganj, New Delhi 110 002, India.
Ph: +91-11-23289259, 23266861, 23266867   Website: www.cbspd.com
Fax: 011-23243014
e-mail: delhi@cbspd.com; cbspubs@airtelmail.in.

Corporate Office: 204 FIE, Industrial Area, Patparganj, Delhi 110 092
 Ph: +91-11-4934 4934   Fax: 4934 4935
e-mail: feedback@cbspd.com; bhupesharora@cbspd.com

Branches

- **Bengaluru:** Seema House 2975, 17th Cross, K.R. Road, Banasankari 2nd Stage, Bengaluru 560 070, Karnataka
  Ph: +91-80-26771678/79   Fax: +91-80-26771680   e-mail: bangalore@cbspd.com
- **Chennai:** 7, Subbaraya Street, Shenoy Nagar, Chennai 600 030, Tamil Nadu
  Ph: +91-44-26680620, 26681266   Fax: +91-44-42032115   e-mail: chennai@cbspd.com
- **Kochi:** 68/1534, 35, 36-Power House Road, Opp. KSEB, Cochin-682018, Kochi, Kerala
  Ph: +91-484-4059061-65   Fax: +91-484-4059065   e-mail: kochi@cbspd.com
- **Kolkata:** 6/B, Ground Floor, Rameswar Shaw Road, Kolkata-700 014, West Bengal
  Ph: +91-33-22891126, 22891127, 22891128   e-mail: kolkata@cbspd.com
- **Lucknow:** Basement, Khushnuma Complex, 7-Meerabai Ma Rg, (Behind Jawahar Bhawan), Lucknow-226001, Uttar Pradesh
  Ph: +0522-4000032   e-mail: tiwari.lucknow@cbspd.com
- **Mumbai:** PWD Shed, Gala No. 25/26, Ramchandra Bhatt Marg, Next to J.J. Hospital Gate No. 2, Opp. Union Bank of India, Noor Baug, Mumbai-400009
  Ph: +91-22-66661880/89   Fax: +91-22-24902342   e-mail: mumbai@cbspd.com

Representatives

- **Hyderabad**   +91-9885175004
- **Pune**   +91-9623451994
- **Patna**   +91-9334159340
- **Vijayawada**   +91-9000660880

Printed at :

Dedicated to

the Teachers and Students

who believe in

Holistic Health Care

The Balance Sheet of Life

The happiness of life is made of little things - a smile, a hug, a moment of shared laughter –

It's not the wealth you amass but what you give to others & the lives
you touch that you take with you for eternity!
Our Birth is our Opening Balance!
Our Death is our Closing Balance!
Our Prejudiced Views are our Liabilities
Our Creative Ideas are our Assets
Heart is our Current Asset
Soul is our Fixed Asset
Brain is our Fixed Deposit
Thinking is our Current Account
Achievements are our Capital
Character & Morals, our Stock-in-Trade
Friends are our General Reserves
Values & Behavior are our Goodwill.
Patience is our Interest Earned
Love is our Dividend
Children are our Bonus Issues
Education is Brands/Patents
Knowledge is our Investment
Experience is our Premium Account.
The Aim is to Tally the Balance Sheet Accurately.
The Goal is to get the Best Presented Accounts Award.
Some very Good and Very bad things ....

✵ ✵ ✵ ✵ ✵

— Anonymous

Contributors

Alka Kalambi

Former Principal

Leelabai Thackersey
College of Nursing
SNDT Women's University
Mumbai, Maharashtra

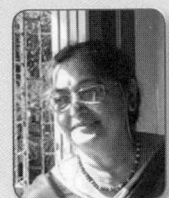

Mamtaz Begum

Professor

BM Birla College of Nursing
Bankrahat Road
Kolkata, West Bengal

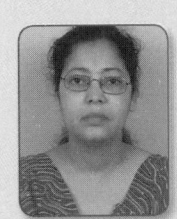

Anil Parashar

Professor and Vice Principal

Pal College of Nursing &
Medical Sciences
Haldwani, Uttarakhand

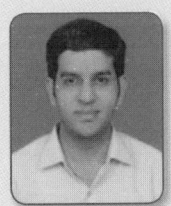

Nagendra Prakash

Academic Advisor

Pal College of Nursing &
Medical Sciences
Anandi Tower, Nainital Road,
Haldwani, Uttarakhand

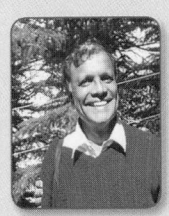

Assuma Beevi TM

Professor and Principal

Govt. College of Nursing
Joint Director at MIMS Academy
Thiruvanathapuram,
Kozhikode, Kerala

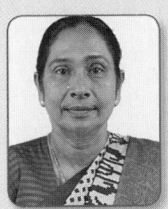

Nancy Fernandes Pereira

Professor and Principal

Leelabai Thackersey
College of Nursing
SNDT Women's University
Mumbai Maharashtra

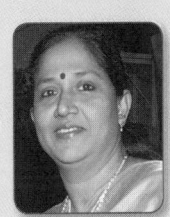

Gitumoni Kanwar

Associate Professor

Regional College of Nursing
Guwahati, Assam

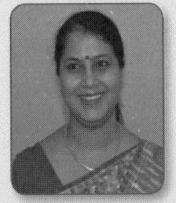

Piti Koul

Professor and Director

School of Health Sciences
IGNOU, New Delhi

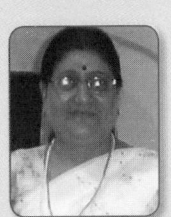

Jagadheeswaran P

Associate Professor

Pal College of Nursing &
Medical Sciences
Haldwani, Uttarakhand

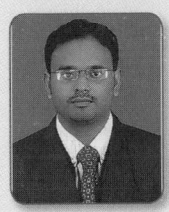

From Publisher's Desk

"Gaining knowledge is the first step to wisdom. Sharing it is the first step to humanity."

The above mentioned lines form the foundation stone of CBS publishers and Distributors Pvt Ltd, the flag bearer in medical publishing. Headquartered in New Delhi, the national capital of India, CBS was established in the year 1972 and it has expanded its roots to grow as a pioneer in the field of medical publishing in Asia. CBS is one of the largest and the fastest growing publishers of medical books in Southeast Asia. We are partners in the education of undergraduate and postgraduate students for we believe in nurturing the brains of medicos since the beginning of their careers in medicine. CBS joins the hands with the medical students as their first choice since the very moment they enter the college with BD Chaurasia's Human Anatomy and CC Chatterjee's Human Physiology. CBS is the proud owner of many bestselling titles like OP Ghai's Textbook of Pediatrics, Manipal's Surgery, KD Chatterjee's Textbook of Parasitology, and the list goes on. CBS has successfully partnered in sculpting the careers of millions of medicos across the world.

Since establishment of CBS Nursing Knowledge Tree last year we have published many successful titles in the field of nursing and we have proved ourselves in the Nursing Fraternity in providing quality education.

Vision and Mission of CBS Nursing Knowledge Tree

CBS Nursing Knowledge Tree is conceptualized with a vision of being the first of its kind to bring the best quality books for education of Nurses. Keeping in mind the changing trends in the Nursing Education, we at CBS have taken up a mission to bring student-friendly and syllabus-based books written by Subject Experts from PAN India without compromising on the Quality of content and presenting it in a Unique manner.

Foundation Stones of CBS Nursing Knowledge Tree

- **Strong editorial support by the leading subject experts and faculties in Nursing from PAN India.** Every manuscript/proposal that is received is critically reviewed by our Editorial Board at various levels to ensure the Quality of content. A book is published only after all the parameters in our process management are satisfied.
- **Special care taken to publish Plagiarism-free matter.** With the copyright laws being highly strict these days, we at CBS are paying extra attention at various stages of publishing a book to crosscheck and avoid any copyright infringement.
- **Books authored by Subject Experts and Senior Faculties all over India.** Every title owned by CBS Nursing Knowledge Tree is written by the senior-most faculties and subject masters from every nook and corner of the country to provide them a bigger platform to share their knowledge and experience amongst budding nursing fraternity.
- **All the books developed as per INC syllabus and needs of the students without compromising on the Quality of the content.** Often students complain that some books are either not covering the complete syllabus or have too much content as compared to the syllabus. In this series, extra care is being taken to develop books strictly as per INC syllabus in the most student-friendly manner.
- **All books being reviewed by Top-notch faculties and Subject Experts to maintain high standards of Quality.** Every title goes through tough grilling regarding the content and the overall presentation by various top subject experts as reviewers. This ensures that only the Quality content gets published.
- **Best International standard layouts for every book.** Every title in CBS Nursing Knowledge Tree is designed and formatted in the best layouts of international standards because we strongly believe that every book deserves to be treated the Best!

- **Additional and Unique features given with every title.** Every title is accompanied by one or the other additional feature to complement the learning of students like—*Workbook, DVD, Last Minute Revision Notes.* We have also included many features like *How to make Most out of this Book, Assess Yourself* that contains questions and MCQs and other special boxes according to the need of the content.

Let's Join Our Hands Together

We can only bring the change that we want to see in Nursing Education with the support and cooperation of leading faculties in all Nursing specialties. If you envision the same, we are happy to welcome you to our panel of contributors and reviewers and let's take up this mission together of creating a Change in Nursing Education.

We crave cooperation from all the students and faculties to provide their genuine feedback on the quality of the books and how we can improve upon the deficiencies in future on the following email id: cbsvpdesk@yahoo.com . Constructive criticism with concrete suggestions for improvement for all our books will be highly appreciated.

Expanding Horizons

We are also highly active in attending various National Level Conferences and Meets organized by various Nursing Societies. We are keenly working to expand our horizons of associations by participating in conferences organized by **SOCHNI, ISPN, NRSI, ICMR, SOMI,** etc. every year. CBS has always been a forerunner and a big supporter of all National level Nursing Conferences. If you have any National and State level conference proposals, we are happy to be the part of these conferences.

Being Social is Our Aspiration

In this era of Social Media, we are happy being social as well by bringing you our Facebook page **facebook.com/cbsnursingtree** of "CBS Nursing Knowledge Tree" to expand our reach to the maximum people in Nursing. It is a platform purely dedicated to bring the important aspects and latest updates and developments in various domains and fields of Nursing. It will be our privilege if you could connect with us and share your knowledge and experiences as well on our Facebook page.

I would like to invite all the readers to come and join us on our facebook page and share some input, information and literature.

With this vision and above features we are happy to announce the release of **Textbook of Nursing Education for BSc Nursing** edited by **Dr Ratna Prakash** and contributed by top subject experts from all over the country!

Bhupesh Arora
Vice President-Publishing & Marketing
(PGMEE & NURSING Division)
CBS Publishers and Distributors Pvt. Ltd.
Email: bhupesharora@cbspd.com
Mobile: (+91) 9555590180

Preface

In the modern era of health care, nursing profession is seemingly emerging as a significant contender. The introduction of advanced technology in curricula and scope for varied areas of specialized practice has opened vistas of opportunities for professional growth.

On the other hand, the health awareness among people is on the rise and keeping at par with the consumers' expectations of care–givers' competency has increased.

Competency in health care inevitably requires integrated use of humanistic attitude, relevant scientific knowledge base and appropriate psychomotor skills in rendering need–based health care. Realization of all these requires *"communication skills"*, whether it is for informative, preventive or therapeutic purposes.

Nursing interventions are based on scientific principles. Also, it is an art of developing interpersonal relationship with persons in need of health care, which helps in understanding their actual needs arising from body-mind relationship in the manifestations of health disorders. In order to achieve excellence in nursing care competency, the students need to be made aware of the role played by *"Communication"* in every aspect of their personal and professional life.

This calls for an altogether renewed outlook on our nursing educational methods, based on the principles of science and art of communication.

On the above reflections, this book on *"Nursing Education"* has been initiated by a group of Nurse Educators and Practitioners, who are futuristic thinkers and are concerned about educating the budding nurses to ensure holistic health care and consumer satisfaction.

The manuscript begins with introducing the students to the concepts of "Communication" as a science and an art, gently leading them to its broader perspectives, including "Understanding their own Self". The content logically flows from "Self" to "Others" and then to the "Clients" of health care. It includes the detail presentation of the technology and techniques of communication, its application to teaching-learning contexts of classroom, clinical and day-to-day life. As a whole this book is an attempt to bring most of the information about "Communication" under a single roof. The language is kept simple, contents are organized in logical sequence considering the principles of education. Throughout its preparation the authors have been vigilant with constant reminder of its users that is our loved students, who are the future torch-bearers of a great profession.

Ratna Prakash

Acknowledgments

Inspired by our students who we felt needed a book which is written in easy language, contains information in points for easy learning and organized following principles of adult learning.

Thanks to the authors, who could find time to pen the chapters, though each one of them is loaded with responsibilities and thus, their every precious minute invested in this book counts.

We are grateful to our parents, spouse and family members who have been with me throughout – encouraging and putting up with our late night toil to squeeze new ideas out of our tired brains.

Our tribute and salutation to our own teachers from school to college to professional education. They have been our ideals and following their foot-steps, we have chosen the vocation of a teacher. Their blessings have been our guiding light to reach the goal.

Our special thanks to **Mr Satish Kumar Jain** (Chairman) and **Mr Varun Jain** (Managing Director), M/s CBS Publishers and Distributors Pvt Ltd for their wholehearted support in publication of this book. We have no words to describe the role, efforts, inputs and initiatives undertaken by **Mr Bhupesh Arora** Vice President- Publishing and Marketing, PGMEE and Nursing Division for helping and motivating me.

We thank Dr Mrinalini Bakshi (Senior Content Developer and Editor) for her editorial support and Ms Nitasha Arora (Project Manager), Ms Neetu Jindal (Asst. Production Manager), Mr Nitish K Dubey (Senior Editor) and all the production team members Mr Ashutosh Pathak, Mr Chaman Lal, Ms Tahira Praveen, Mr Prabhat Ranjan, Mr Prakash Gaur, Mr Phool Kumar, Mr Bunty Kashyap, Ms Babita Verma, Mr Raju Sharma, Mr Manoj Chaudhary and Mr Vikram Chaudhary for devoting laborious hours in designing and type setting of this book.

Syllabus for BSc Nursing

Placement: Second Year   **Time:** Theory– 90 Hours

Course Description: This course is designed to help the students acquire an understanding of the principles and methods of communication and teaching. It helps to develop skill in communicating effectively, maintaining effective interpersonal relations, teaching individuals and groups in clinical, community health and educational settings.

Unit	Time (Hrs) Th.	Time (Hrs) Pr.	Learning Objectives	Content	Teaching Learning Activities	Assessment Methods
I	5		• Describe the communication process • Identify techniques of effective communication	**Review of Communication Process** • Process; elements and channel • Facilitators • Barriers and methods of overcoming • Techniques	• Lecture discussion • Role plays • Exercises with audio/video tapes	• Respond to critical incidents • Short answers • Objective type
II	5		• Establish effective inter-personal relations with patients, families and coworkers	**Interpersonal relations** • Purpose and types • Phases • Barriers and methods of overcoming • Johari window	• Lecture discussion • Role plays • Exercises with audio/video tapes • Process recording	• Short answer • Objective type
III	5		• Develop effective human relations in context of nursing	**Human relations** • Understanding self • Social behavior, motivation, social attitudes • Individual and groups • Groups and individual • Human relations in context of nursing • Group dynamics • Team work	• Lecture discussion • Sociometry • Group games • Psychometric exercises followed by discussion	• Short answers • Objective type • Respond to test based on critical incidents
IV	10	5	• Develop basic skill of counseling and guidance	**Guidance and counseling** • Definition • Purpose, scope and need • Basic principles • Organization of counseling services • Types of counseling approaches	• Lecture discussion • Role play on counseling in different situations followed by discussion	• Short answers • Objective type • Assess performance in role plays situations

Contd...

Unit	Time (Hrs) Th.	Time (Hrs) Pr.	Learning Objectives	Content	Teaching Learning Activities	Assessment Methods
				• Role and preparation of counselor • Issues for counseling in nursing: students and practitioners • Counseling process—steps and techniques, tools of counselor • Managing disciplinary problems • Management of crisis and referral		
V	5		• Describe the philosophy and principles of education • Explain the teaching learning process	**Principles of education and teaching learning process** • Education: meaning, philosophy, aims, functions and principles • Nature and characteristics of learning • Principles and maxims of teaching • Formulating objectives; general and specific • Lesson planning • Classroom management	• Lecture discussion • Prepare lesson plan • Micro teaching • Exercise on writing objectives	• Short answers • Objective type • Assess lesson plans and sessions
VI	10	10	• Demonstrate teaching skill using various teaching methods in clinical, classroom and community settings	**Methods of teaching** • Lecture, demonstration, group discussion, seminar, symposium, panel discussion, role play, project, field trip, workshop, exhibition, programmed instruction, computer assisted learning, micro teaching problem base learning, self instructional module and simulation, etc.	• Lecture discussion • Conduct 5 sessions using different methods and media	• Short answers • Objective type • Assess teaching sessions
				• Clinical teaching methods: case method, nursing round and reports, bedside clinic, conference (individual and group) process recording		

Contd...

Unit	Time (Hrs) Th.	Time (Hrs) Pr.	Learning Objectives	Content	Teaching Learning Activities	Assessment Methods
VII	10	8	• Prepare and use different types of educational media effectively	**Educational media** • Purposes and types of A-V Aids, principles and sources etc. • Graphic aids: chalk board, chart, graph, poster, flash cards, flannel graph, bulletin, cartoon • Three dimensional aids: objects, specimens, models puppets • Projected aids: slides, overhead projector, films, TV, VCR/VCD, camera, microscope, LCD • Audio aids: tape recorder, public address system computer	• Lecture discussion • Demonstration • Prepare different teaching aids projected and non projected	• Short answers • Objective type • Assess the teaching aids prepared
VIII	5	7	• Prepare different types of questions for assessment of knowledge, skills and attitudes	**Assessment** • Purpose and scope of evaluation and assessment • Criteria for selection of assessment techniques and methods • Assessment of knowledge: essay type questions, Short answer questions (SAQ), Multiple choice questions (MCQ) • Assement of Skills: observation checklist, practical exam, viva, objective structure clinical examination (OSCE) • Assessment of Attiudes: Attiude scales	• Lecture discussion • Exercise on writing different types of assessment tools	• Short answers • Objective type • Assess the strategies use in practice teaching session and exercise sessions
IX	5		• Teach individuals, groups and communities about health with their active participation	**Information, Education and communication for health (IEC)** • Health behavior and health education • Health education with individuals, groups and communities • Communicating health messages • Method and media for communicating health messages • Using mass media	• Lecture discussion • Plan and conduct health education sessions for individuals, group and communities	• Short answers • Objective type • Assess the planing and conduct of the educational session

Special Features of the Book

IMPORTANCE OF INTERPERSONAL RELATION IN NURSING

Good interpersonal relation helps to:
- Remove monotony of work environment
- Maximize support from colleagues, supervisors, subordinates, patients and other co-workers
- Improve intradepartmental and interdepartmental communication
- Reduce stress in family life as well as in professional life
- Function effectively in a multidisciplinary team
- Build team through mutual understanding and cooperation
- Improve decision making and problem solving
- Promote self development and wellbeing
- Provide effective patient care
- Promote positive work culture
- Maximize output at personal and group level
- Receive constructive feedback.

> The relevance and importance of every topic in nursing has been separately highlighted in every chapter.

CHAPTER OUTLINE

- Introduction
- Etymological Meaning of Communication
- History of Communication
- Origin of Human Communication
- Petroglyphs
- Pictographs or Pictograms
- Ideographs or Ideograms
- Writing
- Origin of Spoken Language
- Modern Communication system
- Telegraphy and Telephony
- Wireless Communication System
- Digital Communication System
- Communication: Definition and Meaning
- Elements of Communication

> Chapter outline enlists all the topics covered in a chapter.

LEARNING OBJECTIVE

At the end of the Unit, you should be able to-
- Define etymological meaning of communication
- Describe the origin of human communication
- State the definition and meaning of communication
- Describe the elements of communication:
  - The source or sender
  - The message
  - Encoding
  - The medium or channel or transmitter
    - Verbal or oral communication
    - Nonverbal communication
    - Written communication
    - Visual communication
    - Metacommunication
  - The receiver
  - Decoding
  - The response or feedback
- Explain the concepts and theories of communication
- Recognize the facilitators of communication
- Identify the barriers of communication
- Explain the methods of overcoming the barriers of communication
- Describe therapeutic communication
- Explain the importance of research in communication

> Learning objective enlists what a student is expected to learn after the end of the chapter

TABLE 1: The top 15 most effective communication techniques and strategies

S. No.	Techniques and Strategies	Explanation
1.	The silent treatment	Instead of immediately answering or reacting after the other person has talked, remaining silent but being attentive encourages people to open up to give more information than intended
2.	Observation	If we have difficulty in communicating verbally or nonverbally or the situation is not appropriate for that, it is better to observe people who are interacting. We can even ask a good communicator to observe the interactions and give us the information. The observer may or may not be hidden from the persons being observed
3.	Smile	There are many types of smile, that conveys different emotions and meanings. A genuine open smile can make a nervous person feel relaxed, so that he/she can communicate effectively. An artificial smile that does not reaches the eyes can be treacherous. Depending on situations we need to use smile appropriately

Numerous tables and figures have been interspersed to make the concepts easy to memorise.

ASSESS YOURSELF

LONG ESSAY

1. Describe the elements of communication with suitable examples
2. Explain the types and importance of nonverbal communication
3. Explain the importance of effective communication in nursing education and nursing practice, with suitable examples

SHORT ESSAY

1. Describe the modern communication system
2. Explain with suitable examples the facilitators of communication
3. Explain with suitable examples the barriers of communication

Assess Yourself section helps the students to assess their understanding of the chapter.

BIBLIOGRAPHY

1. Etymological meaning of communication (Internet). Available from: https://pragatipath1.files.wordpress.com/2012/02/smc2.pdf
2. History of Communication (Internet). Available from: https://en.wikipedia.org/wiki/History_of_communication
3. King J Barbara. When Did Human Speech Evolve?(Internet). 2013 September 5. Available from http://www.npr.org/sections/13.7/2013/09/05/219236801/when-did- human-speech-evolve.
4. Heidgerken E Loretta. Teaching and learning in schools of nursing. 3rd ed. Delhi: Knark Publishers Pvt. Ltd. Delhi; 1998.

Bibliography provides resources for advanced reading.

Contents

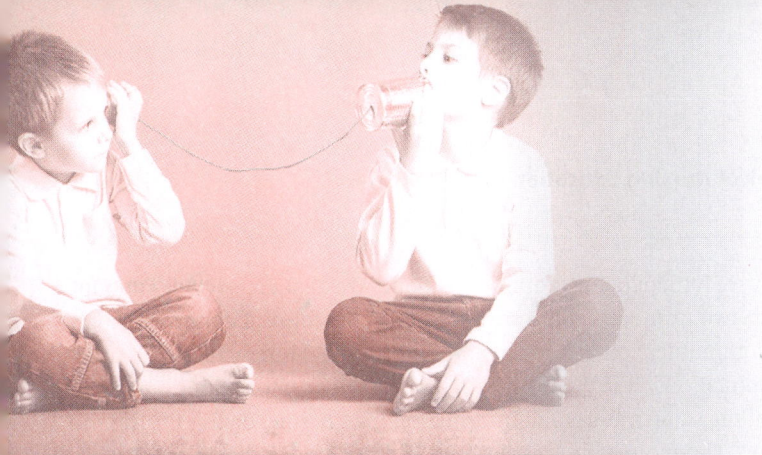

Unit

1

Review of Communication Process

— *Ratna Prakash*

CHAPTER OUTLINE

- Introduction
- Etymological Meaning of Communication
- History of Communication
- Origin of Human Communication
- Petroglyphs
- Pictographs or Pictograms
- Ideographs or Ideograms
- Writing

- Origin of Spoken Language
- Modern Communication System
- Telegraphy and Telephony
- Wireless Communication System
- Digital Communication System
- Communication: Definition and Meaning
- Elements of Communication

📚 LEARNING OBJECTIVE

At the end of the Unit, you should be able to-

- Define etymological meaning of communication
- Describe the origin of human communication
- State the definition and meaning of communication
- Describe the elements of communication:
  - The source or sender
  - The message
  - Encoding
  - The medium or channel or transmitter
    - Verbal or oral communication
    - Nonverbal communication
    - Written communication

  - Visual communication
  - Metacommunication
  - The receiver
  - Decoding
  - The response or feedback
- Explain the concepts and theories of communication
- Recognize the facilitators of communication
- Identify the barriers of communication
- Explain the methods of overcoming the barriers of communication
- Describe therapeutic communication
- Explain the importance of research in communication

INTRODUCTION

Man is a social animal, normally we human beings cannot live alone. We depend on each other for fulfilling our needs. Whenever two or more people are together, some form of communication definitely takes place. Thus, communication is a social and interpersonal interaction. The word 'Communication' has different connotations. It is the transfer of a message or information from one person to other, but the meaning of the same message or information may change depending on the context or situation of the interaction. Therefore it is necessary for all of us to understand and learn the science and art of communication, so as to avoid any miscommunication and misunderstanding. It is all the more essential in health care profession, for the reason that effective communication itself has a therapeutic value.

ETYMOLOGICAL MEANING OF COMMUNICATION

Etymology means a study of origin of the words. The English term *'Communication'* has been evolved from *Latin language*. *'Communis and Communicare'* are two Latin words related to the word communication. *Communis* is a noun, which means common, commonality or sharing. *Communicare* is a verb, which means 'make something' common. According to some scholars **the English word 'Community'** is formed through communication among people who have something common, for example, tribal communities, specific language communities, etc. Hence, communication refers to sharing and it is an act of expressing ideas, feelings, exchange of thoughts or sharing information.

HISTORY OF COMMUNICATION

Origin of Human Communication

Petroglyphs

From available resources, it is known that the human communication originated approximately 500,000 years ago and the symbols for communication were developed approximately 30,000 years ago. The oldest known symbols dating back to the Upper Paleolithic age, created for the purpose of communication were cave paintings, stone carvings, and rock art, known as *Petroglyphs*. There were also wood carving with figures and symbols. The Upper Paleolithic Period that began approximately 40,000 years ago was marked by the development of regional stone tool industries in the oldest known culture of the world. Tools were made up of stone and wood. It took about 20,000 years for human beings to move from the first cave paintings to the first petroglyphs. These paintings and carvings contained huge amount of information. The *first calendar* might have been created about 15,000 years ago. The study of evolution of languages has shown that the specific concepts and words of drawing, carving and writing convey the same meaning or information.

It is possible that human beings of that time had used some other forms of communication, often for *mnemonics* purposes. Mnemonics is a **memory device**; it aids to retain original information in a memory by associating it with a familiar idea or object to make it meaningful. For example, early warning signs of cancer is *CAUTION*, where each alphabet has meaning.

- **C** — Change in bowel and bladder habit
- **A** — A sore that does not heal

- **U** — Unusual bleeding or discharge
- **T** — Thickening or lump in breast or elsewhere
- **I** — Indigestion or difficulty in swallowing
- **O** — Obvious change in growth or mole
- **N** — Nagging cough or hoarseness

There are evidences of a technique of ancient communication also called **Quipus**. In this technique, knots were made with colourful threads of same kind. The number of threads and the specific pattern conveyed a specific information. Ancient Tattoos, when interpreted, were found to contain some meaning. However, very few of those carved stones have survived till today and we can only speculate about their existence based on our observation of still 'existing hunter'-gatherer cultures among some tribes.

The inadequacies of communication needs felt by humans stimulated inventions and eventually resulted in creation of newer forms of communication at every stage of evolution; improving in its variety, longevity and quality. All these inventions were based on the concept of 'symbols'.

Pictographs or Pictograms

Pictographs from the year 1510s were the next step in the evolution of communication. These are different from petroglyphs. The petroglyphs were used to simply show an event, whereas pictographs were used to tell the complete story about the event, with the events arranged chronologically. A **Pictograph** is a symbol demonstrating a thought, an object, an activity, place or events, which are communicated from one person to another by a drawing. It is a form of photo-writing. For example, pictogram of a circle could represent a sun, but not the sun's related ideas as heat, light, day time, etc. Pictograms were used by various ancient cultures all over the world around 9000 BC, when simple pictures were drawn to show the crops or agricultural products. It became gradually popular around 6000–5000 BC. They were the basis of **Cuneiform system of writing** (wedge-shaped characters for writing, found in ancient Mesopotamian and Persian civilizations) and developed further into **Logographic** writing system around 5000 BC. Logograph is a written character that indicates a word or a phrase.

Ideographs or Ideograms

Pictographs evolved into **Ideograms**. These are graphical symbols to express abstract ideas. **Ideographs** could convey more abstract concepts, for example, two sticks mean legs and walking, upward tilt of both corners of lips shows smile and happiness.

Writing

The oldest-known forms of writing were primarily Logographic in nature, based on Pictographic and Ideographic elements. The earliest known form of writing is called **Futhark**. Most writing systems can be broadly divided into three categories: **logographic, syllablic** and **alphabetic** (or *segmental*); however, all three may be found in any given writing system in varying proportions, thus making it difficult to classify a system individually. The first **writing system** was invented probably in the beginning of the Bronze Age i.e. in the later part of 4000 BC. The original writing system was believed to be derived from system of small clay-made objects, which were used to keep count of commodities and developed to include Phonetic elements (the study and classification of speech sounds) by 2800 BC. Finally, this form of writing became a general purpose for **Logograms**, **Syllables** and **Numbers**.

Origin of Spoken Language

About 1.75 million years ago, prehistoric man began to make hand axe with stone, which required more preparation and accuracy than the earlier tool making process. These activities might have required some way to communicate and share ideas with each other. According to scholars, around this time human beings began to talk. Thus, probably tool-making and language skills evolved at the same time.

Modern Communication System

Today we can't imagine a life without radio, telephones, television, etc. and other common gadgets. Most of these modern-day communication systems were invented and developed during the past 200 years.

Telegraphy and Telephony

One of the earliest inventions of importance was the invention of the **Electric Battery** by Alessandro Volta in 1799. In 1837 Samuel Morse made use of this electric battery and invented **Electric Telegraph**. The **first telegraph line** connected Washington with Baltimore and became active in May 1844. **Morse Code** was a channel of communication in which the letters of typed English alphabets were converted to code words of various length and presented by a sequence of dots and dashes, for example, A (.-); B (-...); C (-.-.). In wars, this Morse code was extensively utilized for effective communication. In 1875, Émile Baudot improved the code for telegraphy. In 1858, the **first trans-atlantic telegraphy** was installed connecting the United States and Europe, marking a milestone in the history of technological communication. This became functional from 1866.

Alexander Graham Bell invented **Telephone** in 1876 and established Bell Telephone Company in 1877. Advancement in telephony continued with the development of an **Electromechanical Step-by-Step Automatic Switch** by Strowger in 1897, which was used for several decades. Early versions of telephones were very simple and could communicate within a distance of a few hundred miles. Invention of **carbon microphone and induction coil** during early part of 20th century and the invention of **triode amplifier** by Lee De Forest in 1906 made it possible for telephone signal to transmit sound waves over long distances. In 1915, inter-continental telephone transmission got activated. The First World War in 1914, Great Depression in 1930s and Second World War from 1939 might have been reasons for the long gap in progress of science and technology. The curtain again opened in 1953 when the **first trans-atlantic telephone service** was established between the United States and Europe.

Wireless Communication System

The development of **Wireless Communications** originated from the research works of Oersted, Faraday, Gauss, Maxwell, and Hertz. In 1820, Oersted demonstrated that an **electric current can produce a magnetic field**. In 1831, Michael Faraday demonstrated that a **changing magnetic field can produce an electric field in presence of a conductor.** In 1864, James C. Maxwell predicted the **existence of electromagnetic radiation** and formulated the basic theory that has been in use for over a century. Maxwell's theory was **proved experimentally** by Hertz in 1887. In 1894, **Coherer**, a sensitive device that could **detect radio signals** was invented by Oliver Lodge. He demonstrated a wireless communication over a distance of 150 yards at Oxford, England. Guglielmo Marconi developed ***wireless telegraphy*** in 1895 and demonstrated the transmission of radio signals at a distance of approximately 2 kilometers. Two years later, in 1897, Marconi patented a radio telegraph system and established the ***Wireless Telegraph and Signal Company***. In 1901, Marconi received a radio signal from a distance of about 1,700 miles. The ball of inventions rolled fast.

The invention of the ***vacuum tube*** was especially instrumental in the development of radio communication systems. The ***vacuum diode*** was invented by John Ambrose Fleming in 1904 and the ***vacuum triode amplifier*** was invented by Lee de Forest in 1906. The invention of the vacuum triode made ***radio broadcast*** possible in the early part of the 20th century. ***Amplitude modulation (AM)*** broadcast was initiated in 1920 from the radio station KDKA, Pittsburgh. From that date, AM radio broadcasting grew rapidly across the country and around the world. The ***superheterodyne AM radio receiver***, as we know it today, was invented by Edwin Armstrong during the First World War. Another significant development in radio communications was the invention of ***frequency modulation (FM)***, also done by Armstrong in 1933. After the end of Second World War, FM radio broadcast became popular and developed commercially.

The first ***television system*** was built in the United States by V K Zworykin in 1929. Commercial television broadcasting began in London in 1936 by the British Broadcasting Corporation (BBC). In 1941, the Federal Communications Commission (FCC) officially sanctioned television broadcasting in the United States.

The invention of the ***transistor*** in 1947 by Walter Brattain, John Bardeen, and William Shockley; the ***integrated circuit*** in 1958 by Jack Kilby and Robert Noyce; and the ***laser*** by Townes and Schawlow in 1958, have made the development of small-size, low-power, low-weight, and high-speed electronic circuits possible. These are used in the construction of satellite communication systems, wideband microwave radio systems, and light wave communication systems using fiber optic cables. A ***satellite*** named 'Telstar I' was launched in 1962 and was used to relay television signals between Europe and the United States. ***Commercial Satellite Communication*** services began in 1965 with the launching of the ***Early Bird*** satellite.

Digital Communication System

With the invention of the ***Transistor***, electronic or digital switches became economically viable.

From late 1950s to late 1970s, rapid digital revolution had taken place, which changed the mechanical and electronic technology to digital electronics. The development of ***digital switch*** by Bell Telephone Laboratories in 1960s was another landmark towards advancement in telecommunication system. During the past few decades, numerous important advancements have taken place. Fibro-optic cable lines are replacing copper wires in telephone industries, which can transmit varieties of information including voice, data and video in buses, trains and cars. Cellular radio has been developed to provide telephone services and digital switches have replaced the old electromechanical systems. High-speed communication networks link computers and a variety of peripheral devices around the world.

From the history, we realize that human communication has come a long way from sign language to digital communication system. In this history of development of communication systems, we recognize the contribution of known and unknown scientists, scholars and common people. However, it is the growing needs of human beings that act as a force towards various advancements.

SCIENCE OF COMMUNICATION

Human communication or interpersonal interactions is an art as well as has a verified scientific basis. The sciences involved in Human Communication are *Physical Sciences* (anatomy, physiology) and *Behavioral Sciences*. To be more specific, nervous system and interpersonal or social interactions decide the pattern of communication. Many research studies are going on to understand human communication in the light of scientific evidences.

Physical Sciences

The *nervous system* consists of the *brain*, *spinal cord*, *sensory organs* and the network of *nerves* that connect these sensory organs with the body parts. Together, they control the body functions and our behavioral pattern, by collaborating with each other. Every type of human communication is a specific type of behavior. To understand the scientific basis of how we communicate to each other, we need to understand how the nerve cells (neurons) communicate to each other and transfer messages from one body part to another.

Neurotransmitters

For rapid communication, the neurons send electrical signals to each other along the axons by mechanism of conduction. These electrical signals are known as *action potential*. Communication between neurons takes place at synaptic junctions, by the process of *neurotransmission*.

All the functions of our brain depend on the adequate and timely release of *neurotransmitters*. These are small chemical molecules, which act as medium to transmit messages/information from one brain cell to another across a *Synapse* (gap of about 50 nm between two neurons). Neurotransmitters are stored in small bubble-like structures, called **vesicles**. Each vesicle has a single type of neurotransmitter, for example, dopamine, relates to our memory and mental skills like intelligence; serotonin, regulates our mood, etc.

When a nerve impulse (message) reaches at the end of a nerve fiber, a neurotransmitter is released from the end of one neuron (known as presynaptic terminal). It travels through the synapse and gets attached to the receptors on the next neuron in the series (known as postsynaptic terminal) (Fig. 1). Some neurotransmitters (glutamate, aspartate etc.) are stimulatory or excitatory in nature; they bind to

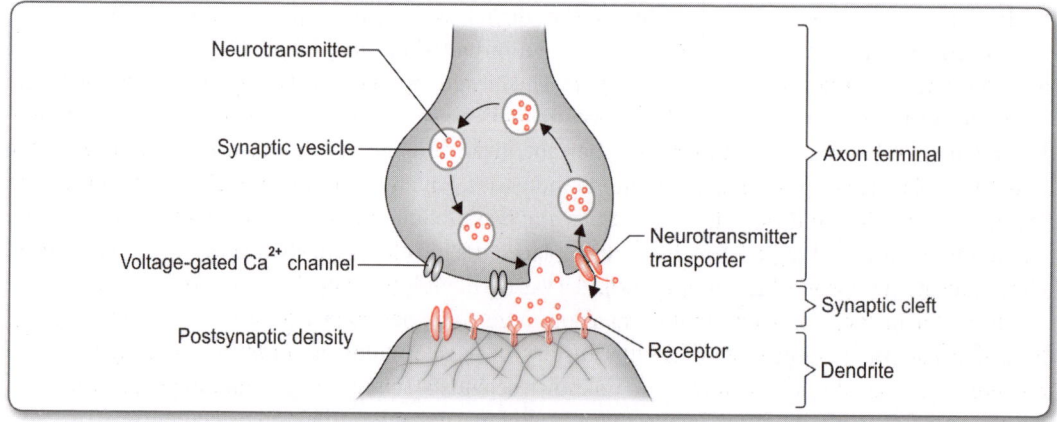

Fig. 1: Communication through neurotransmitters between the nerves

the nerve receptors at the postsynaptic terminal and generate an electrical impulse (action potential), which stimulate the neuron. Some others gamma aminobutyric acid (GABA), glycine etc. bind to the post-synaptic terminal nerve receptors, but inhibit or prevent the production of electrical impulse, thus preventing the neurons to act or slowing the speed of action.

In short, neurotransmitters can change the activities within our nervous system by changing their chemical stimuli. This in turn can change our behavioral pattern. Any problem for the adequate and timely release of neurotransmitters would lead to defective communication.

Sensory Organs

Normally we all have five sensory organs, which help us to communicate. These are senses of sight, hearing, smell, taste and touch. There are many complex processes continuously taking place inside our body to communicate messages or information to and fro through these sensory organs. Let us understand, how this works.

Sight

There are visual signals, which include our facial expressions, gestures and postures. These are called 'body language'. We receive these visual signals by using our sense of sight in eyes.

When we see something, the light rays from the object fall on the pupil of the eye. The light rays crosses the lens of the eye, the upside down image of the object is formed, which shines on the retina at the back of the eye. Retina contains rods and cones cells, which are photoreceptive and they help us to see the detailed image of the object and colors. The optic nerve sends a message of this image to the brain, where the picture is turned to right way up. Our eyes help us to judge the distance of the object, the brain tells us what is the meaning of this image and what should be our response to the object we are seeing.

Seeing objects with two eyes gives much better understanding of the situation than seeing with only a single eye, thus affecting communication.

Hearing

Hearing of the sounds made by speech/talking is the most common way of human communication. The three parts of the ear are the Outer Ear, Middle Ear and Inner Ear.

The compressed air pressure is much higher inside the ear than outside environment. As the sound wave enters the outer ear, the difference in air pressure is smoothened by the funnel shaped pinna. The sound wave then passes through the auditory canal, (which amplifies the low pitch sounds) and hits the ear drum (tympanic membrane) which marks the beginning of the Middle Ear. The pressure from the sound wave makes the ear drum vibrate.

The middle ear consists of three small thin bones (malleus, incus, stapes); the oval window, the round window and the Eustachian tube. In the middle ear, the sound becomes louder and clear and travels to the inner ear through the oval window. The inner ear consists of the cochlea (a snail-like structure containing fluid and hair fibers), the vestibules (contains fluid and hair fibers, helps the body to maintain balance or equilibrium) and the auditory nerve, which is connected to the auditory center of the brain. The round window makes the fluid in the cochlea to move, setting the thousands of hair fibers (approximately 24,000) to motion, which send electric impulses to the auditory nerve. The hair fibers in the cochlea are all connected to the auditory nerve. The receptor cells then send these electric impulses signals along the auditory nerve to the brain. In the brain, these electric impulses are translated into specific meaningful sounds, which we hear and understand.

The Eustachian tube's work is to equalize the air pressure on both sides of the eardrum, to prevent increased air pressure in the ear. If the air pressure is not equalized, the ear drum cannot vibrate properly, thus reducing the hearing ability and causing ineffective communication.

Taste

There are four different types of taste buds on our tongue. The front buds are responsible for sweet taste, side ones are for sour, bitter taste is experienced at the back of the tongue and salty taste can be felt all over the tongue.

Though directly the sense of taste may not be linked to human communication, its indirect influence on social interactions while tasting food has great impact on communication. Throughout the world, in all communities, food plays an important role in human relationship. Choice of the ingredients, the manner of preparation and the way food is served and the body language while taking food conveys messages non-verbally, which are sometimes stronger than the verbal speech. For example, during festivals, many people together prepare, serve and eat food together, which helps to develop a positive relationship and healthy communication.

Touch

Our skin (integumentary system) is the largest organ of the body and contains more than four million sensory nerve receptors with hundreds of nerve endings on every square inch surface. They function like an antenna receiving streams of messages continuously from all sources coming in contact to the body such as softness-hardness, hot-cold, pain-pleasure etc. When they are squeezed, the cell layers rub against each other and send electrical signals to the brain, then we feel the touch.

It is the first sense organ developed *in utero* and is an important non-verbal communication technique. The most sensitive areas are lips, back of the neck, fingertips, and the sole of the feet. The middle part of our back is the least sensitive area. We communicate our feelings by touching people. Shaking hands, hugging etc. shows our happy and friendly feelings; we put our arms around to console a person who is upset. Touch can reduce mental stress by lowering the level of the hormone cortisol. Touch stimulates the brain to release endorphins, which help to reduce pain. Even blood pressure and heart rate can be reduced by touch.

As natural as our mother's touch, **therapeutic touch** is a technique to help people to relax, relieve anxiety and pain, and help them heal faster. It is based on ancient **healing** practices. It is thought to promote healing by balancing the body's biochemical environment. **Dolores Krieger**, a professor at New York University School of Nursing, and **Dora Kunz**, a natural healer, developed therapeutic touch in the early 1970s.

Smell

Just like the sense of taste, the sense of smell is a part of our chemosensory system. The olfactory sensory neurons (5–6 million yellowish cells) located in a small patch of tissue high up inside our nasal passages. When we breathe, air passes through nostrils and travels down the back of the mouth and to throat and sticks to the mucus membrane of the nose. The small hairs in the nostrils, called sensory hairs sense the smell or odor and send the message to the brain where the smell is recognized.

Sense of smell is important in social interactions, though it differs from culture to culture. Smell can influence our moods, emotions, immunity, endocrine system and overall health. Smell also triggers memories very effectively. In our day to day life, we use fragrant flowers and incense sticks to express positive emotions as love, respect etc. Different perfumes are believed to be used to arouse different kinds of emotions. Good smell from food increases appetite. In contrast, the smells of smoke from a fire communicates danger. Sense of smell is a powerful instrument for nonverbal communication.

Sensory Distortion

The messages or information can be distorted by sensory distortion. Physical health problems such as pain, discomforts, level of consciousness, defective sensory organs etc. are common causes for distortion of messages. Psychological disorders, which cloud the thought process are also responsible for distortion. If the received messages are distorted, the responses will not be correct as well, thus creating confusion in the communication system. Any mechanical defect in the mechanized communication is another reason for this confusion. Many a times our mind distorts or changes the information received consciously, to fit into our own expectations and desires for our own benefits.

Perception affects communication. Perception is the processing, interpreting, selecting and organizing information, giving it a meaning and responding accordingly. Different people interpret the same information differently depending on their own mental condition at that time. For example, two of us meet someone for the first time – one of us thinks the person is smart, intelligent and well learned. The other one thinks that the person is egoistic, showing off his knowledge and over confident. Both of us may be wrong and the person may be very different. Perceptions are result of our past experiences, culture and personality, which seeks reasons for our own actions or responses to communication. Perceptions can lead to distortion of messages, which are biases or judgements of others.

Behavioral Sciences

The concepts of Social Sciences and Psychology are integral parts of human communication. Human to human interactions are very complex because of our differences in personal traits, culture, external environment and the present context of interaction. However, human beings are social animals and therefore cannot live in isolation without interacting with each other. During social interaction, we receive both conscious and unconscious social signals from others' expressions, gestures, postures, actions, and intonation that decides the quality, pattern and outcome of the interaction.

Although verbal communication is often stressed in the analysis of social interaction, a major part of human-to-human interaction is nonverbal. Only 7% of the meaning of verbal communication comes from the spoken words. The remaining understanding breaks down as: 50% from facial expression and 38% from the way how the words were spoken.

In our day-to-day interactions, we usually categorize people according to their gender, skin color, dresses, profession, language, religion, etc. and thus, the initial interactions are judgmental and prejudiced. If the relationship continues and the both parties are psychologically comfortable with each other, they gradually understand each other as they are and the interactions become informal, nonjudgemental and genuine. In a successful communication, the interacting persons should keep an open mind and try to understand each other's responses without distorting the true meaning of the message.

COMMUNICATIONS

Definition and Meaning

The word *Communication* has a different meaning for different people. The meaning may change according to the situation. The word has been defined by several authors; there are as many as 95 well known definitions. For our purpose, few simple and clear definitions are mentioned here.

- "Communication is not just interaction, it is carrying a message or information from one person to another"—**Teaching and learning in schools of nursing. Loretta E. Heidgerken. 3rd Ed. Knark Publishers Pvt. Ltd. Delhi, 1998**
- Webster dictionary defines it as, "the art or action of imparting or transmitting".
- "Communication refers to the process by which information is transmitted and *understood* between two or more people. Understanding is the most important point in any successful communication". **Organizational Behaviour. McShane Steven L, Mary Ann Von Glinow, Radha R. Sharma. 3rd Ed. Tata McGraw-Hill Publishing Co. Ltd., New Delhi, 2006**
- "Communication is the process of exchanging information and understanding between people". **Organisational Behaviour. K. Aswathappa. 8th revised edition. Himalayan Publishing House. Mumbai, 2008**

   From the above statements we can recognize some common points which are essential parts of the communication process. These are known as *Elements* of communication.

ELEMENTS OF COMMUNICATION

There are seven major elements or components, which are essential for the process of human communication. These are:

- The Source or Sender
- The Message
- Encoding
- The Medium or Channel or Transmitter
    - Verbal or Oral communication
    - Nonverbal communication
    - Written communication
    - Visual communication
    - Meta-communication
- The Receiver
- Decoding
- The Response or Feedback

The above elements indicate that there is a person or a device to initiate and send a message, the message travels through a medium or channel and is received by another person or a device. A response or feedback completes the system.

Source or Sender

It is the origin or encoder of the message, who wants to send a message or share an idea or information. The source or sender may be a human being such as teacher in a class or a written material like a book or a mechanical device like an alarm clock. The characteristics and abilities of the source or sender are important influences on the quality and effect of communication. Therefore, human sender has to be conscious, should have a clear voice and speech, should understand accurately the message to be sent and its importance. The instrument or device as a sender must be in proper working condition to encode the message.

Message

There are *three types* of messages, depending on its *purpose* of sending:
- **Information:** These are communication of ideas and knowledge.
- **Feelings:** These are communication of concerns, reactions, pleasant or unpleasant feelings, interest, attitudes, likes and dislikes etc.
- **Orders and Requests:** These are orders or requests to do certain activities. For example, Institutional rules and regulations are an order and application for sanctioning leave is a request.
  (**Understanding Organizational Behaviour. Udai Pareek. Oxford University Press, New Delhi, 2004).**
  The message needs to be clear and the medium of its transmission has to be appropriate to prevent any distortion or deviation of the message.

Encoding

In human communication, the message can be of numerous forms, it may be abstract feelings, which are only mentally conveyed or it may be concrete or actual factual information. Therefore, to transfer the message to others, the message requires the use of symbols, gestures, actions or pictures. This process of conversion of the subject matter of the message to symbols, actions, pictures etc. is termed as Encoding. Only after encoding, a message can enter a Medium or Channel of communication.

Medium or Channel or Transmitter

Medium is the way we communicate or the way a message is transmitted. Medium or channel of communication is very important, as each channel has different advantages and disadvantages. For example, announcement to a village public about an exhibition on 'Preventive Measures of Tuberculosis' by a written letter or a printed leaflet may be clear to some people who can read it, but for others broadcasting through a microphone would be more effective, also it may be less costly. On the other hand, to convey technical or complex information, telephonic conversation may not be clear. Rather it is better to use a written or printed document. It gives time for the receiver to understand the message and act accordingly.

Now a days, many communication channels are available to us, such as, face-to-face conversation; telephone calls, cell phone text messages (Short Message Service); Electronic Mail (email); radio and television; written letters; printed materials; Internet including social media such as Facebook and

Twitter etc. The medium of communication may be *classified* as *Verbal, Nonverbal, Written and Visual* communication mediums. Now let us discuss about them one by one.

Verbal or Oral Communication

Verbal communication is the process of exchanging information or message between two or more persons through spoken words. Sound waves carry the words to and fro. It is used in our daily human interactions, in speech, classroom lectures, and phone calls or in formal and informal discussions. If the transmission system is perfect, the message of the sender and the receiver is the same. For example, clarity of speech, clear audible voice and no physical barrier between the sender and receiver of the message can transmit the message as it is without any distortion.

It is important that the body language including facial expressions of the sender of the verbal message is appropriate or matching with the meaning of the message. For example, while conveying good news, a smiling face is more appropriate than a crying face. Face-to-face and Eye-to-eye contact between the sender and receiver of the message makes the meaning very clear. The body language accompanying a verbal communication also can indicate the interacting persons' personality and relationship, to some extent.

Nonverbal Communication

It has been estimated that human communication is approximately 20% verbal and 80% nonverbal, so if we are saying something to a person but our body language is saying different things, then we are not getting our message across. The purpose of communication is lost.

In our day-to-day life whenever we are with others, unknowingly we give out indications or signals about what is in our mind. Similarly we also receive signals from others who are present around us. Here the communication is wordless, hence soundless and is called a nonverbal communication. Our body speaks many things. Our body language including facial expression, gestures, posture, the way we dress, the way we talk, eye contact, how we behave, even our body odor – all communicate some meaning, send strong messages to others. Even when we are silent, not speaking, we are still communicating nonverbally and expressing our emotions. Nonverbal communication uses all our five senses, is natural, unconscious and represents our true feelings and purpose, shows our true self. However, consciously we try to hide our true feelings, sooner or later it gets revealed through our behavior of which we are not aware.

Many a times what we speak out and our body language convey different meanings. In such situations, the receiver of the message often believes our nonverbal message and decides to act accordingly.

Types of Nonverbal Communication and Body Language

It is important to understand nonverbal communication, as its influence on verbal communication is great and makes a communication effective or ineffective. There are different types of nonverbal communication, such as, **Facial Expressions, Body Movements and Postures, Gestures, Eye Contact, Touch, Space and Voice**. Let us see what these body languages depict.

Facial Expressions

It is generally believed that 'face is the mirror of mind'. Human facial muscles are so flexible that with slightest change of movements we can express numerous kinds of emotions. Most of the facial expressions are common all over the world among different cultural groups, e.g., happiness, sadness, anger, disgust, surprise, fear, affection, etc. (Fig. 2).

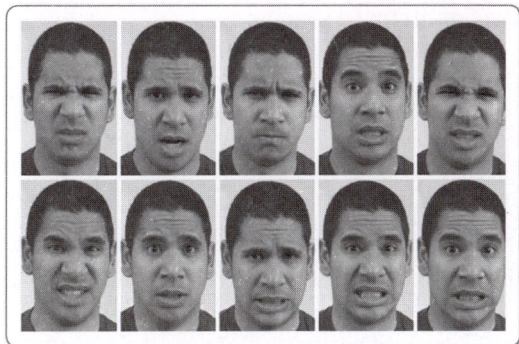

Fig. 2: Facial expressions

Body Movements and Postures

Our body posture i.e., the way we sit, stand, lie in bed and very subtle movements, communicates many messages. For example, open arms indicate welcome; crossing arms across chest, when the weather is not cold, and leaning away from the person - signals putting up a barrier between us and the other person (Fig. 3).

Gestures

Gestures are specific meaningful movements of our hands and legs, which are different in different cultures. Most gestures are learnt from our family members, friends and society, some if repeated for a long time become habit. These animated actions may be conscious or unconscious movements. For example, calling someone by waving hand or saying 'ta ta', using hands while speaking or arguing with others etc. We need to be careful to use gestures appropriately in different circumstances, otherwise our nonverbal communication would be misinterpreted.

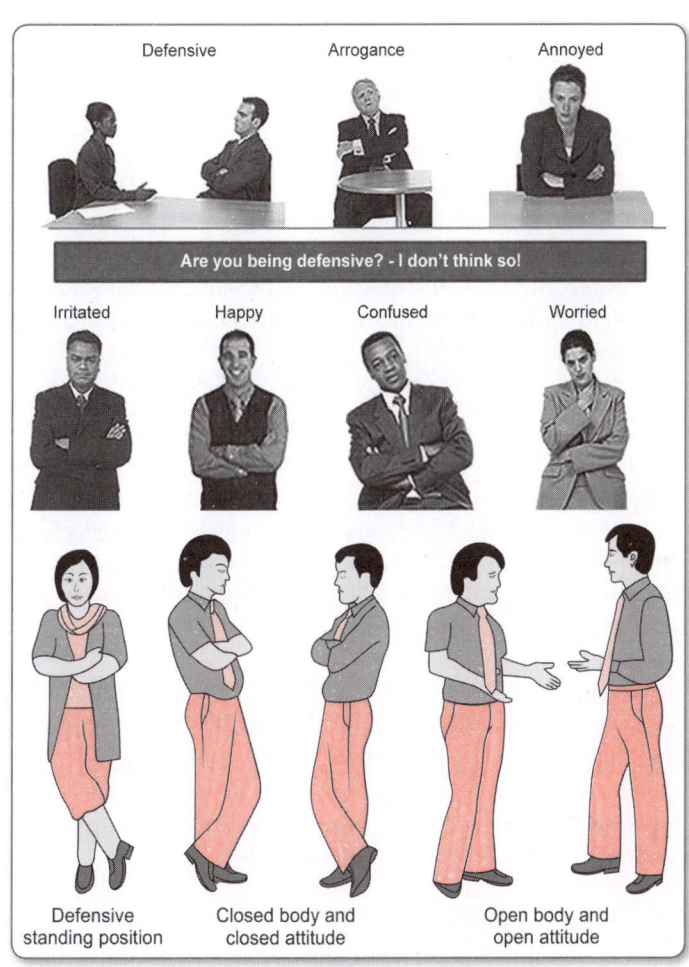

Fig. 3: Body postures

Eye Contact

It is generally believed that on our face, eyes are the main mirrors of our mind because all emotions can be expressed through our eyes. There are smiling eyes, sad eyes, cruel eyes, etc. Most of our nonverbal communications are with the signals of our eyes. The way we look at someone can communicate many things: our interest to meet someone; affection, unfriendliness or attraction. Eye contact is also important in maintaining the flow of conversation and for measuring the other person's attention and response. If a teacher while teaching in a class, looks at all students and occasionally makes eye contact with each student in turn, the students' attention is drawn to the subject of teaching and their minds get concentrated in listening to what the teacher is saying.

Touch

We communicate a great deal through touch. For example, an affectionate hug of parents; a warm handshake of a friend; a gentle touch to console a grieving person; an appreciating pat on one's back, all convey meaningful messages.

Space

Every living being needs a physical space of its own and that is its comfort zone, more so for human beings. With conscious observation, we can understand how much the distance between two interacting persons has impact on their relationship and signals the nature of their communication. For example, when two persons are sitting or standing very close and talking amicably, it indicates intimate informal relationship and the communication is on some common matters. Similarly, while communicating, persons in formal relationship will position themselves in a comfortable distance maintaining each other's personal space.

Voice

The pitch and tone of our voice while speaking, i.e., how much loud or how much soft is our voice, suggests the nature of the communication. Voice indicates affection, interest, anger, sarcasm, confidence, etc. characteristics of a communication. Teacher's voice modulation or making variation in tone is important to maintain the students' attention to listen to the class.

Written Communication

This is suitable for recording and presenting technical details, sometimes it is easier to follow written words than verbal communication. Written documents are important to maintain permanent records in all life situations. These are handwritten letters, lawful documents, drawings, pictures, posters, e-mails, printed materials, internet information etc. In hospitals, patients' health related notes are important legal documents. The content of the written message or information must be clear, legible and to the point for effective communication.

Visual Communication

In a classroom teaching, the written teaching-aids such as Over-Head-Projector Transparent Sheets; the liquid crystal display (LCD) Projector Slides are written visual information. For public information, written information such as posters, placards, leaflets, graphs, charts, banners, maps and logos are used, these all are visual communication. Colors used for visual messages or information need to be appropriate for the message conveyed.

Metacommunication

It is a process of analyzing the content of communication, the actual meaning of a particular word, a phrase or a sentence. It requires intuition or insight to understand others' feelings; it is an important way to establish and maintain interpersonal communication. For example, just before an important subject examination teacher notices a particular student, who is very sincere in studies and in all previous examinations has performed very well. The student appears tensed and disturbed. The teacher asks whether he is confident about the examination, he replies verbally that he is confident, but he does not look at the teacher directly, fidgeting with his pen and in general looks distressed. This nonverbal message alerts the teacher. The teacher takes the student to her office, makes him comfortable, offers a glass of water to drink and opens up conversation by asking, "You say you are confident, but you look tensed. Would you like to tell me what is troubling you?" The student reveals that his father has suddenly fallen ill this morning and is hospitalized. He is worried and unable to remember what he has studied. An interpersonal relationship has been established between the teacher and the student, which helps in further exploration of the situation and actions can be taken accordingly. This is Metacommunication.

The rule of **'ABCDE'** can be followed for all types of communication to make it effective - A stands for **Accurate**; B for **Brief**; C for **Clear**; D for **Direct** and E for **Elimination** of unnecessary jargon from the message. For effective communication, a person needs to be efficient in all the above types of communication.

Receiver

It is a human being or a technical device, which receives the message and tries to decipher or interpret the meaning. We use our intelligence to understand the meaning of the message, the technical device does the same by its working system.

Decoding

The receiver converts the message to meaningful symbols and words and this process of conversion is known as decoding. The human decoder, knowingly or unknowingly, may add his own emotions, experience and opinion to understand and decode the message. Therefore, there is a chance that the message gets deviated from its actual intention. For example, all gossips or rumors are not true; we need to check its reality before we decide to act.

The technical device can decode a message objectively as it is, if it is in perfect working condition. However, if there is any defect in the device or instrument, the decoded message may be misleading. In healthcare area, we depend on instruments like sphygmomanometer to measure blood pressure, thermometer to measure body temperature etc. devices. We need to check its working condition before using, to make correct healthcare decisions. Similarly, our professional skills need to be precise to get correct measurement of the health parameters.

Response or Feedback

The receiver responds to the source or sender to ensure that the message has been received and understood correctly as it is. This is a very important element of communication system. The success of the communication is judged on the extent of accuracy of the feedback, therefore it has to follow the rule of ABCDE. In healthcare area, our feedback to our clients' queries about their own health conditions goes a long way to determine their health behavior and health action.

These elements of communication are interrelated and interdependent on each other and mostly occur in a recurring chain. If any of the elements is defective or stops functioning, the chain is broken, the message is not transmitted as intended. In human interactions, we need to be alert to identify and control our medium or channel or method of communication, so as to prevent the distortion of the message sent. That brings us to the Theories and Models of communication.

CONCEPTS, THEORIES AND MODELS OF COMMUNICATION

The elements of communication are *concepts* or ideas, thoughts and notions, which explain all matters related to communication. Concepts are used to develop a theory. When the concepts are systematically arranged in a definite structure and they present a clear view of the matter or knowledge, a theory is created. These concepts are open for exploration and examination for proving their authenticity. A theory gives direction to understand an event.

Communication Theory proposed by S.F. Scudder (1980) states that "All living beings communicate, although the way of communication is different. The universal law of communication theory says that all living beings, whether they are plants, animals or human beings, all communicate using sound, speech, body movements, gestures, etc. to share their feelings and information. Communication is necessary for survival".

Communication Theories in Nursing

There are many theories that explain communication in Nursing. Among these, Peplau's Interpersonal Relations Theory is commonly used in practice.

Peplau's Interpersonal Relations Theory

This theory focuses on the nurse-client relationship in the context of therapeutic environment. Also it takes into consideration the factors influencing nurse-client communication such as attitudes, beliefs, and health care practices in the culture of the community. The theory defines four stages of the relationship aiming to achieve the common goals of care. These are—

- **Orientation phase**: The nurse engages the patient in treatment, and the patient is able to ask questions and receive explanations and information. This stage helps the patient develop trust and is where first impressions about the nurse and health care system begin to evolve. Factors influencing orientation phase are given in Fig. 4.
- **Identification phase**: The patient and nurse begin to work together. These interactions provide the basis for understanding, trust and acceptance as the patient becomes an active participant in treatment.

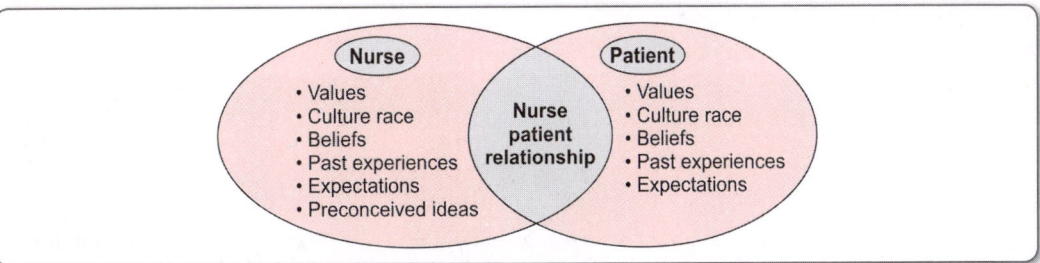

Fig. 4: Factors influencing orientation phase

- **Exploitation phase**: The patient takes advantage of all services offered, exploiting the nurse-patient relationship to address treatment goals.
- **Resolution phase**: As a result of effective communication, the patient's needs are met, and he or she moves toward full independence. The patient no longer needs help, and the relationship ends.

Models of Communication

A model is a symbolic representation of interrelated and meaningfully connected concepts, which explains an idea. Communication is a Process, in which all the interrelated elements are linked to each other. These links explain and give direction to the communication process, horizontally (linear) or vertically; in single or multiple relationships. A model of communication is a visual and structural representation of the communication process. Linear model and Berlo's Sender-Message-Channel-Receiver models of communication are given in Figs 5 and 6.

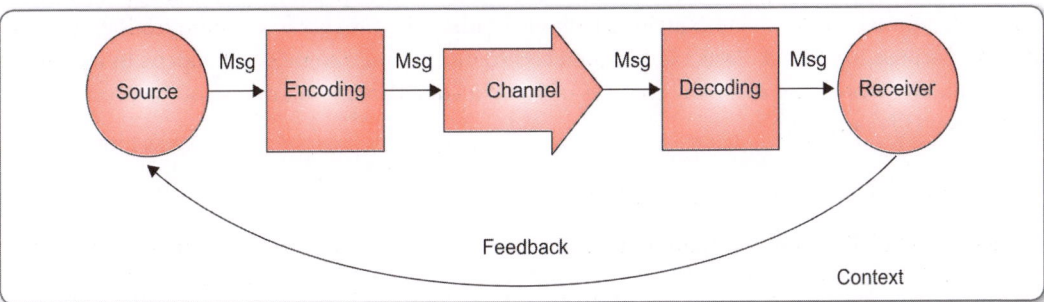

Fig. 5: Linear model of the communication process and the elements of communication

PRINCIPLES OF COMMUNICATION

Effective communication needs to follow certain guidelines, which are established truths. There are most common and important five principles:

Interpersonal Communication is Inescapable

Human beings are social animals, therefore, can't live normally without communicating. When two people are together, there has to be communication, verbal or nonverbal. It is used in our day-to-day life among family members, friends, relatives and all others we come in contact. Sometimes the communication is started with a purpose, while at other occasions, it is instant and casual.

Interpersonal Communication is Irreversible

Once the message has been communicated, verbally or non-verbally, it cannot be taken back, whatever may be the effect on the interacting persons. Therefore, to maintain a good interpersonal relationship, we need to think before we communicate about the message content, situation, medium and all other important factors that affect relationship.

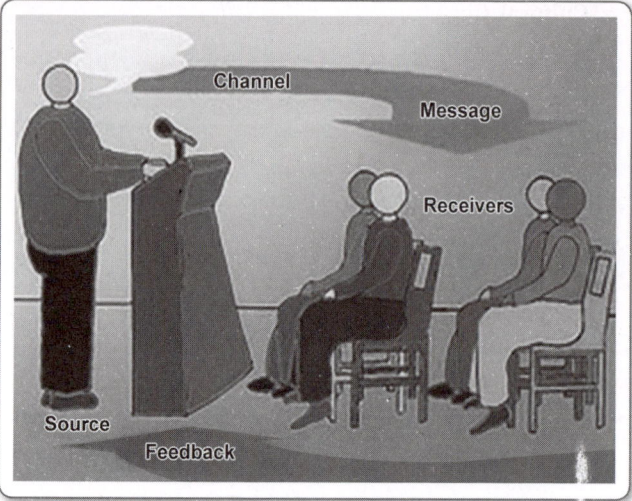

Fig. 6: Berlo's sender-message-channel-receiver model of communication

Interpersonal Communication is Complicated

There are many things involved even in smallest communications. The situation, relationship and mind-set of the interacting persons, the subject matter, environmental factors and the medium of communication. If all these are matching with each other, the process of communication is proper and the purpose is fulfilled. Particularly, when communication or interaction happens in a group to solve an issue or breaking news, the chances of complications are more because of the presence and involvement of many people.

Interpersonal Communication is Contextual

- **Psychological Context** of the interacting persons: The need for communication, values, personality, attributes, etc.
- **Rational Context**: The reactions of the interacting persons to one another are different in an organizational set up like a workplace. Here, the psychological context is different, but all involved are focused on the same issue.
- **Situational Context**: The place where the interaction is taking place. Here, the mass media plays an important role to govern our behavior. For example, during a cricket match, the Mob Behavior is influenced by the media presentation of the game. We develop our understanding of the other people from the TV and Radio news, debate etc.
- **Environmental Context**: The surroundings, i.e., time of the day, weather, noise level, how comfortable the physical environment is, etc. Thought process gets affected by the environmental elements, some distract and others may facilitate smooth interactions.

- **Cultural Context**: Beliefs, values, social norms, attitude, mannerism, customs etc. There are differences in cultural practices, which may cause misunderstanding among the interacting persons. For example, in Western world people easily smile at the strangers as a friendly gesture. But in India, strangers especially persons of opposite genders smiling at each other is generally not socially accepted.

People usually remember:
- 10% of what they read
- 20% of what they hear
- 30% of what they see
- 40% of what they hear and see

FACILITATORS OF COMMUNICATION

These are the characteristics, which support effective communications. The main facilitators identified are as follows:

Personal Qualities of the Human Source or Sender of the Message

Empathetic Understanding

Empathy is to put ourselves in other's situation and understanding their feelings. It is to identify with others during interaction. This gives confidence and strength to the relationship of the interacting persons. Empathetic understanding requires ability for attentive listening and conveying understanding without making any judgment of the other's feelings.

Recognizing Others

All humans need to be recognized by others, more desirable if it is by someone special. We recognize a person by a word of concern, appreciation or by signaling nonverbally familiarity and closeness. Teacher recognizing a student's effort to improve academic performance works as an incentive to motivate the student to achieve greater heights.

Goal-Oriented Communication

When the sender and receiver of a message are in amicable relationship and have a common goal, the communication is effective and successful. For example, when we help a person to rehabilitate, whose one leg has been amputated, the goal of achieving a near-normal independent life becomes the ultimate goal of both parties involved. Then together can plan rehabilitation activities that are realistic.

Type and Condition of the Mechanical Source of the Message and the Receiver

The mechanical device used in transferring message needs to be appropriate to the need for communication and in perfect working condition. Microphones used as a Public Address System (PAS) transmitting a recorded message need to produce clear and loud sound to attract people's attention.

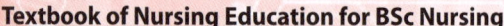

Type and Quality of the Message and the Communication Channel

It has been discussed earlier that effective communication is possible by following the rule of ABCDE while constructing the message to be sent. The type of the message and channel of communication need to be suitable to each other. For a long distance communication in remote places where digital communication services are not available, trying to send a message through a Cell Phone is useless.

Personal Qualities of the Human Receiver

The intended receiver of the message needs to have adequate and accurate message receiving capacity. The human receiver must control influencing the received message by his own emotions, information and opinion. The effective feedback by the receiver is equally important as transmitting message by the sender.

External Environment

This is the situation or context in which the communication is taking place. For successful communication, the environment needs to be free from unnecessary noise, should be comfortable for the human sender and receiver. Possible interference by the radioactive particles to electronic communication has to be considered while selecting the place to establish such kind of stations for technical communication process.

It is important to know that the context of the communication should be understood by all involved. The participants need to be on the same 'mental wavelength' and they should have the common intent for an effective communication.

BARRIERS OF COMMUNICATION

There are several barriers, which can interfere or prevent the natural flow of communication. The identified common barriers are discussed below—

- **Language Barriers:** Barriers related to different meaning of words, symbols and sentences. **These are:**
  - Words and symbols with different meaning and the meaning changes when the situation changes. All languages have these characteristics. For example, *date* is a fruit and also it means a calendar date.
  - Incorrect translation of the message when the interacting persons' known languages are different
  - Technical jargon. For example, pyrexia is simply fever
  - Body language and gesture, which do not match the meaning of the message
  - Assuming or judging the message instead of taking it as it is. The actual meaning gets changed
  - Adding own emotions to the message sent, which changes the language
  - Defective hearing and speech
  - Too long message or with too many points in verbal communication. Also, sender tries to send too much information in very short time
  - Written message is in long complex confusing sentences, too long and lack of organization in writing

- Spoken message is vague: For example, "meet me tomorrow at 8." The listener again has to ask whether it is morning or evening 8.

- **Paralanguage:** This is when verbal and nonverbal communication in a same message creates misunderstanding. It is the way we emphasize certain words or phrase with body language and tone, which changes the meaning completely. For example, "Come to my birthday party". Understanding the actual meaning of this simple sentence depends on the closeness of the relationship; situation of interaction and emotional condition of the persons involved.

- **Cultural barriers:** Words and symbol have different meaning in different cultures and communities. For example, in one culture holding hands between men and women shows a good relationship and accepted by society, while in other cultures, the same holding hands is considered against cultural practice.

- **Psychological or Personal Barriers**: Lack of confidence while speaking; poor language skill; fear of reprimand or censor; lack of motivation; poor interpersonal relationship; poor listening skills, intellectual capacity etc. Poor memory to retain whole information correctly also affects communication.

- **Physical Barriers:** It includes, noise; very soft or very loud voice; distance between the sender and receiver; selection of wrong channel; physical environment as too warm or too cold weather; lighting of the place; uncomfortable meeting place; uncomfortable chairs etc. act as distractions in effective communication. Sometimes in informal relationship, even a table in between may be a hindrance to free communication.

- **Defective technical gadgets** as channels of communication

- **Attitude:** Assuming and taking it for granted that the other person knows something about the information, hence it is enough to tell only the main points. For example, while teaching senior students, teacher may assume that they know the basics. Always it may not be true. Also the trust between the sender and receiver of the message - distortion of the message is possible if there is mistrust between the interacting persons. Time pressure may overlook some parts of the message, receiver of the message may be preoccupied with some other thought.

- **System Policies**: Organization or institution may have the following policies which may hinder free flow of communication. Employees' status forms a barrier, thus affecting the feedback –
  - Line of authority and communication:
    - Vertical line of communication: means the message or instruction is passed from the person in top position to the persons in lower positions according to their level or designations. The lowest category employee has to go through his higher level persons step by step to communicate to the top boss. In this the communication is uni-directional (single direction).
    - Horizontal line of communication: in this system all persons of same level or position communicate to each other on equal footing. Here the communication is multi-directional.
  - Facilities: Telephone, Internet, Stationeries and adequate time are required for daily communication in a work place

- **Stereotyping**: This is judging and labeling a person as strict, nonsincere, good-bad, friendly etc. For example, city people communicate with villagers in a superior manner assuming and stereotyping them as illiterate and uncivilized.

- **Selective hearing**: It is when a person is only pretending to listen to other's talk, but not sincere in trying to understand the actual meaning or has no intention to act on the message. For example, a child is busy in playing with friends, parents are telling him to stop playing and get ready for study time. The child hears the message but continues playing. When parents come to take him by force, he says that he has not heard his parents call.

To have an effective communication, it is necessary to break all these barriers. Let us see how.

Methods of Overcoming the Barriers of Communication

To overcome the barriers of communication, we have to think about all the elements of communication. The source or the sender and the receiver of the message need to be physically, mentally and intellectually sound so that proper encoding is done. If machines are used for communication, they need to be in a perfect working condition. A complete communication system must have a feedback mechanism, which is the evidence of a successful communication.

Apart from the above-mentioned there are "**Seven Cs**" for effective communication, similar to the ABCDE rule of communication:

1. **Completeness**: A message should convey all facts and add any extra information, so that there is no need for further questions or queries.
2. **Conciseness**: A brief message using minimum possible words is better than an elaborate explanation. It makes communication cost-effective in terms of manpower involved, money required and time taken.
3. **Consideration**: A message needs to be suitable for the sender's and receiver's level of understanding. Also, the sender should consider the situation and emotional condition of the receiver for proper decoding of the message and feedback.
4. **Clarity**: A message with a focus or goal with a few clear points is received without distortion. Especially in public communication, one clear message at a time is successful in achieving the goal.
5. **Concreteness**: Message needs to be factual and to the point for easy transmission and preventing misinterpretation.
6. **Courtesy**: For effective communication, the sender needs to be polite, attentive and listen sincerely to the receiver's opinion of the message. These are the basis for good interpersonal relationship.
7. **Correctness:** The language of the message should be grammatically correct and with matching nonverbal signs.

A good successful communicator observes the situation, listens, is empathetic, enthusiastic, honest, patient, has language skills, sense of humor, smiles, respects other's opinion, never stops learning and most importantly has a balanced ego.

TECHNIQUES OR ART OF COMMUNICATION (Table 1)

TABLE 1: The top 15 most effective communication techniques and strategies

S. No.	Techniques and strategies	Explanation
1.	The silent treatment	Instead of immediately answering or reacting after the other person has talked, remaining silent but being attentive encourages people to open up to give more information than intended
2.	Observation	If we have difficulty in communicating verbally or nonverbally or the situation is not appropriate for that, it is better to observe people who are interacting. We can even ask a good communicator to observe the interactions and give us the information. The observer may or may not be hidden from the persons being observed
3.	Smile	There are many types of smile, that conveys different emotions and meanings. A genuine open smile can make a nervous person feel relaxed, so that he/she can communicate effectively. An artificial smile that does not reaches the eyes can be treacherous. Depending on situations we need to use smile appropriately
4.	Honesty	Effective communication is mostly based on mutual trust. But in circumstances where being honest and giving correct information may be harmful to others involved, we should carefully frame the content and communicate in a manner appropriate to the situation. For example, breaking bad news to a patient's family about his health condition – we need to plan properly, so that the family has time to cope up to the information. It requires counseling skills
5.	Choice of language	The words we use for communication, spoken or unspoken, can either make or break a relationship. The hurt and pain inflicted by an improper language is more severe than a weapon. Hence, we need to choose our language carefully in any interaction, considering the circumstances and persons involved in communication. For example, in a group work, we need to use 'we', 'us', 'our' etc. so that all members feel a sense of belonging and cooperate to achieve the common goal. On the other hand, if we have to convince someone about a point, 'I' and 'me' can be used to emphasize on the matter. For example, making a sick person to agree for a painful lab test to make final diagnosis
6.	Asking question	An interaction can be started and continued by asking relevant questions. Depending on the situation questions can be – • **Closed-ended**: The purpose is to get only simple 'yes' or 'no' answers. These are used to get basic information, which do not need explanations. For example, did you sleep well? • **Open-ended**: The information, which needs some detail. For example, how did you have this accident? How much pain you feel? Questions need to be focused to a point, such as, "On a scale of zero to ten, show me how much better you feel today?" Asking questions verbally is an art, properly chosen non-verbal body language can make a question clearer to get a correct information
7.	Listening	Listening is not just hearing. An effective communication requires active listening by both interacting parties. Listening is to hear the information with attention, mentally analyzing and understanding the meaning. For example, we may hear a child crying, but when we try to understand why he is crying, that is listening. This is a part of counseling skill

Contd...

S. No.	Techniques and strategies	Explanation
8.	Response or Feedback	Any communication cannot continue unless all persons involved respond or give feedback to each other verbally or nonverbally. Giving feedback is a way of confirming that the message has been received. Response can be obtained by asking open-ended or close-ended question. For example, after placing the patient with pain in a position supposed to be comfortable, we need to ask whether really he is comfortable or not. To get a clear response, all the elements of communication need to be in proper order
9.	Empathy	Empathy means placing ourselves in other's situation, so that we can feel how he is feeling. All are not skilled in communicating clearly verbally or nonverbally. Factors like shyness, speech defects etc. may hinder in transfer of message from the sender to the receiver. Unless we have empathy, we will not be able to understand the message the person is trying to convey. Empathy requires paying attention to listen to the other's communication and get its deep and real meaning. For example, a student may be unable to express his/her family problem, which is disturbing his/her concentration to learn. The teacher needs to have empathy to counsel the student, so as to strengthen him/her to cope up with the situation
10.	Enthusiasm	Showing enthusiasm by being attentive and showing interest in what others are saying is to encourage the person to communicate clearly and completely. A few positive words or body language like appropriate facial expressions and eye contact are way of showing enthusiasm. Showing impatience, boredom or interfering unnecessarily signal that one is not interested to continue interaction.
11.	Sense of Humor	Except some rare people, all human beings like to laugh. Laughing releases endorphins that relieves stress and thus improve the mood for conversation. But the use of humor should be appropriate to the situation. We cannot crack joke when a person is anxious or sad. It would rather harm the relationship between the interacting persons.
12.	Stress management	Communication cannot fulfill its purpose if the persons involved are under stress. In a situation where the interacting persons are argumentative over an issue or their viewpoints are very different, it is better to stop the conversation temporarily till the interacting persons can think clearly with cool head. Sometimes, a third party is required to smoothen the situation.
13.	Speak equally	In order to get an attentive audience or cooperation from the persons communicating, sometimes it is necessary to speak on equal terms, so that all feel the satisfaction of participating in the conversation. For example, using the words as 'we', 'ours' etc. creates a sense of equality and the purpose of communication is achieved. Especially in a group discussion, all should be given equal opportunity to voice their opinion as the group-leader controls the focus of discussion.
14.	Reading books	A book means any good reading material which increases and updates our knowledge of daily life. Adequate knowledge on the subject makes conversation easy and free flowing
15.	Never stop learning	Communication is a science. With the rapid changes in the socio-economic-political scenario, its field is ever advancing with the invention of newer dimensions. Hence we need to keep learning the newer techniques. For example, a couple of decades back, lecture method was predominant in classroom teaching. Now a days, the use of over-head and LCD projectors has added a different outlook. Today, it is not only 'teaching', it's 'teaching-learning' sessions where learning takes place through teacher-student interactions. Group discussions have become popular tools for learning. Effective communication requires appropriate attitude, knowledge and skill.

Human communication has become very complicated these days owing to our complex life styles and advances in technology. People have become very sensitive and less tolerant to each other. This results in misunderstanding, chaos and conflict. Practicing these techniqies of effective communication would help us to maintain good interpersonal relationships and help everyone involved to achieve the real purpose of communication which is beneficial to all.

THERAPEUTIC COMMUNICATION

It involves interaction between the sick person and healthcare professionals. Nursing is a science and an art. Art involves the quality of a nurse, which helps a sick person to recover quickly from illness. Therapeutic communication includes:

- **Active listening**: Open and relaxed posture, eye contact and genuine expression
- **Showing empathy**: Understanding and acknowledging each other's feelings. Showing honest attention and interest to what the other is saying can gain the client's trust
- **Giving hope**, which is realistic: For example, "As per our knowledge and experience, we will see you well within two months. But you should also feel optimistic and give us this time to do our best for you. We appreciate your courage and patience".
- **Providing and clarifying information** about his illness and recovery, maintaining the ethical limit. Explanation is required at every stage of therapy, so as to assure the person of a competent caring communication system.
- **Touch:** Therapeutic touch is a topic of research in healthcare. It has been proved that touch has many meanings and a meaningful touch at an appropriate place, time and context helps in the recovery of a sick person.
- **Sharing observations**: by saying," You look happy today, any good news?" It makes the person feels good.
- **Sharing feelings**: In a counseling situation, counselor has to share some feelings with the counselee. This encourages him/her to open up his problem. This is known as *Self-Disclosure*. However, the ethical limit must be maintained
- **Paraphrasing**: It is restarting another sentence using a word or phrase from the other's talk. For example, the student says, "I cannot concentrate in my studies". The teacher starts by asking, "You say you cannot concentrate in your study. Have you tried to analyze, why you cannot concentrate?"
- **Confrontation**: Making the client aware of his own attitude and behavior. For example, "You said you would stop smoking, but still you have not made up your mind to do that."
- **Summarizing**: It is important to summarize the whole conversation or counseling session to make sure that the client has understood the advice or health instructions.

NEUROLINGUISTIC PROGRAMING

The Unit on Communication is not complete without some knowledge about neurolinguistic programing (NLP).

The Achievers

Arunima Sinha, 26, is the first Indian woman to climb Mount Everest on her prosthetic legs (artificial legs). On May 21, 2013, she was awarded Padmashree. On 11th April, 2011, on her journey from

Lucknow to Delhi, she resisted a group of robbers, who tried to snatch her gold chain. The robbers threw her out of the running train. Another train coming on the parallel track ran over her legs. Her left leg had to be amputated below knee and a rod was fixed in her right leg from the knee to ankle. People sympathized with her, but she was determined to win over her fate and achieve her goal of climbing Himalayan Mountains. She wrote, "The moment I decided to conquer the Mount Everest, my inner sense of handicap or disability faded away. Now, it was a matter of time to show the outer world what I was made up of."

There is a saying, "What we think, we become". There are ample instances showing that if we think and believe in ourselves that 'we can' – yes, we can succeed in most difficult tasks.

History and Origin of NLP

NLP is an approach to communication, personal development and psychotherapy. It was developed during the early 1970s by an information scientist and a linguist, John Grinder and Richard Bandler, respectively at the University of California at Santa Cruz. They observed that people with similar background of education, years of experience etc. had achievements of various levels, some were high achievers, some mediocre, while others were unfocussed. On investigating about how successful people communicated, they observed that successful people had a definite pattern of thinking, which helped them to achieve the desired goal. On this basis they developed a theory stating that, *"the brain can learn the healthy patterns and behaviors which brings about positive effects on people's physical and emotional status and thus, changing their attitude and behavior"*. This concept is known as Neurolinguistic Programing and is extensively used in psychotherapy. Later, Grinder and Bandler refined the linguistic patterns used by therapists to successfully influence people's behaviors towards positive outcome.

What is NLP?

NLP proposes that all behaviors are the results of our neurological process. Our behavior gets demonstrated through the way we communicate. NLP is a method of influencing behavior through the use of language. It is a collection of techniques and strategies, which explores the connection between neurological process of human communication, language used and experience-based behavior, which brings desirable achievements. It often includes auto-suggestions, self-hypnosis or hypnosis in its program. NLP focusses on the method of communication, not the content of behavior (Fig. 7). Let us understand the real meaning of three parts of NLP.

- **Neuro**: Refers to the part of the nervous system that helps to send, receive, store and reciprocate information. NLP is established on the knowledge that we experience in the world through our senses and the sensory information gets translated into thought process, consciously and subconsciously. Thoughts activate the neurological system, which in turn affects our physiology, emotions and behavior.

- **Linguistic**: Means the language of the content of communication, verbal or non-verbal, which is being sent to and fro. Linguistics in NLP is the study of how our words and body language influence our experience in interpersonal interactions. The same language we use for ourselves in perceiving our life events, thus either making us happy or sad about the events.

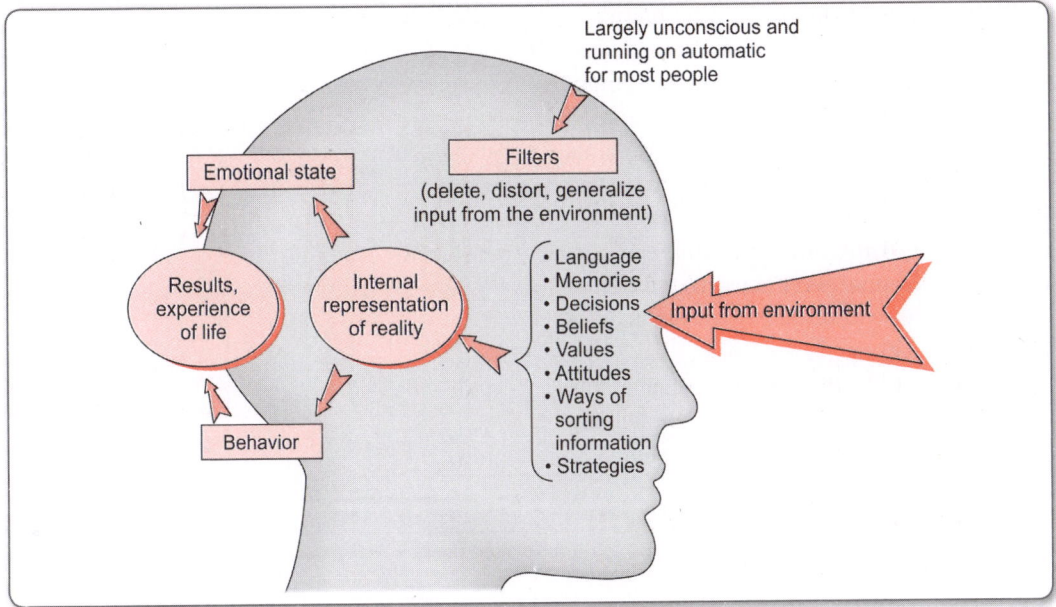

Fig. 7: Neurolinguistic programing

- **Programing:** The way the brain manipulates and changes the content of the communication, on the basis of past experience or in connection to some other related experiences stored in our brain. This results in changes in our thinking pattern and demonstrated behavior. It is based on the learning theory and explains how our experiences influence our way to think, make decisions about the response or behavior and get the anticipated results. We all have potentials to use our internal capacity to succeed. NLP helps to make us aware of that potentials. The NLP skill has to be learnt.

The basic principle of NLP is that the words or language we use reflect our inner subconscious perception of our problems, which direct our attitude towards it. If the language we use are inaccurate or with negative suggestion, it will create a deep-seated problem, that itself becomes an obstacle for our goal achievement. Our attitude, in fact, decides the direction our life will take. We are responsible for our happiness.

For an example, a person with speech defect may subconsciously accept the problem as incurable. Teasing in school and by others add to the feeling of dejection. So, he does not participate in any common event where he has to talk. Gradually he isolates himself from his peer groups and others and develops inferiority complex and psychological depression. This makes him demotivated to progress in common terms, he starts failing to achieve his even ordinary goals. NLP can bring him out of that and make him aware of his own potentials, his attitude about himself changes, self-esteem gets a boost and he gets self-motivated to progress.

The Process of NLP: A Model (Fig. 8)

By learning and practicing NLP, we can be aware of our full potentials and utilize it for achieving our desired goals of life. Also, we can help others to attain their goals through this specific technique of communication. Many research studies are underway to establish the facts about NLP.

- **Rapport**: Creates mutual trust among interacting persons.
- **Sensory Awareness**: Sometimes without anyone telling us, we can sense the mood of the interacting persons. By NLP training, we can sharpen our senses, so that we can understand the situation instinctively.
- **Outcome Thinking**: Involving in any communication keeping in mind the outcome or end-result helps us to achieve the purpose or goal.
- **Behavioral Flexibility**: means being able to change our behavior, if it is not helping us to attain our goal of communication.

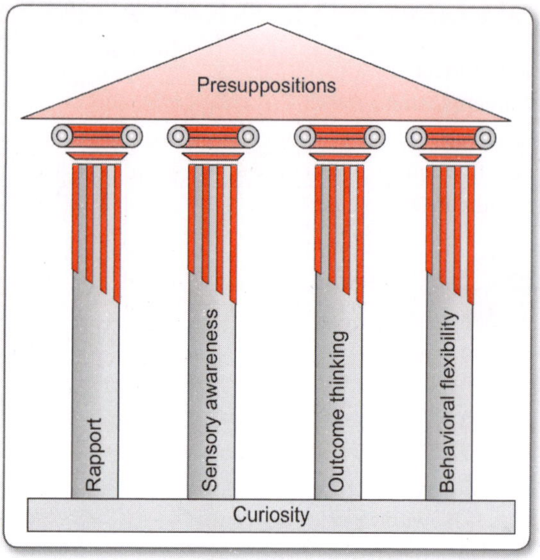

RESEARCH ON COMMUNICATION

Research on Communication has its origin in behavior sciences, as social relationship

Fig. 8: Pillars of NLP

plays a role in deciding the type of interactions in all situations. Healthcare professionals work and deal with human health and life. The close interdependent relationship between body and mind has long been established. In healthcare settings, important research projects reveal intricacies of human communication, which help in identifying the deep delicate unspoken facts influencing our health, illness and recovery.

In a hospital, as the patients await respite or recovery from sickness, their hospital experience has two distinct dimensions—the discomfort caused by their illness and treatment; and the interaction or communication with the care-givers. The nature of this interaction greatly determines the extent of patients' discomfort and therapeutic outcome.

In a research study of Nurse-Patient Communication including 150 patients and 50 nurses of a multispeciality 2000 bed hospital, the major facilitators and barriers of communication were identified. The facilitators were 1:3 Nurse: Patient Ratio and nurses' positive and hopeful attitude towards patients' recovery, even when the patients were critically ill. The main barriers were found to be restrained hospital policies and functional assignment for nurses, which limited their duration of interacting time with individual patients. The patients' socio-economic background and common language spoken by both nurse and patient had no significant impact on the quality of communication.

Our responses and actions depend on our attitudes and habits. The goal of any kind of education is to develop appropriate *'attitude'* in students, which influences their personal qualities and interpersonal skills. It is our attitude towards our work, people and society which makes us efficient and successful. The interrelated factors determining attitude are **3Es**, i.e., **Environment**, **Experience** and **Education**.

A Management study in Harvard University found that a person gets a job, 85% of time because of his attitude and only 15% time because of his smartness and knowledge.

SUMMARY

This unit includes a brief history of communication, the elements, step-by-step process, communication concepts, theories and models. Also the techniques of communication, facilitators and barriers of effective communication and methods to overcome barriers are discussed. The significance of effective communication in education is presented in examples. The importance of communication in healthcare setting is evidenced by research studies.

ASSESS YOURSELF

LONG ANSWER QUESTIONS

1. Describe the elements of communication with suitable examples
2. Explain the types and importance of nonverbal communication
3. Explain the importance of effective communication in nursing education and nursing practice, with suitable examples
4. Describe the modern communication system
5. Explain with suitable examples the facilitators of communication
6. Explain with suitable examples the barriers of communication

SHORT ANSWER QUESTIONS

1. Etymological meaning of communication
2. Any two definitions of communication
3. Types of message
4. What is encoding?
5. Importance of the channel of communication

SHORT NOTES

1. Petroglyphs
2. Pictograph
3. Origin of spoken language
4. Verbal or oral communication
5. Meta-communication
6. Models of communication
7. Methods of overcoming barriers of communication
8. Therapeutic communication
9. Importance of effective communication in nursing profession

Contd...

MULTIPLE CHOICE QUESTIONS

1. The oldest known symbols dating back to the Upper Paleolithic age is:
   A. Ideographs
   B. Petroglyphs
   C. Pictograph
   D. Telegraph

2. Human communication involves the following, EXCEPT:
   A. Acoustics
   B. Behavioral sciences
   C. Linguistics
   D. Physical sciences

3. The types of message are:
   A. Feelings
   B. Information
   C. Orders
   D. All of the above

4. The process of analyzing the actual meaning of the content of communication is:
   A. Decoding
   B. Encoding
   C. Meta-communication
   D. Visual communication

5. The stages of Peplau's Interpersonal Relations Theory are:
   a. Communication phase
   b. Exploitation phase
   c. Identification stage
   d. Orientation phase
   A. a, b, c
   B. b, c, d
   C. c, d, a
   D. a, b, d

6. The contexts of Interpersonal Communication are:
   a. Cultural context
   b. Environmental context
   c. Psychological context
   d. Social context
   A. a, b, c
   B. a, b, d
   C. a, c, d
   D. b, c, d

7. Normally people remember ---- % of what they hear and see:
   A. 10%
   B. 20%
   C. 30%
   D. 40%

8. Language barriers in communication includes:
   a. Defective hearing
   b. Paralanguage
   c. Poor memory
   d. Technical jargon
   A. a,b,c
   B. b,c,d
   C. a,b,d
   D. c,d,a

9. Techniques of communication include all EXCEPT:
   A. Empathy
   B. Enthusiasm
   C. Honesty
   D. Intimacy

10. NLP focusses on the following EXCEPT:
    A. Experience-based behavior
    B. Method of communication
    C. Neurological process of communication
    D. Meta-communication

ANSWERS TO MCQS

1. (B)	2. (A)	3. (D)	4. (C)	5. (B)	6. (A)	7. (D)
8. (C)	9. (D)	10. (D)				

BIBLIOGRAPHY

1. Etymological meaning of communication (Internet). Available from: https://pragatipath1.files.wordpress.com/2012/02/smc2.pdf

2. History of Communication (Internet). Available from: https://en.wikipedia.org/wiki/History_of_communication

3. King J Barbara. When Did Human Speech Evolve?(Internet). 2013 September 5. Available from http://www.npr.org/sections/13.7/2013/09/05/219236801/when-did- human-speech-evolve.

4. Heidgerken E Loretta. Teaching and learning in schools of nursing. 3rd ed. Delhi: Knark Publishers Pvt. Ltd. Delhi; 1998.

5. L Steven McShane, Glinow Von Mary Ann, Sharma R Radha. Organizational Behaviour. 3rded. New Delhi : Tata McGraw-Hill Publishing Co. Ltd ;2006.

6. Aswathappa K . Organisational Behaviour. 8th revised ed.Mumbai: Himalayan Publishing House; 2008.

7. Pareek Udai .Understanding Organizational Behaviour. New Delhi: Oxford University Press; 2004.

8. B Julia George. Nursing Theories. 6th ed. New Delhi: Dorling Kindersley India Pvt Ltd; 2011.

9. W Danique. Communication Process Model (Inernet).2011 october22. Available from http://cape-commstudies. blogspot.in/2011/10/communication-process.html

10. Berlo's Sender-Message-Channel-Receiver Model of Communication. Available from https://en. wikipedia.org/wiki/Models_of_communication

11. S Samiksha. 4 Different Types of Barriers to Effective Communication. Available from: http://www.yourarticlelibrary.com/business-communication/4-different-types-of-barriers-to-effective-communication/1004/

12. Chand Smiriti. 7 Major Elements of Communication Process. Available from: http://www. yourarticlelibrary.com/business-communication/7-major-elements-of-communication-process/25815/

13. Communication Barriers - Reasons for Communication Breakdown Available from: http://www. managementstudyguide.com/communication_barriers.html

14. What is Communication? Available from :https://www.skillsyouneed.com/ips/barriers- communication.html

15. Barriers to Communication. Available from:http://communicationtheory.org/barriers-to-communication/

16. Models of Communication. Available from https://en.wikipedia.org/wiki/Models_of_communication

17. Defining Communication Theories. Available from http://www.mhhe.com/mayfieldpub/westturner/student_resources/theories.htm

18. Communication Theory. Available from: http://www.managementstudyguide.com/communication-theory.htm

19. The Top 15 Most Effective Communication Techniques and Strategies. Available from: http://bettermindbodysoul.com/effective-communication-techniques/

20. Amarin Tawfiq, Rasheed Al- Adel. Methods of Communication A Field based project submitted as a requirement for the Organizational Behavior.Available from http://www.leadersoutlook.com/Article. aspx?id=1495andlang=enArticle Title or Author:

21. Seven C's of Effective Communication. Available from: http://www.managementstudyguide.com/seven-cs-of-effective-communication.html

22. Therapeutic Communication. Available from: http://www.studentnursejourney.com/part-i-therapeutic-communication-techniques/

23. Maheswari Anisha. Educational Technology. 3rd ed. Indore: N.R. Brothers; 2011.

24. Chakraborty Ratna. Nurse-Patient Communication. Unpublished Thesis.

25. Prakash Ratna. Soft Skills: Not Hard to Learn. NITTE Journal; 2008.

26. Stone d., Bruce Patton, Sheila Heen, Difficult Conversations: How to Discuss What Matters Most. Penguine Books; 2000

27. McMaster Michael D., John Grinder. Precision: A New Approach to Communication: How to Get the Information You Need to Get Results. California: Grinder DeLozier Associates; 1994

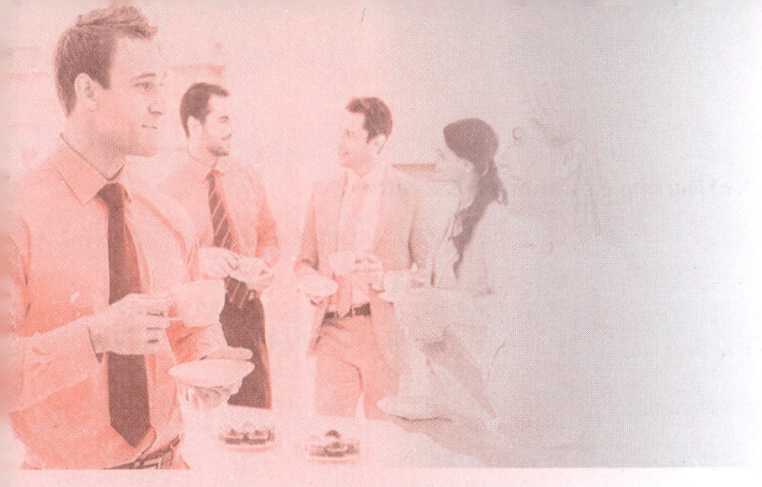

Interpersonal Relations

— *Alka Kalambi, Mamtaz Begum*

CHAPTER OUTLINE

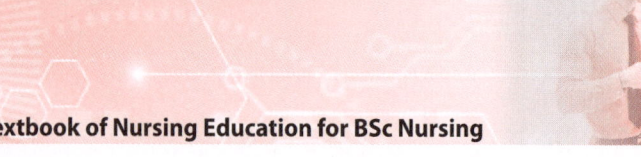

📖LEARNING OBJECTIVES

The learner will be able to-

- Define Interpersonal relation
- Recognize the reason of forming interpersonal relationship
- Describe the characteristics of interpersonal relation
- Discuss the purposes of interpersonal relation
- Describe the types of interpersonal relation
- Enumerate the stages of interpersonal relationship development
- Discuss the phases of interpersonal relationship
- Define interpersonal skill
- Describe the interpersonal skill required for professionals
- Classify interpersonal response traits
- Identify different types of interpersonal behavior while dealing with people
- Illustrate the theories of interpersonal relationship
- Recognize the barriers of interpersonal relationship
- Discuss the methods of overcoming barriers of interpersonal relationship
- Describe the concept of Johari window model
- Discuss the stages of Knapp's relationship model
- Recognize the importance of interpersonal relationship in nursing
- Explain the way of improving interpersonal relationship at workplace

INTRODUCTION

As a social being, every individual develops number of relationships throughout their lifetime. The name and nature of the relationship may be different but each relationship is developed on some social context to satisfy the desires and needs of individual. When individual's needs are similar, they come together and committed to satisfy their needs. Stronger the commitment of two people, longer will be the duration of relationship. Other than commitment, some common characteristics should be present between the individuals, which initiate the relations. Based on individual needs, people develop relationship between two or more people and it is essential for performing primary and secondary roles. To perform professional role, every professional needs to know interpersonal relations and they should apply the skill wisely in day to day life. A shopkeeper needs to maintain good interpersonal relation with customers for maximizing the sales; similarly a nurse has to maintain good interpersonal relation not only with patients but the other health team members too for providing better care as a professional.

DEFINITIONS OF INTERPERSONAL RELATIONSHIP

- Interpersonal relationships are social associations, connections, or affiliations between two or more people with a varying degree of intimacy, developed for attaining mutual goal.
- An interpersonal relationship is a close association or acquaintance between two or more people that ranges in duration from brief to enduring and based on inference, love, solidarity, regular interactions in professional field, or some other type of social commitment.
- Interpersonal relationship refers to close association between individuals, who share common goals.
- Interpersonal relationship can be defined as the association between two or more people that range from temporary to lifetime and personal to professional.

WHY WE FORM INTERPERSONAL RELATIONSHIP?

- **Appearance**: At the beginning of forming relationship, people are attracted to the appearance of an individual. Individual with pleasant appearance, good physical structure and appropriate personal hygiene is more likely to be attracted by others. After initial meeting and progression of relationship, physical structure become less important.
- **Similarity**: People like to form relation with those who have similar characteristics such as language, attitude, belief, cultural habits, etc. People are attracted towards similarity because it is easy to predict and validate the unknown characteristics.
- **Complementarity**: Sometimes two individuals with opposite characters are attracted because their opposite traits complement each other and satisfy their needs.
- **Reward**: According to the exchange theory an individual wants to be related with others as he expects some rewards out of the relations either at the same or less cost of dealing.
- **Competency**: People like to be associated with those who are competent. Very high level of competency is not desirable because it makes one uncomfortable.
- **Proximity**: We form relationship with people who are nearer to us and can interact frequently. Proximity allows getting information and benefit that motivates an individual to form relationship.
- **Disclosure**: When two people disclose personal information to each other, they come to know the similarities and dissimilarities. Self disclosure also helps in developing trust that increases connectivity and dependency.

CHARACTERISTICS OF INTERPERSONAL RELATION

- **Involvement of two or more people**: At least two people should be involved in developing interpersonal relation. Interpersonal relation exists between two people of same sex or opposite sex. For example, friendship between two boys or girls; interpersonal relation also exists within a group of student nurses who are studying in same class.
- **Interaction**: When an interpersonal relation is established between two or more people, they interact with each other. More or less interaction is necessary to initiate, develop and continue the relation. While interacting with each other if open and direct communication is used, it progresses faster. In a healthcare organization, nurse and patient interact with each other on various occasions to develop interpersonal relation.
- **Gradual process**: Development of interpersonal relation is a gradual process. Interpersonal relation develops between two or more people when they interact frequently and come across developmental stages.
- **Dynamism**: Interpersonal relation is dynamic in nature because it changes continuously throughout its developmental phase. It may last from shorter to longer period of time with a varying degree of intimacy.
- **Intimacy**: A varying degree of intimacy is observable in interpersonal relation. In the relationship between soul mates, intimacy may be very close, where as intimacy among club members may not be that much close.
- **Variety of context**: Interpersonal relationship takes place in a great variety of contexts such as family, clubs, schools, colleges, work place, etc.

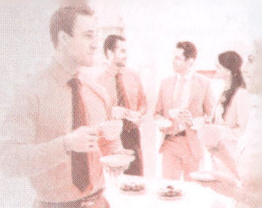

- **Common goals or objectives**: The people who intend to develop interpersonal relation always have some common set of goals, which may or may not be achieved during the lifespan of interpersonal relations.
- **Helping relationship**: Interpersonal relationship is a helping relationship in which both are helped in terms of gaining knowledge, ideas and confidence; there by functioning well.
- **Disclosure**: People involved in interpersonal relation discloses personal information that allow to know each other.
- **Honest communication**: Honest communication is the basis of interpersonal relationship that develops trust.

PURPOSE OF INTERPERSONAL RELATION

- **To help each other**: Interpersonal relation is necessary to help each other at home, workplace, community and other variety of context. As a social being, humans like to live together in a family, community, workplace or other units of society. In every social unit, there is a division of work, role, responsibilities and functions. To perform individual role, responsibility and smooth functioning of social unit, individuals need to help each other.
- **To develop personal identity**: To grow and develop personal identity, interpersonal relation is necessary at every stage of life since childhood to adulthood.
- **To maintain and improve functioning status**: Every human being has some function which may vary with their age, personal quality, capability, cultural practice, role and responsibility. To carry out basic function as well as other additional functions an individual need to maintain interpersonal relation with different group of people in society. When a nurse does his/her professional function, he/she needs to maintain interpersonal relation with the supervisor, subordinates, colleagues, physician, administrator, patient, family members of patient, and other health team members. To provide best nursing service, best performer needs to maintain professional functioning status and poor or good performer needs to improve his/her professional functioning status.
- **To promote maturity**: Interpersonal relation is a necessary requirement for promotion of maturity at individual level as well as group level.
- **To adapt to the continuous changing environment**: As we expect development for us as well as for the organization, we need to accept the change also. Many a times, changes come unexpectedly in the internal and external environment of an organization. With the occurence of any kind of change either planned or unplanned we need to adapt to it; failure to adapt makes the survival in the environment difficult. Interpersonal relation plays important role in faster adoption or quick adjustment. After completion of training period, when a student nurse joins in an organization, her role is changed. To adjust to the new role, she needs to maintain good interpersonal relation with her supervisor, colleagues and co-workers.
- **To explore individual potential**: Every individual is not aware of his potential. They receive feedbacks from the people with whom they interact in terms of positive and negative aspects of individual qualities and their hidden qualities as a result of interpersonal relationship.
- **To cope with stress**: In case of stress, interpersonal relations help us to cope with it effectively by seeking support from them.

TYPES OF INTERPERSONAL RELATION

- **Family and Kinship relationship**: The people staying together in a family are bound either by bond of blood or marriage. Kinship refers to the relationship of people that develops either by virtue of blood relation or by marriage. There are two types of kinship: *Consanguineous kinship* and *Affinal kinship*. In consanguineous kinship, people are related by blood. For example, relationship between parent and children. Kinship due to marriage is called affinal kinship. For example relationship between father-in-law/mother-in-law with daughter-in-law or son-in-law.

  Based on degree of the relation, kinship is classified as primary, secondary and tertiary kins (Fig. 1).

  - **Primary kins**: When people are close and relation is direct. For example, parent and child, husband and wife, sister and brother, etc.
  - **Secondary kins**: Secondary kins are those which are related to primary kins. For example, father's brother, mother's sister, sister's husband, etc.
  - **Tertiary kins**: When somebody is related to the secondary kin. For example, husband of sister-in-law.
- **Friendship**: Friendship refers to a freely chosen association where relationship is based on acceptance, trust, love, respect and commitment.
- **Romantic relationship**: It is the deep connection between two people where both support and accept each other unconditionally; share their attitudes, visions, dreams, strengths and vulnerabilities, thereby enriching each other's lives.
- **Soul mates:** Soul mates are the peoplewho connect in every way and at every level so deeply that the bonding brings greater happiness and satisfaction, which is not comparable to any other relationship.
- **Work relationship**: It is the relationship among people as team members, mentor-mentee, supervisor-subordinate, co-workers, and Work friends. It develops through interaction in the workplace. Work relationship may be professional or personal.
- **Professional relationship**: It is the relationship that develops on specified condition among people related as employer-employee, co-professional, professional-client, professional-public, professional-professional, where both the groups have some degree of responsibility and loyalty to each other.

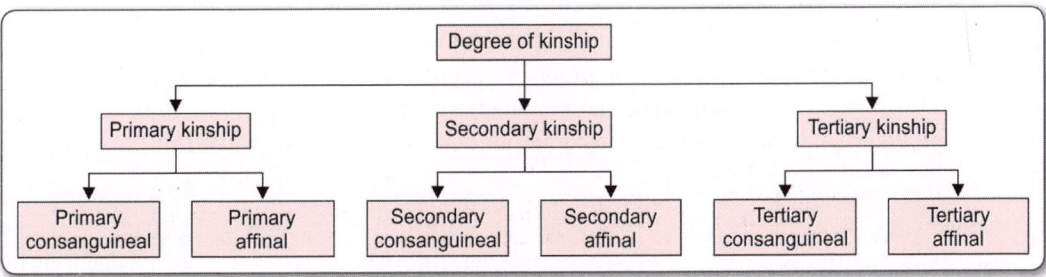

Fig. 1: Degree of kinship

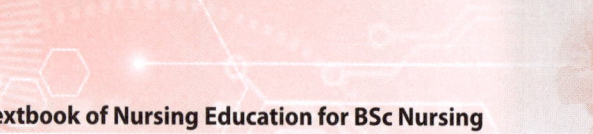

- **Formalized intimate relationship**: Generally, it is a long term relationship that develops among people through law and public ceremony and brings special status in society. For example, marriage and civil union.
- **Non-formalized intimate relationship**: It is also a long term relationship where intimacy exists without conditional responsibility or loyalty. For example, loving relationship, living together etc.
- **Platonic love**: An intense feeling of two people creates powerful attachment that is purely spiritual in nature, and is called platonic love.

STAGES OF INTERPERSONAL RELATIONSHIP DEVELOPMENT (Fig. 2)

According to the psychologist George Levinger, relationship development process is not sudden; it develops gradually through five definite stages that include Acquaintance, Build up, Continuation, Deterioration and Termination stage.

Stage I – Acquaintance

It is the first stage of relationship development process when two people meet with each other and get attracted. At the first meeting, they recognize the need to know each other and decide to start a relationship.

Stage II – Build Up

In the second stage of relationship, the feeling of being strangers disappears and people trust each other. Trust is the basis of build up stage and it helps them to come close. They depend on each other so that relationship is continued for a longer period. Build up stage is characterized by closeness of two people, feeling of passion, dependency, etc. People from similar background and interest tend to involve faster in a relationship than people having diverse backgrounds or interests.

Stage III – Continuation

Continuation stage or third stage is based on the commitment of two people. As the people get committed, relationship becomes stronger and lasts for a prolonged period. Trust and transparency is essential to continue the relationship forever.

Stage IV – Deterioration

All the relationships may not reach this stage but when two people cannot adjust with each other relationship is deteriorated. Adjustment problem may arise due to misunderstanding, lack of compatibility, trust, love and care. Some sort of maladjustment can be compromised by one or both the partners, but when both donot intend to compromise, then it turns towards end.

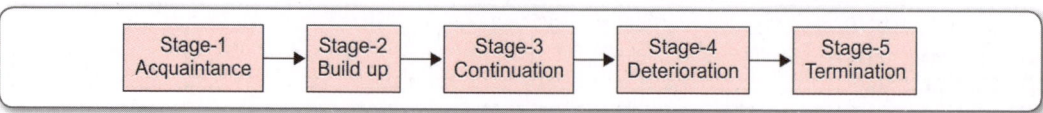

Fig. 2: Interpersonal relationship developmental stage

Stage V – Termination

It is the last stage of a relationship, when relationship exists no more. In the deterioration stage, both persons understand about its negative ending. Relationship is usually terminated due to separation, death of one partner or divorce.

FACTORS ESSENTIAL FOR BUILDING INTERPERSONAL RELATION

Certain that the progress, maintenance, continuity and outcome of interpersonal relationships depends on the following factors.

- **Respect**: In developing interpersonal relationship, respect is essential. Two persons should respect each other's opinions, views and emotions. Disagreement of any fact, opinion or views is also possible to express respectfully.
- **Mutual goal setting**: The persons involved in interpersonal relationship must share common goals or objectives. Mutual goal setting is one of the essential factors in developing interpersonal relationship.
- **Similar interests**: Similar interests of two persons make them to set common goals and progress them towards mutual agreement. When interests of two people are different, then the line of thinking also goes in different directions and mutual goal setting is not possible.
- **Attachment**: To develop a healthy interpersonal relation, two individuals must be attached to each other. When both the individuals consistently show the concerns for safety, security and protection for each other, attachment develops.
- **Transparency**: Individuals in an interpersonal relationship must be transparent to each other. Transparency is declined when either of them is unable to share information, avoids to share information or hides information. In a relationship, if the individuals become more transparent, trust increases and the strength of relationship also increases.
- **Trust**: Literally, trust is the "assured reliance on the character, ability, strength, or truth of someone or something". It is not a pre-existing condition in a relationship; it is created by both individuals through openness, direct communication, keeping promises, truthfulness, being empathetic and loyal. An infant develops trust for the caregiver when all needs are met consistently and mistrust develops if needs are not met, inadequately met or excessively met.
- **Empathy**: Empathy is the ability to understand the thoughts, feelings or emotions of someone. In an interpersonal relationship, one individual should understand the feelings, emotion and needs of the other before expressing it. Mental connection increases if both are empathetic to each other.
- **Interpersonal attraction**: According to the traditional definition in social psychology, "Interpersonal attraction is a positive attitude or evaluation regarding a particular person". Interpersonal attraction indicates the degree of positive attitude of one individual towards the other. It is recognized through: tendency to approach the person (behavioral attitude), positive beliefs about the person (cognitive attitude), and positive feelings for the person (cognitive). The predictors of interpersonal attraction are physical appearance, personality, status, familiarity, peer approval, similarity in attitudes and likes.
- **Interpersonal compatibility**: Interpersonal compatibility is the long term interaction between two or more individuals and when both have a feeling of comfort, satisfaction and enjoy each other's

company. Interpersonal compatibility exists in both cases when two individual have similar or dissimilar attitudes and likings. Individual with similar characteristics become compatible because of similar views towards an issue or decision that exerts greater happiness and less conflict. On the other hand, individual with opposite characters get attracted and become compatible because they could be complement to each other.

- **Interpersonal communication**: It is the process of communication between two or more individuals when exchanged ideas, views or information is understood clearly by each of them through constant awareness. Effective interpersonal communication helps to establish interpersonal relationship.

- **Cooperation**: Cooperation is the working together for common purpose or goal with the willingness of assistance to each other. Cooperation facilitates in developing interpersonal relationship between two or more persons.

- **Empowerment**: Empowerment can be defined "as a multidimensional social process that helps people gain control over their own lives. It is a process that fosters power in people for use in their own lives, their communities and in their society, by acting on issues they define as important."- Page N and Czuba CE. In a relationship, when an individual is empowered by the other, it makes the connectivity stronger for developing interpersonal relationship.

PHASES OF INTERPERSONAL RELATIONSHIP

According to Hildegard E. Peplau, nursing is viewed as an interpersonal process where nurse and client interact with each other for achieving common goals. In the theory of interpersonal relations, man is defined as an "organism that lives in an unstable equilibrium". Man "strives in its own way to reduce tension generated by needs." There are four levels of anxiety: mild, moderate, severe and panic. Among these four levels of anxiety, client may exhibit the features of any one level that is recognized by the nurses. After recognizing the level of anxiety, client's needs are met through the process of interaction and common goals are attained by following sequential phases (Fig. 3).

- **Orientation phase**: It is the first phase of relationship between the nurse and client. Orientation is the function of this phase initiated by the nurse by providing information, explanation and answering client's question. In this phase, client seeks professional assistance by sharing perception. Nurse's role includes: responding to clients, helping to identify problems and informing about services.

- **Identification phase**: In this phase, the client identifies the person who can help him and the nurse allows the expression of his feeling. Appropriate nursing assistance is identified to reduce client's anxiety. Clients have a feeling of belongingness as they rely on nurses. Client develops confidence to deal his/her problem as tension reduces and hope increases.

- **Exploitation phase**: In the third phase of interpersonal relation, professional assistance is provided to client. The client takes the full advantage of provided service. Client's dependency is progressed towards independency.

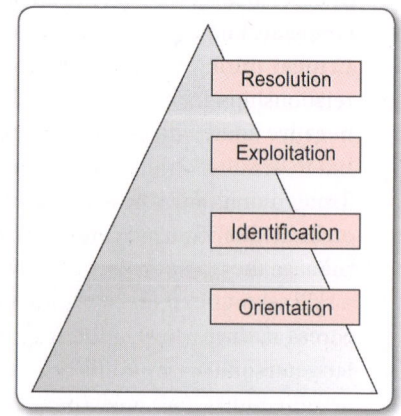

Fig. 3: Phases of interpersonal relation

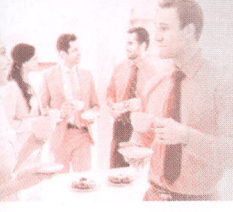

- **Resolution phase**: It is the last phase of interpersonal relation where relationship is terminated. Clients need is met through mutual interaction in the previous phase. In this phase, client becomes independent and healthier, emotional balance is maintained by nurse and client, thereby no need arises to continue the relationship.

INTERPERSONAL SKILLS

Interpersonal skills refers to the set of abilities that enable a person to interact positively with others.

Interpersonal skills are important for every individual for their personal life, family life, social life and professional life. It is an acquired skill, learned through observing and experiencing interaction of parents, family members, peers, member of society and other public figure. Good or healthy interpersonal skill helps an individual to play her/his role satisfactorily in any part of society. It enables a person to minimise interpersonal stress, conflict thereby positive adaptation with a changing environment.

Interpersonal Skill Required for Professionals

A professional should have self confidence and positive attitude for developing interpersonal relation. Self confidence indicates realistic confidence in one's own judgment, ability, power, etc. An individual having self confidence does not requires wrong representation of self for impressing others. People with increased levels of self confidence can trust on their own capabilities and are also being trusted by others. Attitude towards any person or fact is considered positive when feelings or emotions remain optimistic or favorable towards that person or fact. An individual with positive attitude can avoid worries and negative thought, cope easily with daily life processes and motivate others thereby likely to be attracted more. The following interpersonal skills are necessary for a professional.

- **Communication skills**: A good communicator is not only able to read, write and speak but also has the ability to understand others and makes others understand himself. Good communication skills give the greater advantage to an individual for developing interpersonal relations through effective interaction.
- **Cooperation and Coordination**: Cooperation and coordination both are essential for developing interpersonal relation. As a member of any social group or professional association, needs to cooperate and coordinate; otherwise interpersonal relation does not develops.
- **Critical thinking and Problem solving skills**: As our life is not directed with a straight line, relationships are also not formed in one day. It has certain phases of ups and downs; positive and negative endings. In every interpersonal relation, problem may arise at any point of time, which has to be solved by thinking critically or using different techniques of problem solving skills.
- **Time management skills**: With an increase in the number of interpersonal relations, the roles of an individual also increases. Moreover to develop, maintain and continue a relation, he/she has to manage the time. The people who are able to manage the time are able to perform multiple tasks; a skill set required these day for a multirole performer.
- **Stress management skills**: Stress is common for every professional but it is high among nurses, surgeons, pilots and traffic controllers. Through effective stress management, one may feel happy, sensitive and approachable to others; thereby developing and maintaining interpersonal relations becomes easier.

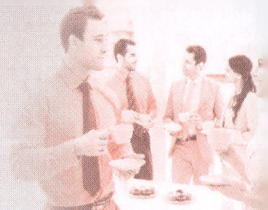

- **Flexibility**: Ability of being flexible is an important interpersonal skill by which an individual meets a diverse group of people, handles their problems, protects their security and becomes favorable.
- **Ability to accept constructive feedbacks**: Every human being commits mistakes, therefore, criticism is expected. People need to acquire the skill of tolerating criticism and accepting constructive feedback, which maximizes group acceptance.
- **Strong work ethic**: Having strong work ethics or adaptability with ethical culture makes a person more attractive for others and hence, enhances interpersonal relations.

INTERPERSONAL RESPONSE TRAITS

As a social being every individual interacts and develops relationship with multiple people in the society. They exhibit some characteristic pattern of responsiveness, which is influenced by heredity and environmental factors. This distinctive pattern of response to other people in society is known as interpersonal response traits. Interpersonal response traits helps: to understand social behavior of a person; to describe his/her sociability; to predict actions and ability of interpersonal relationship development. Some of the primary interpersonal response traits are categorized into three major dispositions: *role disposition*, *sociometric disposition* and *expressive disposition* (Table 1).

Role Disposition

There are four primary interpersonal response traits that come under role disposition category. An individual may have one or more interpersonal response traits under this category. Each interpersonal response trait has two extreme poles.

- **Ascendance**: An individual with interpersonal response trait of ascendance always puts self forward and defends his rights. The individual is not socially timid.

TABLE 1: Some primary interpersonal response traits with opposite poles

Role dispositions	
Ascendance	Social timidity
Dominance	Submissiveness
Social initiative	Social passivity
Independence	Dependence
Sociometric dispositions	
Accepting of others	Rejecting of others
Sociability	Unsociability
Friendliness	Unfriendliness
Sympathetic	Unsympathetic
Expressive dispositions	
Competitiveness	Non competitiveness
Aggressiveness	Non aggressiveness
Self consciousness	Social poise
Exhibitionistic	Self effacing

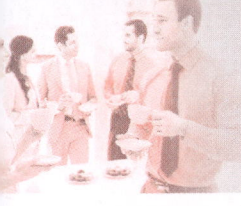

- **Dominance**: Dominance interpersonal response traits is characterized by strong will power, higher self confidence level and assertiveness. A leader with dominance interpersonal response traits would like to give orders and directions.
- **Social initiative**: The individual is socially active; actively involves in group activities; takes the charge over the group; makes suggestions at meetings; and is very organized.
- **Independence**: Generally, they don't depend on others. They do their own planning, rely on their own abilities and are considered as self sufficient.

Sociometric Disposition

Individuals who have more positive interpersonal response traits or high score on these four sociometric dispositions are likely to develop faster interpersonal relation with other person.

- **Acceptance of others**: The individual shows non-judgemental attitude towards others, recognizes and appreciates best qualities of others, and is trustworthy.
- **Sociability**: The individual is outgoing, likes to participate in social affairs and become an integral part of it.
- **Friendliness**: With interpersonal response trait of friendliness, an individual is able to approach others easily and is also recognized as highly approachable by others. They are warm and open to others, hence, are engaged in many interpersonal relationships.
- **Sympathetic:** These people are concerned about others feeling and show kindness as well as generous behavior towards others.

Expressive Disposition

In this category, all four response traits indicate an individual's interpersonal functioning style. Individual may be competitive or non-competitive; aggressive or non-aggressive; self-consciousness or social poise; exhibitionistic or self effecting.

- **Competitiveness**: An individual with the interpersonal response traits of competitiveness considers every relationship as a contest and sees others as rivals. They are non-cooperative in nature.
- **Aggressiveness**: An individual with this trait is quarrelsome, negative and attacks other directly or indirectly. This group of people is not liked by others.
- **Self-consciousness**: An individual with these response traits feels uncomfortable when he/she meets unknown or different group of people. He/she hesitates to speak in public places, do not come forward in group discussions and think that everybody is watching.
- **Exhibitionistic**: An individual who tries to attract others attention through dress and behavior. They want to be recognized by the behavior, which is not natural.

Interpersonal response traits were classified by Karen Horney into three categories discussed below (Fig. 4):

- **Moving towards people**: People under this category show a marked need for affection and approval in their life. They want to be liked, loved, and appreciated by others especially by their partner. The partner may be husband, wife or friend who will take care of them and takes their responsibility every time, whether it is good or bad times.

- **Moving against people**: This group of people are success oriented, achievers, and use other people for their own purpose. They are very calculative in developing relationships and think about the gains and loss.
- **Moving away from people**: Individuals under this category do not want to be attached with anybody. Self sufficiency and privacy remain first priority for them.

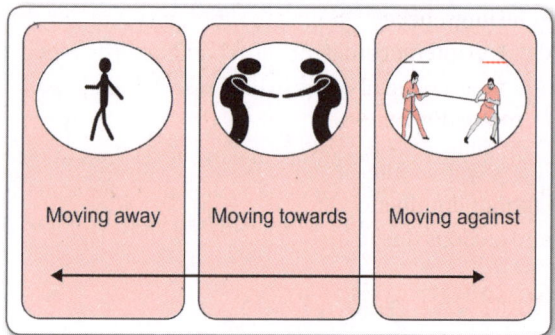

Moving away   Moving towards   Moving against

Fig. 4: Interpersonal response traits based on Karen Horney's classification

INTERPERSONAL BEHAVIOR

Interpersonal behavior is the interaction between two or more persons using verbal and/or nonverbal communication.

Types of Interpersonal Behavior (Table 2)

Assertive Behaviour

It is the behavior observed during interaction between two or more persons, when one is attempting to protect own's rights without violating other's rights. Assertive behavior is demonstrated through direct communication; placing demand at right place, person and time and appropriate expression

TABLE 2: Comparison of three types of interpersonal behavior

	Non-assertive	Assertive	Aggressive
Characteristics of behavior	Does not express own feelings, opinion and demand	Expresses opinion, feelings, and ideas freely and demands directly and appropriately (to the right person, right place and right time)	Express opinion, feelings, ideas and demand inappropriately (violating others right)
Feelings of the individual who behave	Anxious, angry, feeling of disappointment, and resentment	Confident, hopeful, feeling good	Self-righteous, superior, late feeling of embarrassment
Feelings of others people about themselves	Feeling of superiority or guilt	Respected, valued	Humiliated, hurt
Feelings of others people about the individual	Pity, disgust, irritation, annoyed	Respect, rely	Angry, annoyed, disrespectful
Outcome	Non-accomplishment, building up of anger	Accomplishment	Chances of wish fulfillment
Payoff	Avoids unpleasant situation, avoids conflict, tension, confrontation	Respected by others, improved self confidence, develops and maintains relationships	Feels superior

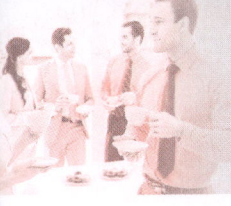

of feelings, beliefs and opinions. Assertive people have higher level of self confidence and are able to develop interpersonal relationships quickly.

Non-assertive Behavior

It is a type of interpersonal behavior observed when one fails to stand up for his own rights with or without domination of others. A person who demonstrates non-assertive behavior may feel hurt, sad and anxious due to inability to protect own rights.

Aggressive Behaviour

It is the behavior observed during interaction between two or more persons when one is attempting to protect his own rights by violating other's right. The person who is engaged in aggressive behavior often tends to humiliate, dominate and disrespect others; and shows verbal and/or physical aggression. Aggressive behavior may be spontaneous, impulsive and proactive.

THEORIES OF INTERPERSONAL RELATIONSHIP

Social Exchange Theory

Social Exchange Theory was proposed by George Casper Homans in the year 1958. Social exchange theory is based on the concept of "give and take". People engaged in a relationship always have one or the other expectation. As relationship is never one sided, both the partners expect something out of the relationship. Every individual invests their time and energy to form relationship and expects to fulfil their needs. When one finds that the invested time and energy is equal or less than the benefit or the outcome of relationship, then he/she starts to compare the relationships with others. When comparison comes, people do not want to put the best efforts, which is fatal for the continuation of the relationship.

Uncertainty Reductions Theory

Charles R. Berger and Richard J. Calabrese proposed *Uncertainty Reductions Theory*. The theory explains relationship between persons who are not known to each other and their strangeness or stress is reduced as they close.

There are three stages in the process of uncertainty reduction and relationship development.

Stage-I: Entry Stage

In the entry stage, two individuals try to know each other through self disclosure. They collect information about their interest and hobby; likes and dislikes; social and economic status, etc. Based on information collection and self disclosure, bond is strengthened and it moves to the next stage.

Stage-II: Personal Stage

In the second stage of relationship formation, both the individuals become more interested to know each other about their attitude, beliefs, values, behavior, etc. If the strangeness has disappeared they are able to collect more personal information.

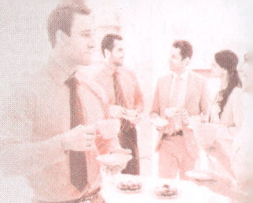
Stage-III: Exit Stage

The future of the relationship is decided in the personal stage. If both the partners feel comfortable and compatible, they then are committed to a long term relationship otherwise they terminate their relationship.

BARRIERS OF INTERPERSONAL RELATIONSHIP

Meaning

Barriers of interpersonal relationship are the factors that interrupt the development and promotion of interpersonal relation between individuals.

Personal Barriers

The factors related to the individuals' physical, emotional and intellectual characteristics that interrupt in development, progression and maintenance of interpersonal relationship is referred as a personal barrier.

- **Physical appearance**: Individuals with ugly look and unhygienic appearances are not attracted by others; thereby unlikely to be invited for making interpersonal relations.
- **Lack of interest**: Individuals with less or no interest in others develop interpersonal relations with fewer member of society and strength of relationship also weakens.
- **Feeling of insecurity**: An individual who has a feeling of insecurity never trusts or depends on others, as a result it becomes difficult for him/her make long lasting relationship.
- **Feeling of inferiority**: The people who perceive themselves inferior always hesitate to approach others, thereby, difficulty arises to start a relationship.
- **Poor or ineffective communication**: People with poor communication are unable to express their own views or opinions, therefore face the difficulty to understand others. This ineffective communication is related with misunderstanding, conflict, and disharmony and does not facilitate the development or maintenance of interpersonal relations altogether.
- **Inappropriate self esteem**: It indicates overestimation or underestimation of self or the inaccurate belief and evaluation of self. People with inappropriate self esteem tend to behave aggressively or nonassertively, which is not liked by others.
- **Rigid attitude**: Individual with rigid attitude are unable to consider others views, unable to accept change and they face difficulty to meet new people or unfamiliar gatherings, which act as an obstruction in making relationship.
- **Non-caring attitude**: Lack of caring attitude is less impressive to others for interpersonal attraction. Caring is demonstrated through concern of one individual to other, attention and proactive approach in offering helps to the other individual.
- **Disrespecting others**: People who respect individuality and rights of others, develop rapport that is essential at the beginning of every relationship. Disrespect towards others generates negative feeling and avoidance, thereby not facilitating interpersonal relations.
- **Dishonest and lack of loyalty**: People cannot depend on the individual who is not loyal or shows dishonesty during one or more occasion along their interaction. Dishonest person cannot protect rights of others, thereby is easily rejected by their partner.

- **Self-centeredness**: Individuals who are self centered always intend to satisfy their own needs and give priority to their own desires without considering partner's need. People of this category are less bothered by others problems and are less attached to anybody.
- **Fear of rejection**: Fear of rejection may develop in an individual as a result of previous experience of rejection, personal incapability, etc. An individual with fear of rejection does not comes forward during a group discussion with his/her ideas or views. He/she does not approach others and remains less responsive when approached by others.
- **Inappropriate level of dependency**: Too high or too low dependency level causes obstruction in interpersonal relation. If one of the partner shows over dependency or less dependency, dissatisfaction arises and both the individuals become unconnected.
- **Lack of commitment**: If people are not committed to the relationship, the connection gradually weakens and the relation is terminated.
- **Mental disorders**: Individuals having preexisting psychological issues or mental disorder is considered as a personal barrier in interpersonal relations. A number of interpersonal skills (communication, critical thinking, problem solving skill) are lost in some mental disorder (personality disorder, manic depressive psychosis, schizophrenia etc.). Therefore, the individual is unable to develop or maintain the relationship.

Situational Barriers

Situational barriers are the factors that are art of personal control and arise as a result of complexity of lifestyle and environment. Some of the situational barriers are discussed here.

- **Lack of time**: Time is one of the important factors that influences interpersonal relations. Individuals need to spend quality time to develop and maintain relationships. As a multirole performer, every person should wisely schedule their activities. However, uneven distribution of time or lack of time minimizes interaction between people and needs are not fulfilled. Prolonged unsatisfactory needs cause frustration and week connectivity.
- **Absence of physical proximity**: The closer the physical proximity, higher the chances of interaction. Frequent interactions promote interpersonal relations but increased physical distance is a hindrance for interpersonal relationship.
- **Adverse environmental condition**: Interpersonal and extrapersonal environment both may be adverse due to some unavoidable circumstances that obstruct connection of two or more people. Interpersonal environment becomes adverse when too many problems remain unresolved or too many challenges are encountered. Extrapersonal environment becomes adverse due to natural calamities, disaster or scarcity of resources.
- **Lack of space**: Every individual needs some personal space for intrapersonal interaction, growth and development. Lack of personal space restricts natural thinking and desire to be close; thereby inhibits development and maintenance of relationship.
- **Space invasion**: Value of personal space may differ from person-to-person, but generally individuals like to protect it. Space invasion causes some psychological and physical effects to the individual, who experiences it. When someone experiences space invasion, he/she becomes responsive with limited movements, reduced eye contact, defensive position, stopping conversation, etc. Space invasion restricts interpersonal interaction and does not facilitates development and promotion of interpersonal relations.

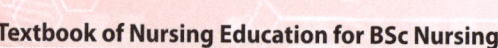

- **Complex interactional setting**: Interactional setting is physical and social environment where interaction takes place. Due to complexity of setting people may be detached from each other therefore connection remains weak.
- **High density of individuals**: Density increases when number of individual is increases in a given environment. People who exposed in an environment with high density of individuals often respond differently due to higher level of anxiety and stress. Inappropriate response like irritation, aggression and hostility does not facilitate normal interaction as well hindering to relationship development.

Sociocultural Barriers

Social and cultural factors has influence in interpersonal relations development. As people from similar sociocultural background are easily attracted to each other and tend to make relationship, similarly sociocultural diversity is a barrier of interpersonal relations.

- **Stereotypes**: In every culture, there are certain norms, beliefs, customs, and practices. These cultural norms and beliefs are so deeply seated in ones existence that many a times our judgements towards other individuals become wrong. With a wrong judgement, we can't communicate effectively and ineffective communication is a greater difficulty in establishing relationships. Due to stereotypical thinking, our views and opinion towards any person or event are incorrect.
- **Ethnocentrism**: It is the tendency of people to judge other groups according to the cultural values of one's own group. Ethnocentric view or behavior are not only barriers of effective communication, they also inhibit interpersonal relations. People from different ethnic groups have different values, attitudes and beliefs that are reflected in their behavior. Individual as a member of one ethnic group may dislike values of the other ethnic group. When intolerance or non-acceptance arises at individual level, it may act as a greater barrier for interaction as well relationship development.
- **Social diversity**: As long as society is there, social class will also exist because it created by people. Individuals from different social class having different status, express emotion differently, and attachments among family members are different. Recognizing this fact many people avoid interpersonal relations with somebody who is unable to adjust after developing relation.
- **Language diversity**: Language plays an important role in our day to day life. We use language to express our thoughts and ideas and similarly receive from others. To understand each other, use of language is very common. Interpersonal relationship does not develop without knowing each other. If spoken language is uncommon, it does not facilitates development and promotion of interpersonal relations.

METHODS OF OVERCOMING BARRIERS OF INTERPERSONAL RELATIONSHIP

Method used in Overcoming Personal Barriers

- **Attractive physical appearance**: Individual may not be tall or fair but general fitness, posture, hygiene, dressing and grooming brings attractiveness in personality. Dressing and grooming would be appropriate with personality, situation and season.

- **Genuine interest towards people**: Individual may show genuine interest through his/her concern, caring attitude, patient hearing and proactiveness.
- **Effective communication**: People are not born with good communication skill. They are learned over time and experience. To communicate effectively one should: know the language; clear perception about audience; appropriate use of channel; good organization of content, etc. Appropriate level of emotions along with timely delivery of message and feedback are two important factors that should never be neglected. Using simple words and listening before responding are the two important techniques one can remember to improve communication skill. Communication could be more effective, if we avoid the following seven barriers (Fig. 5).

1. **Criticizing**: Criticism involves judgmental statements that usually put down a person instead of not knowing the view of others and correcting wrong action or mistakes. For example, "You should look more happy". "You are not very good in painting".

2. **Labeling**: It is a barrier to communication because it categorizes people. We forget the unique characteristics of an individual and label him or her as – "You are useless"; "Substandard people...". These kinds of labeling destroy interpersonal relationship.

3. **Diagnosing**: It involves stating the cause based on own perception. Some examples of the diagnosing barrier are: "You have done this because of jealousy", "Because of your carelessness, you missed the train."

4. **Praising**: Praising may be a communication barrier if not used appropriately. We need to praise a person's behavior not the person. Sometimes, inappropriate praising makes the person

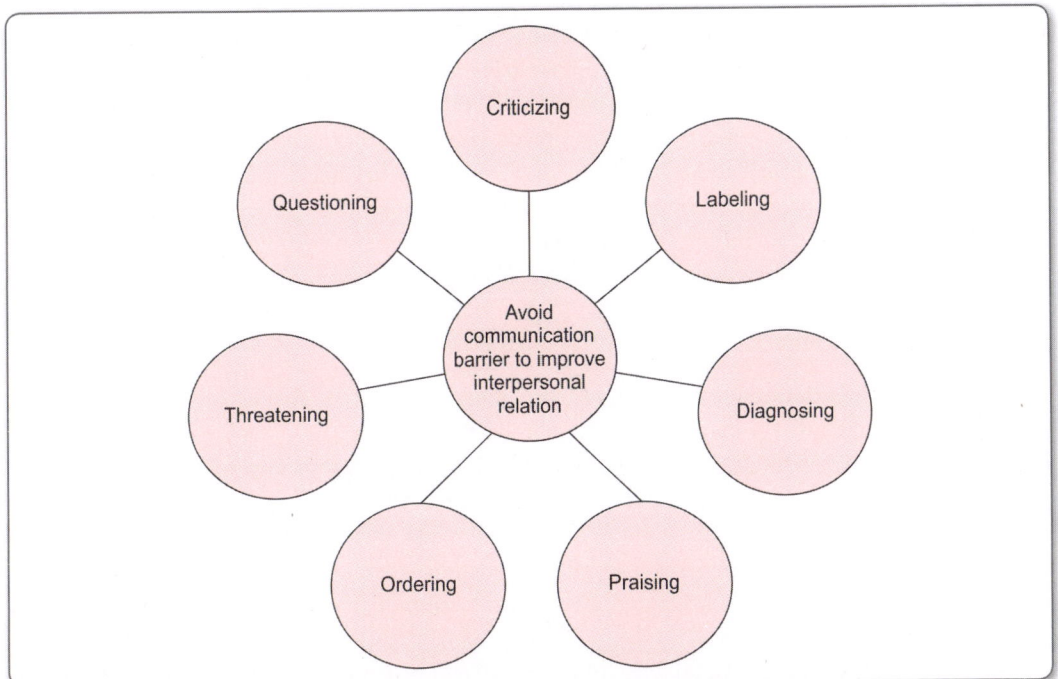

Fig. 5: Seven barriers of communication that inhibits interpersonal relations

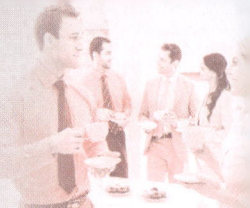

specially children dependent on our praise and also encourages manipulative intention. For example, "You are a wonderful person because you brought a nice gift for me."

5. **Ordering**: Ordering is a way to control people's behavior by applying power. To maintain or improve compliance authoritative power is used but its long term effect is poor. It leads to resentment and makes the person resistant to change. In teacher student relationship also, instead of repeated order we need to make them understand their responsibility.

6. **Threatening**: An order is converted to threat when it has emphasis on punishment. When a threatening statement is used, people may follow it because of fear but if resentment increases, it kills relationship. For example, "If you are unable to rank in first semester, your schooling will be terminated".

7. **Questioning**: Inappropriate questioning is a barrier of effective communication. For example, " Why do you disobey me?" "Why do you always mistakes?" Using inappropriate questions, we ignore the person's needs or intention.

- **Being flexible**: Many a times, we need to be flexible while interacting with people considering their uniqueness. Adopting flexibility, an commit individual becomes more tolerable that facilitates interpersonal relations.

- **Providing constructive criticism**: In interpersonal relation, criticism is a barrier but it can be avoided. During the process of communication, feedback is used by the receiver as well as sender but it should be constructive in nature. Constructive feedback is accepted easily and it indicates personal level of communication that facilitates development of interpersonal relation between two people.

- **Being loyal and honest**: Being loyal and honest is always important towards the partner, group members and everybody. It is a social responsibility also. People can rely and trust on an honest and loyal person that promotes interpersonal relation. Loyalty and honesty is demonstrated through: telling truth, keeping promises, protecting rights of other, being impartial etc.

- **Being aware towards self and others**: People who are aware of their needs, aspirations, strengths and weaknesses and also understand others, they interact effectively. Awareness minimizes misunderstandings and conflicts but maximizes self concept and confidence, thereby enabling people to develop. To improve self awareness, reflective thinking is important.

Method used for Overcoming Situational Barriers

- **Simplicity of interactional environment**: The setting where interaction will take place should be simple and familiar to the partner or group members.

- **Scheduling activity:** Indidividuals should plan their activity, thereby making it possible to avoid interruption during interaction or incident like postponing meeting etc.

- **Time management**: Everybody, either homemaker or professional, must manage their time. Inappropriate time management causes role dysfunction, stress and disharmony in relationships.

- **Appropriate organization**: Group member should be responsible to collect and utilize resources appropriately.

- **Special arrangement**: In case of adverse environmental situations, special arrangement in terms of accommodation, comfort, safety and security is important.

Method used for Overcoming Sociocultural Barriers

In healthcare organizations, nurses need to interact with many people from diverse sociocultural background. If we donot have the intercultural awareness, it becomes difficult to make interpersonal relations with colleagues, patients, family members, and other health team members. There are some ways by which we can develop intercultural awareness and overcome the cultural barriers.

- **Admitting ignorance**: Acknowledging one's own ignorance is the first step of learning others culture.
- **Developing awareness of own culture**: Individuals need to realize about their own cultural values, beliefs and practices that he/she likes and dislikes.
- **Being non-judgemental**: Sometimes we perceive wrong because of our ignorance. Therefore, it is better not to be judgemental.
- **Developing empathy**: Realizing others' view by standing at their place prevents us from committing wrong action or inappropriate use of words.
- **Growing interest to know others' culture**: Study your own and others' cultures to understand behavioral differences.
- **Validating your assumptions**: After gathering enough information, we can validate our assumptions that guide our behavior.
- **Putting sincere effort to adopt and adapt**: If we constantly check ourselves at every occasion, a habit is formed that facilitates in the development of interpersonal relations.

JOHARI WINDOW MODEL

Johari Window

"Johari Window is a model to evaluate the extent of open and authentic communications between individuals."

The model is related to communication and self awareness and was developed by American psychologists, Joseph Luft and Harrington Ingham in 1955. Combining the first name of two authors Joe and Harry it is called as 'Johari'.

Concept in Johari Window

The model has four important quadrants namely: *open area*, *hidden area*, *blind area* and *unknown area* (Fig. 6).

	Known to others	Not known to others
Known to self	Open	Blind
Not known to self	Hidden	Unknown

Fig. 6: Johari window model

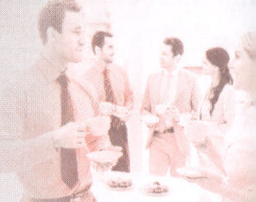

Open Area/Arena

It is the space that indicates an individual's awareness about self and is also known by others. Every individual has certain characteristics including strength and weaknesses. The open area represents how much is known to the person himself/herself and by others. Each individual should aim to increase the open area, which facilitates self awareness and allows in receiving feedback from others. Increased open area helps to promotes interpersonal relations, and improves personal development and team development (Fig. 7).

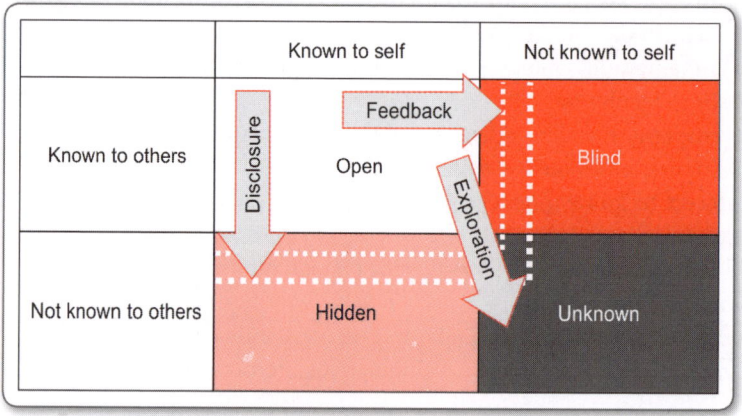

Fig. 7: Increasing open area in Johari window

Hidden Area/Facade

This area is known by the individual but unknown to others. Person may have some feelings, emotions, qualities, talent, information or typical interpersonal response that are purposely hidden by the individual and not disclosed to others. Too much hidden areas do not facilitate the development of interpersonal relations. The individual should share information to the person on whom they trust and depend. Supervisor can encourage self disclosure to reduce hidden area.

Blind Area/Blind Spot

It is known by other individuals but unknown to self. It is not an effective or productive area for the individual as well as the group. The individual should aim to solicit information or get a feedback from peers and group members, thereby inculcating good qualities and quit bad habits. Supervisor also takes the initiation to reduce blind area by giving constructive feedback.

Unknown Area/The Unknown

The area is unknown by the individual and not known by others also. This space can be occupied by some traumatic past experience, feelings, hidden talent, aptitude etc. The space of unknown area can be reduced through self discovery or collective and mutual discovery. Supervisor or manager also creates an environment (job enrichment) that encourages self discovery. The individual may be unaware about repressed feelings in subconscious mind where counseling is effective.

Importance of Johari Window Model

It describes the process of giving and receiving information, which improves self awareness between individual and group. It helps to understand relationship, self development and group development (Fig. 8).

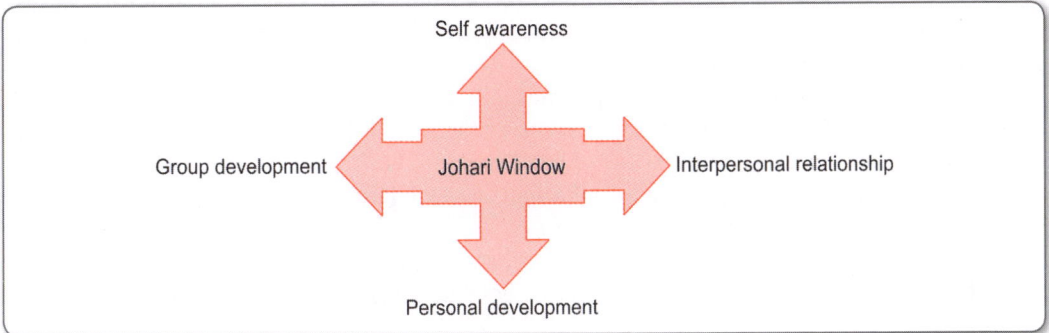

Fig. 8: Importance of Johari window

KNAPP'S RELATIONSHIP MODEL

Mark L Knapp, born on July 12th, 1938, is the developer of theoretical model for relational enhancement which explains the interpersonal relationship development between two people.

According to Knapp's relationship model, there are ten different stages, which explain the progression and deterioration of relationship. These ten stages are grouped under two main concepts coming together and coming apart (Fig. 9).

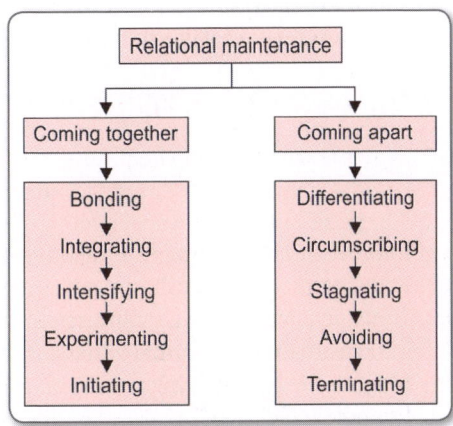

Fig. 9: Knapp's relationship model

COMING TOGETHER

- **Initiation**: It is the first stage of relationship development. In this stage, both the individuals like to impress each other. Physical appearance has important role in this stage, therefore people become more concerned to project themselves with appropriate level of presentatation.

- **Experimentation**: The stage of experimentation is also called as probing stage. In this stage, people explore information about each other. They analyze the gathered information to identify similarities of interest. Most of the times they decide either to continue or discontinue the relation.

- **Intensifying**: It is the more serious stage of relationship when people become less formal. Each one tries to nurture and strengthen their relationship using varieties of techniques. They expect commitment to continue the relation.

- **Integration**: In the stage of integration, intimacy is increased between the people. People become closer than before and progress towards next stage.

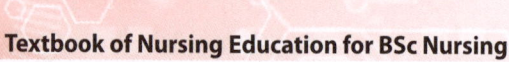

- **Bonding**: After the stage of integration, people become more confident and depend on each other. They like to be recognized by others regarding the relatedness or by the name of relation.

Coming Apart

As relationship may progress towards maturity, it may progress towards deterioration as well because of conflicts and misunderstandings. When relation fails to persist, it is called as coming apart. There are five stages in coming apart.

- **Differentiating**: In a relationship, if people think individually without involving the partner, it leads to weakening of the bonding gradually. It may start because of some internal or external pressure. In this situation, both the partners develop a feeling of dislike.
- **Circumscribing**: In this stage people set the limit of their interaction. They remain busy with their own space and activities.
- **Stagnation**: The relationship is deteriorated further and is characterized by poor communication, lack of interest and feelings. In this stage, relation neither progresses towards positive end, nor gets terminated. It remains stagnant.
- **Avoidance**: After the stage of stagnation, people purposefully avoid each other. They are not at all willing to keep a contact and avoid all forms of communications.
- **Terminating**: It is the last stage of coming apart. In this stage, relationship is completely terminated. In the termination stage, partnership or friendship is broken with loads of negative feelings.

IMPORTANCE OF INTERPERSONAL RELATION IN NURSING

Good interpersonal relation helps to:
- Remove monotony of work environment
- Maximize support from colleagues, supervisors, subordinates, patients and other co-workers
- Improve intradepartmental and interdepartmental communication
- Reduce stress in family life as well as in professional life
- Function effectively in a multidisciplinary team
- Build team through mutual understanding and cooperation
- Improve decision making and problem solving
- Promote self development and wellbeing
- Provide effective patient care
- Promote positive work culture
- Maximize output at personal and group level
- Receive constructive feedback.

HOW TO IMPROVE INTERPERSONAL RELATIONSHIP AT WORKPLACE

- **Avoid treating office as your home**: Professional behavior is expected in the workplace. Organizational policy, rules, regulations, and standards should be followed by everybody. It is better to avoid somebody if not tolerable instead of misbehaving or fighting.
- **Give space to your colleagues**: Excessive curiosity needs to be avoided. Overhearing someone's conversation is unprofessional.
- **Avoid spreading rumors at workplace**: Spreading rumors spoils the organization's culture. The person who spreads rumors loses the trust of others.

- **Share correct information with others**: Correct and valuable information is needed to be shared with each other.
- **Avoid sharing all your secrets with co-workers**: Secrets can be shared with the person who cares for you.
- **Avoid partiality**: Impartial nature is desirable by team members and it helps to build your rapport.
- **Avoid blaming**: An individual needs to take the responsibility of his/her own actions.
- **Never be aggressive to others**: An individual needs to learn assertiveness. Aggressive behavior creates disharmony.
- **Admit ignorance**: Admitting ignorance is desirable than committing mistakes that may harm one or more individual.

SUMMARY

An interpersonal relationship is the association between two or more people with varying degree of intimacy and continued for mutual goal attainment. Formation of interpersonal relationship depends on the level of proximity, similarity or complementarity of two persons, their level of competency, information disclosure and expectation of rewards. Development of interpersonal relations among people serves many purposes including: improvement of functional status; development of personal identity; promotion of maturity; adapting with changing environment; exploring individual potential; coping with stressors and helping each other. Interpersonal relationship has some characteristic features such as interaction, involvement, dynamism, intimacy and common goals. Beside these, it is also observed that people involved in interpersonal relationship communicate honestly to each other, disclose some sort of personal information and it develops in variety of social contexts. The name of interpersonal relationship may be different but the characteristics are similar in family relationship/kinship, friendship, romantic relationship, soul mates etc. Interpersonal relationship is developed following five sequential stages: acquaintance stage, build up stage, continuation stage, deterioration stage and termination stage. All the stages of development are influenced by some factors. According to the nursing theorist, Hildegard E. Peplau the process of development of interpersonal relationship includes four phases: orientation, identification, exploitation and resolution. To develop effective interpersonal relation, people should have some skill and positive interpersonal response traits. Based on one's acquired skills, some typical behavior is demonstrated by them like assertive, non assertive and aggressive. People with aggressive behavior face more problems in maintaining effective interpersonal relation.

According to the Social Exchange Theory, two or more people make interpersonal relation with the desire of fulfillment of needs and engaged persons act as giver and taker. The concept of uncertainty reduction theory is different. It explains that stress or strangeness is reduced while engaging in relation. The dynamic nature of interpersonal relationship indicates that it is not continued to same level. There are some factors that hinder interpersonal relations that are categorized into personal, situational and sociocultural. All these hindering factors can be avoided with conscious approach of personal and interpersonal label. Situational factors can also be controlled to some extent by modifying environmental characteristics. The importance of self awareness in interpersonal relation is better understood using Johari window model but the Knapp's relationship model explains about progression and deterioration of interpersonal relationship. Importance of interpersonal relation is recognized by the professionals. It has several importance in nursing also.

ASSESS YOURSELF

LONG ANSWER QUESTIONS

1. Define interpersonal relations. Describe different types of interpersonal relations. Classify the barriers of interpersonal relation and discuss each type with suitable example.
2. Classify interpersonal relationship. Discuss the phases of interpersonal relation. Explain why interpersonal relationship is important in nursing.
3. Write down the concept of interpersonal relationship. Describe the characteristics of interpersonal relationship. Explain the stages of interpersonal relation development.

4. What is interpersonal behavior? Classify interpersonal behavior. Discuss the skills necessary to develop and maintain good interpersonal relationship.
5. What is Johari window? Discuss the concept of Johari window. Write down the importance of Johari window in the process of interpersonal relation.

SHORT ANSWER QUESTIONS

1. State the purposes of interpersonal relationship.
2. Describe the characteristics of interpersonal relationship.
3. Describe the factors essential to build up interpersonal relationship.
4. Classify interpersonal response traits.
5. List out the different types of interpersonal skill.
6. Which type of interpersonal behavior is desirable and why?
7. Describe the personal barrier of interpersonal relationship.
8. How to overcome sociocultural barrier of interpersonal relationship.
9. Describe the concept of social exchange theory.
10. What are the seven barriers of communication that inhibit interpersonal relation?

SHORT NOTES

1. Phases of interpersonal relation
2. Importance of interpersonal relation in nursing
3. Stages of interpersonal relation development
4. Uncertainty reduction theory
5. Johari window
6. Situational barrier of interpersonal relation
7. Interpersonal response traits
8. Method used overcoming interpersonal barrier of interpersonal relation
9. Implication of Johari window
10. Method used to improve interpersonal relation in workplace

Contd...

MULTIPLE TYPE QUESTION

1. **Interpersonal relationships are social associations, connections, or affiliations between two or more people with a varying degree of**
   A. Power
   B. Intimacy
   C. Possesion
   D. Importance

2. **People like to be associated with others, who are:**
   A. Competent
   B. Emotional
   C. Highly sensitive
   D. Talkative

3. **Individual develops interpersonal relation with others as they expect some rewards. It is the concept of:**
   A. Johari model
   B. Knapp's relationship model
   C. Social exchange theory
   D. Uncertainty reduction theory

4. **According to Hildegard E. Peplau, the third stage of interpersonal relation is:**
   A. Orientation
   B. Identification
   C. Intervention
   D. Exploitation

5. **Assertive people attempt to protect own right without:**
   A. Violating other's right
   B. Considering other's right
   C. Controlling own temperament
   D. Controlling other's temperament

6. **Interpersonal response traits in the category of expressive disposition, indicates an individual's interpersonal:**
   A. Functioning style
   B. Expression style
   C. Style of attitude
   D. Style of behavior

7. **When someone experiences space invasion, become responsive with:**
   A. Flexible position and relax mood
   B. Reduced eye contact and flexible position
   C. Reduced eye contact and defensive position
   D. Defensive position and relax mood

8. **In Johari window, open area is the space indicates an individual awareness about:**
   A. Self
   B. Self and known by others
   C. Others
   D. Others and not known by self

9. **Interpersonal relationship helps to:**
   A. Decision making
   B. Problem solving
   C. Decision making and problem solving
   D. Searching and problem solving

10. **The tendency of people to judge other groups according to the cultural values of one's own group is known as:**
    A. Stereotypes
    B. Social diversity
    C. Language diversity
    D. Ethnocentrism

ANSWERS TO MCQS

1. (B)	2. (A)	3. (C)	4. (D)	5. (A)
6. (A)	7. (C)	8. (D)	9. (C)	10. (D)

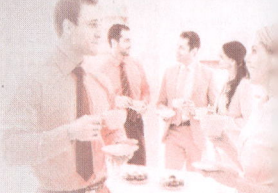

BIBLIOGRAPHY

1. Krech D, Crutchefield RS, Ballachey EL. Individual in society:a textbook of social psychology. Tokyo, Japan: Mcgraw-Hill international book company; 1982.

2. Morgan CLT, King RA, Weisz JR, Schopler J. Introduction to psychology. New Delhi, India: Tata Mcgraw Hill edition; 1993.

3. Stuart GWS, Laraia MT. Principle and Practice of Psychiatric Nursing. 8th ed. St Louis, Missouri: Mosbey; 2005.

4. Tomey AM, Alligood MR. Nursing Theorists and their work. 5th ed. St Louis, Missouri: Mosbey; 2002.

5. Neeraja KP. Textbook of Nursing Education. New Delhi, India: Jaypee; 2003.

6. Sharma SK, Sharma R. Communication and Education Technology in Nursing. New Delhi,India: Elsevier; 2012.

9. Abosi CO, Alao AA, Okoye NN, Yoloye TW. Psychological foundation of education: Heineman Semester Series. 2015. http://eprints.covenantuniversity.edu.ng/1115/1/Psychology%20And%20Social%20 Behaviour.pdf

10. Aron A, Lewandowski G. Interpersonal Attraction, Psychology of. International Encyclopedia of the Social & Behavioral Sciences., 2001. Available from: www.sciencedirect.com/topics/page/ Interpersonal_attraction. Accessed July 27,20`7.

11. Page N, Czuba CE. Empowerment: What Is It. JOE October 1999; 37(5). Available from: https://joe.org/ joe/1999october/comm1.php. Accessēd July 22 2017.

12. Benoit D. Infant-parent attachment: Definition, types, antecedents, measurement and outcome. Paediatr Child Health. Oct 2004; 9(8): 541–545. Available from: https://www.ncbi.nlm.nih.gov/pmc/ articles/PMC2724160/. Accessed June 20.2017.

13. Capps MA. Characteristics of a sense of belonging and its relationship to academic achievement of. texas.2003. Available :http://oaktrust.library.tamu.edu/bitstream/handle/1969.1/1584/etd-tamu-2003C-EDAD-Capps-1.pdf?sequence=1&isAllowed=y.Accessed June 18 2017.

14. Theories of interpersonal relationship. Management study guide. Available: http://www. managementstudyguide.com/interpersonal-relationship-theories.htm. Accessed 16June 2017.

15. Uebergang J .7 of 12 Relationship-Deadly Barriers to Effective Communication. Available: http://www. selfgrowth.com/articles/7_of_12_Relationship-Deadly_Barriers_to_Effective_Communication. html.Accessed July 2 2017.

16. Definition of 3 types of interpersonal behaviour. Available: http://www.sandiego.edu/student-leadership/documents/3%20types%20interpersonal.pdf. Accessed July 2 2017.

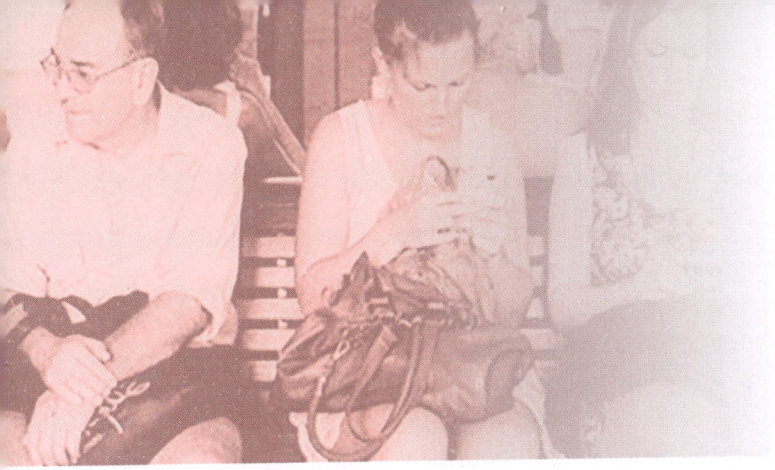

Unit 3

Human Relations

— Nagendra Prakash, Ratna Prakash

CHAPTER OUTLINE

- Describe the Concept of "Understanding Self":
- Expansion of Human Relations During Life Stages of Human Growth and Development
- Social Attitude, Social Behavior, Motivation
- Social Attitude and Social Behavior
- Motivation –
- Individual and Groups
- Team Work
- Human Relations in Context of Nursing
- Unit Summary
- Self-Evaluation Questions
- Bibliography

LEARNING OBJECTIVE

At the end of the Unit, you should be able to-

- **Describe the concept of "Understanding Self"**
  - How self-concept evolves
  - Stimulus-response and evolution of personality
  - Self-concept and self-identity
  - Self-concept and self-image
  - Self-concept and inner conversation
  - Understanding oneself
  - Reflective thinking as a tool to understand 'self'
  - Self-concept and life roles
  - Comparison of positive and negative Self-Concept
  - How to help develop positive Self-Concept
- **Expansion of human relations during life stages of human growth and development**
  - Infancy and childhood – learning family relationships (dependent role)
  - School age and adolescence – learning social relationship through peer group influence (dependent role)
  - Adulthood – creating own nest (establishing independent relationship)
  - Old age – stable relationship
  - Evolution of inner-self (immature to mature relationship)
- **Social attitude and social behavior**
  - Meaning
  - Categories
  - Difference between social behavior and social attitude
  - How social behavior and social attitude are inter-related
  - Factors influencing social attitude and social behavior
  - Social attitude, social behavior
- **Motivation**
  - Meaning
  - Factors influencing motivation –
  - Motivation and human needs
- **Individual and groups**
  - What is a 'group'
  - Types of group
  - How groups are formed through social relationship
  - Group dynamics and human relations
  - Roles and responsibilities of an individual in a group
  - Group behavior and communication

- **Team work**
  - What is a 'team'?
  - What we need to build a team (7 cs) –
    - Clear goal
    - Communication (Interpersonal)
    - Collaboration (spirit of)
    - Competence (of the members)
    - Commitment (of the members)
    - Coordination (of different functions of the team)
    - Control (by Team Leader)
  - Role of an individual in a team (do's and don'ts)

- **Human relations in context of nursing**
  - Nursing – a humanistic profession
  - Self concept, self image and nursing
  - Significance of human relations in nursing practice
  - Nurse-client communication
  - Nurse as a member of the 'health team'
- **Unit Summary**
- **Self-Evaluation Questions**
- **Bibliography**

INTRODUCTION

Our life moves around a central axis, which is made up of all relationships we create or get involved with others in the family and environments close by or far away. How these relationships grow and flow has an immense influence on the way our life is directed and monitored. This unit brings about our responsibility towards making this influence positive by understanding our own self; developing appropriate acceptable social attitude and behavior throughout the stages of growth and development.

Group or team work is the essence of nursing profession, which needs healthy interpersonal relationship and a common focus. This makes learning about Human Relations in multifaceted contexts of nursing a front-runner in the Nursing Education curriculum.

UNDERSTANDING SELF

Human self has many dimensions; the in-born qualities are only a part of it. Over the years, the self gets influenced by others through interactions and gradually develops to a self, which is typical of that individual. Therefore 'understanding self' is to understand all these aspects, that make us unique.

How the Self-Concept Evolves

At birth, normally the human child does not have the ability to talk, express feelings or perform activities. During the early stages, the child can't recognize objects or individuals, even the mother or the other care-givers. During continuous contact with the mother, the child is exposed to the external stimuli such as mother's appearance, touch, voice and gradually, he learns to recognize and respond to mother's and other stimuli. The presence and absence of mother's contact makes the child to experience the presence or absence of other stimuli. Thus, mother becomes the first and the main initiator of the child's identity of relationship with herself and others in the environment.

Stimulus-Responses and the Evolution of Personality

In the process of stimulus-response, child's thought process begins to evolve. As he starts recognizing mother, he begins to recognize himself. He learns to identify mother as the "other" and himself as "I" or "Me". This marks the beginning of identification as "I" or "me" as oneself and mother as the other self. The "I" or "me" is the self-concept that starts unfolding in the process of relationship with mother, which has a great influence in development of the child's personality.

Subsequent addition of every experience of relationship with other family members such as father, siblings, other family members, relatives etc., leads to the expansion of self-concept and building up of personality.

Thus, the overall self is the result of the sum of self-concepts that get formed in relationship with all the individuals. This self-concept is the core determinant of his personality and the type of social being he is.

Now we know that the self-concept is the result of stimuli-evoked responses. Some responses are consciously learnt and some are unconscious.

For example, if somebody gives a toffee to a child. The mother tells the child to say, "thank you". The child opening his hand to receive the toffee is the response and the expression of "thank you" is the manner of response. This manner of response is learnt in human relationships.

When the toffee is given, the child may like to open the cover immediately and put it in his mouth, which is an instinct. But mother tells him to say "thank you" first, which is based on **Social Conditioning**. Most of our responses to stimuli are socially conditioned. Even the stimuli that evoke biological response get modified by social conditioning.

The self and self-concept consist of socially conditioned responses to life situations. In the process of making the socially conditioned responses, each person learns to behave. The social conditioning may be similar to all, but how much a person accepts it is unique and the way of expressing it is also unique to each person. This is known as his 'personality'.

Self-Concept and Self-Identity

The human relationship consists of mutual responses and the responses create an experience of self-identity.

In the process of growing up, as the child learns to respond to others on the basis of socially conditioned relationship, he is influenced by the responses of others to his own. The child's self-identity begins to form on the basis of these mutual responses. Thus self-concept and self-identity are related to the quality of human interactions experienced by the child.

Self-Concept and Self-Image

The self image is the outcome of all experiences and identification with the people around. If one gets appreciation for his actions and achievements often, the self-identity and self-image becomes positive. On the contrary, if one gets adverse comments for the actions often, the self-image becomes negative. The early childhood experiences and the peer group relationships are very important determinants of our self-concept, self-image and self-identity.

Self and Inner Conversation

The self-concept determines how an individual functions in a group. As the self-concept evolves in relationship with people, the individual starts reflecting within himself his own responses with others and vice versa. This leads to an inner conversation with oneself. In this, the individual imaginatively assumes himself in two roles and engages in conversation between them.

For example, a teacher is taking class. During this, he is able to mentally observe both his act of teaching as well as students' response to his class. After the class, he recollects and reflects on his teaching and students' responses; two roles - each observing the other.

This capacity of inner conversation within oneself is the unique ability of human beings. Without self-concept, this inner conversation (reflective thinking) is not possible. It is an important fact that self-concept and reflective thinking mutually promote each other and develop the whole self.

Understanding Oneself

The self image is the result of the nature of a person's relationship with other members of the group and develops in relation to the images of others. His self image also reflects the group image. If the group image changes, the self image of the members also changes accordingly without them being aware of it.

Reflective Thinking as a Tool to Understand Self

Self- reflection is an important exercise to understand self. Understanding oneself gives a capability to the person to exercise control on oneself and discover ways to modify the self-image. This process helps to discover one's own capacity and progress to achieve the set goals.

For Example, a nursing student's academic performance remains only average in spite of trying very hard, which makes her depressed with self-pity. However, her teachers observe that in the clinical practice, her overall skill is above average. With guidance from teachers, the student reflects on all her abilities, which makes her clinical performance better. She is surprised to discover that she has so many innate abilities that make her a competent clinical nurse. This finding gives her a lot of confidence and her *self-concept, self-identity and self-image (also called as self-esteem)* gets enhanced.

Self-Concept and Life Roles

The core of the self that is acquired in early childhood is the gender role. The child assumes the roles by observing the others in the family. Usually, a girl child identifies with the mother and through this identification, she acquires the role of a daughter, sister, wife, mother, etc. Each role when learnt becomes a part of the self-identity. For example, a girl when interacts with her parents, her entire self becomes the daughter as if she has no other identity. The same daughter while interacting with her brother assumes the role of the sister and so on. This change in role happens automatically without any conscious effort of the person. Self-concept and self-identity are made up of all the roles the person performs. With the change of the role, the self-concept and self-identity also changes. The seriousness of the role identification of a person depends on how much importance he gives to that role. His thoughts and behaviors are governed by these roles or identities, and ultimately determine the self-image. The way he dresses up, his walking, interaction etc. gets influenced by his life role.

Hence, the loss of any life role may lead to a loss of self-concept, self-identity and self-image. Some people can cope up with this loss by adopting alternative role, others succumb to the loss. For example, a father in the role of the only earning member of the family assumes the role of the provider and protector. His self-concept, self-identity and self-image are shaped accordingly. After retirement from job, as his role changes, so as his self. Many people fall sick after retirement, others join some groups or organizations and adopt another role as coping mechanism, and they remain comparatively healthy.

Our self-concept, self-identity and self-image are associated with the perceived recognition/status or acceptance we have by the group we belong to. If there is a difference between this perception and reality, the self-concept, self-identity and self-image undergo considerable changes leading to disturbance in the person's emotional status. For example, because of some reason, the student leader suddenly finds himself disliked by the group members. This loss of status may affect his mental health. On the contrary, sudden elevated status of a person in the group may make him egoistic.

All the above discussions on self-concept lead to the following conclusions:
- Self-concept is not present at birth; it is developed through social relationships.
- Self-concept begins to evolve in early childhood and develops through experience of various life situations.
- Individual's perception of his own 'self' may be different from others' perception about him.
- Self-concept gets refined by reflective thinking.
- Self-concept expands as one begins to assume different life roles.
- Individuals perceive different aspects of their self at different times as they get exposed to various experiences. This makes self-concept dynamic.
- Changes in any life role may lead to loss of self-concept, self-identity and self-image. Healthy coping mechanism can protect the person's mental and physical health.

The above points suggest how various factors determine the components of self-concept. Understanding oneself is like pealing an onion. As we start pealing each layer of onion we discover that the whole onion is made up of many layers of skin with a central seed. Similarly in understanding 'self' as we keep analyzing and removing each layer by reflective thinking, we discover that the 'self' is made up of several layers of 'identity', with a core of our intellect, thoughts and emotions. Understanding or being aware of this core is **Understanding Self** (Fig. 1). We understand ourselves better when we recognize how the negative feelings like anger, jealousy, hatred, dislike etc. arise in us and our ability to control them.

Human self is gradually evolved from birth and is a continuous process till the end of interactive life. There are many personal, inter-personal and social factors which play important roles in formation of human self. These are—

- Relationship with people
- Life-situation and life-experiences
- Role identity and role change

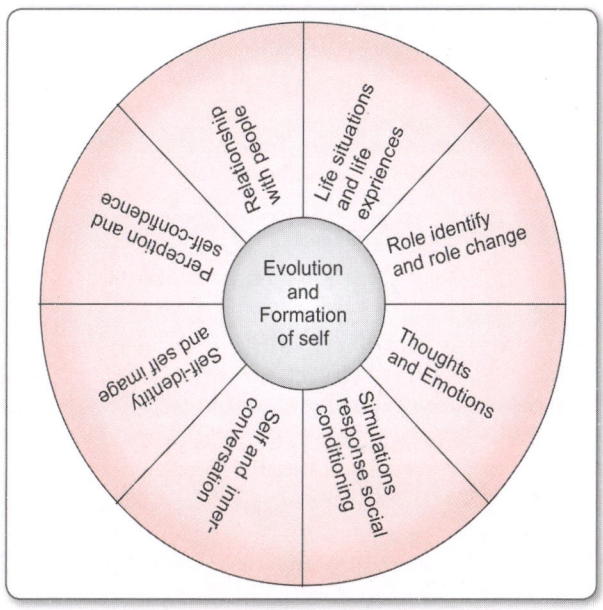

Fig. 1: Understanding self

- Thoughts and emotions
- Stimulus-response, social conditioning
- Self and inner-conversation
- Self identity and self-image
- Perception and self-concept.

Understanding self is to understand first ourselves in relation to the above factors. This self-analysis or introspection helps us to understand others, with whom we interact. Understanding self also helps us to understand our client's problems and needs. That makes 'Nursing' a holistic service.

There are positive self-concepts that give us confidence, coping ability to all situations, a mature personality and healthy relationships with people with whom we interact. Negative self-concepts lead to inferiority complex, maladjustment to life situations, weak and conflicting personality. In this, either the person becomes socially withdrawn leading to emotional problems or if leads to unsocial behavior (Table 1).

TABLE 1: Differences between positive and negative self concepts

Positive self-concepts	Negative self-concepts
Persons have a clear idea of what they should achieve and why they should achieve the goal	No goal and if the goal is fixed, persons have no clarity of how to achieve
Try to set goals independently or with the advice of others who are successful in that area	Depend on others to fulfil their needs and attaining set goal
Persons with positive self- concept can link their self-image or self-esteem with appropriate activities to achieve the set goal	Because of lack of self-confidence, they are indecisive about the activities to achieve the set goal. Also, they doubt their own capacity and others' advice about the activities and keep worrying
They can decide on ways to achieve the set goal. If they experience barriers, they try out alternative ways till the goal is attained. They don't easily give-up	Give up the actions and even the goal itself with little trying, if they experience barriers
Failure in getting desired results makes them to search for the reasons in their own activities and they try to rectify with alternate methods	Failure in getting desired results of any attempt to achieve the set goal makes them to blame others
They try to establish contact with those who are successful in attaining this goal	Find faults with the people who are successful and avoid them
Appreciate others who keep progressing to attain the goal	Find faults and feel jealous of others who are progressing towards attaining the goal
Can overcome their own physical or other difficulties with determination to achieve the set goal. Once the problems are resolved, they start working with full attention	Keep complaining about their difficulties, depend on others to help them to overcome difficulties. Even after the problems are resolved, they take time to resume activities or give up the goal itself
Take up goals that can be achieved and proceed to next after each goal is attained	Keep talking big and dream about high goals, but do not attempt to work towards attaining the goals
Appreciate the hard work and courage of the subordinates, help them to achieve the set goals. Believe in team-work	Magnify others' defects and try to find ways to explain why it is not possible to achieve the set goals with this type of subordinates. They cannot adjust in a team

Behaviors that promote negative and positive self concepts are enlisted in Table 2.

TABLE 2: Behaviors that promote positive and negative self-concept

Behavior that promotes positive self-concept	Behavior that promotes negative self-concept
Appreciating those who work hard to achieve. Like team work, seek honest ways to attain goals	Comparing self with others and self-pity. Dominating others, comfortable with dishonest ways to attain goals
Learning from others success. Having confidence on own abilities. Action-oriented	Happy at others' failure. Doubting own abilities. Wasting time day-dreaming
Continuously trying to acquiring skills that help improvement. Keeping company with good role-models who are successful in achieving goals	Does work only how much is just enough, nothing extra. Keeping company with persons who do not like to work hard to achieve set goals

Every failure can be a step to success if we do not repeat the same mistakes. If one wants to be successful in reaching the goal, one should ensure that his/her own attitude and behavior is not a barrier.

EXPANSION OF HUMAN RELATIONS DURING LIFE STAGES OF HUMAN GROWTH AND DEVELOPMENT

Erikson's Stages of Human Development

- Infancy and Childhood – learning family relationships (dependent role)
- School age and Adolescence – learning social relationship through peer group influence (dependent role)
- Adulthood – creating own nest (establishing independent relationship)
- Old age – stable relationship
- Evolution of inner-self (immature to mature relationship)

Human relation is a relationship or connection between two persons. It shows how an individual is related or connected to another. It implies how people interact and cooperate with each other when they come together in a group to achieve objectives. In the context of an organization, like hospital, human relation is about how people come together in a work-like situation and later, form a workgroup (team) with some motivation and cooperate to achieve organizational goals effectively. From an academic viewpoint, human relations involves studying the human behavior at a workplace and then use systematic knowledge to analyze and suggest necessary efforts required to maintain and enhance the performance of humans.

It is to be remembered that human relations also involve an ethical and moral sense. It includes recognizing, respecting and also safeguarding the dignity of every individual along with his or her's sincere efforts and valuable contribution made for the achievement of given objectives. Every healthcare professional should have a thorough understanding about human relations. The study of human relations along with a clear understanding of its essentials helps us to understand:

- Our psychology and that of others with whom we interact
- Why our belief-systems, religions, attitudes, prejudices and behaviors, create problems sometimes in our personal, professional and social life

- Which crucial steps we must take to mitigate and solve relationship-related problems in our life
- How to utilize the obtained knowledge appropriately and implement the learned skills to build, improve, enhance and maintain healthy relationships with others to achieve our goals in a smooth manner without any conflicts and hindrances.

It is interesting to learn how the human relations develop through our developmental period from birth to death. The famous developmental psychologist Erik H. Erikson (1902-1994) was best known for his theory on social development of human beings. The Table 3 depicts the various stages of human life in terms of social development. This will help us to understand the human relations in a better way.

TABLE 3: Social development of humans during various stages of life

(Approx. age) Stage and Psychosocial crisis	Significant relations	Psychosocial modalities	Psychosocial virtues	Maladaptations and malignancies
(0–1) Infancy Trust vs mistrust	Mother	To get, to give in return	Hope, faith	Sensory distortion, withdrawal
(2–3) Toddler Autonomy vs shame and doubt	Parents	To hold on, to let go	Will, determination	Impulsivity, compulsion
(3–6) Preschooler Initiative vs guilt	Family	To go after, to play	Purpose, courage	Ruthlessness, inhibition
(7–12) School-age child Industrious vs inferiority	Neighborhood and school	To complete, to make things together	Competence	Narrow virtuosity, inertia
(12–18) Adolescent Identity vs role-confusion	Peer groups, role models	To be oneself, to share oneself	Fidelity, loyalty	Fanaticism, repudiation
(20–45) Young adult Intimacy vs isolation	Partners, friends	To lose and find oneself in a another	Love	Promiscuity, exclusivity
(30–65) Middle aged adult Generatively vs Stagnation	Household, co-workers	To make, to take care of	Care	Overextension, rejectivity
(50+) Old adult Integrity vs despair	Mankind or "my kind"	To be, through having been, to face not being	Wisdom	Presumption despair

According to Robert Owen, "Human Relation is interaction and cooperation of people in a group." The human interaction primarily starts with mother or immediate caregiver and later expands to others in the family and community.

Infancy and Childhood – Learning Family Relationships (Dependent Role)

The human relation commences during the prenatal period itself. The interactions that happen outside the womb are believed to influence the future interactions of the fetus. The cognitive development during infancy and childhood also play a very important role. Jean Piaget (1896-1980) explained the cognitive development of the humans through different age groups. Cognition refers to all mental activities associated with thinking, knowing, remembering and communicating. Since birth, babies of all cultures develop an intense bond with their care givers. Infants prefer familiar faces and voices. They coo and giggle when they receive their mother's or father's attention. After 8 months, they develop stranger anxiety. They greet strangers by crying and try to reach near the parents or care givers. By 12 months, infants cling tightly to a parent when they are frightened or expect separation. After the reunion, they show their happiness by smile and hugs. This is the origin of attachment. Body contact is a very important factor in attachment along with familiarity. This is the time when they develop a sense of trust- a sense that world is predictable and reliable. Our early attachment forms the foundation of our adult relationships and our comfort with affection and intimacy. At this time, we are dependent on our primary care givers for most of our needs.

Do parental neglect, family disruption or day care affect children's attachments and thereby the human relations in future? To a greater extent, the answer is yes. Self concept—"the understanding and evaluation of who we are", also develops through attachment. Parenting style like giving space to children in open discussions, also influences the child's human relations.

School Age and Adolescence – Learning Social Relationship through Peer Group Influence (Dependent Role)

During school age, the peers and neighborhood play a vital role in the human relations and social development of the child. Moreover, teachers and elders also can become a role model for them in their communication style. The peer group helps them to develop the sense of "We" instead of "I and me" and thereby, the cooperation and working in a group. Plays are the foundation stones where we understand our specific roles to be performed to achieve the organizational goal or common goal. Reasoning power is achieved to a greater extent by this time. The ability to discriminate the right and wrong, good or bad or the basic forms of morality are also developed from school age itself. Adolescence is the period of forming an identity, which is very important in developing social relations. Parents and peer relations also play a vital role in shaping the social interactions at this time. Even though most people have a great sense of autonomy, they are dependent on their family for their financial and other needs. Thus, the role of the parents is inevitable in shaping the human relations of a school-going child and adolescent. Making the children understand and share their responsibility in their families and taking their participation in decision making in family-related matters improves their self esteem and will influence accountability in social interactions to a greater extent.

Adulthood – Creating Own Nest (Establishing Independent Relationship)

It is true that many differences exist between young and old adults, which are created by significant life events. A new job means new relationships, new roles, new expectations, new challenges and new demands. This is the time period of finding a partner and starting a new life. Marriage indeed brings joy of intimacy and the stress of merging one's life with another's. The birth of a child introduces new responsibilities and in turn alters the focus of one's life. Two basic aspects of our lives dominate adulthood. Erikson called them as *Intimacy and Generativity*. Intimacy refers to form close relationships and generativity is being productive and supportive to future generations. Even though researchers use multiple terms to explain this, like affiliation and achievement, attachment and productivity, commitment and competence, it simply means that a healthy adult is one who can love and work.

Old Age – Stable Relationship

This stage is the extension after 65 years till death. By this age, people have limited goals and abilities. The crisis in this stage is the integrity v/s despair in which the person finds meaning in memories or instead looks back at life with dissatisfaction. The term *Integrity* implies emotional integration; it is not accepting one's life as one's own responsibility. It is not based on what has happened but, how one feels about it. We have seen that the elderly people live with a sense of satisfaction that they have wonderfully used their resources and mentored the younger generation. Sometimes the youngsters also feel whether the old age can be determined by the chronological age because in social interactions elderly population is very active. It should also be noted that this period of life is characterized by stable and mature relationships.

If a person has found meaning in certain goals, or even in suffering, then the crisis has been satisfactorily resolved. If not, the person experiences dissatisfaction, and the prospect of death brings despair. The declining physical health conditions, decreased income, death of spouse, etc. worsen these feelings.

EVOLUTION OF INNER-SELF (IMMATURE TO MATURE RELATIONSHIP)

Havighurst (1953) prepared a developmental model, in which he has presented the list of developmental tasks from birth to old age. Every cultural group expects its members to master certain essential skills and acquire certain approved patterns of behavior at various ages during the life span. Havighurst has labeled them developmental tasks.

According to him a developmental task is "a task which arises at or about a certain period in the life of the individual, successful achievement of which leads to happiness and to success with later tasks, while failure leads to unhappiness and difficult with later tasks".

During infancy, which is the shortest developmental period and is time for radical adjustment. The new born infant must make four major adjustments to postnatal life viz., to temperature changes, to sucking and swallowing, to breathing and to elimination. During infancy and early childhood the tasks are learning to take solid foods, learning to walk and talk, learning to control the elimination of body wastes, learning sex differences and sexual modesty, getting ready to read, learning to distinguish right and wrong and beginning to develop conscience.

In late Childhood the tasks are learning physical skills necessary for ordinary games, building a wholesome attitude toward oneself as a growing organism, learning to get along with age-mates, beginning to develop appropriate masculine or feminine social roles, developing fundamental skills in reading, writing and calculating, developing concepts necessary for everyday living, developing a conscience, a sense of morality, and a scale of values, developing attitudes towards social groups and institutions and achieving personal independence.

During adolescence, the tasks include achieving a new and more mature relation with age-mates of both sexes, achieving a masculine or feminine social role, accepting one's psyche and using one's body effectively, desiring, accepting, and achieving socially responsible behavior, achieving emotional independence from parents and other adults, preparing for an economic career, preparing for marriage and family life, acquiring a set of values and an ethical system as a guide to behavior-developing an ideology.

In early adulthood, the task are getting started in an occupation, selecting a mate, learning to live with a marriage partner, starting a family, rearing children, managing a home, taking on civic responsibility and finding a congenial social group. In middle age, the tasks are achieving adult civic and social responsibility, assisting teenage children to become responsible and happy adults, developing adult leisure-time activities, relating oneself to one's spouse as a person, accepting and adjusting to the physiological changes of middle age, reaching and maintaining satisfactory performance in one's occupational career and adjusting to aging parents.

In old age, the tasks are adjusting to decreasing physical strength and health, adjusting to retirement and reduced income, adjusting to death of spouse, establishing an explicit affiliation with members of one's age group, establishing satisfactory physical living arrangements and adapting to social roles in a flexible way. If we closely look at these developmental tasks, we can come to a conclusion that our social relations develop from a very immature to very stable and mature relationship through infancy to old age.

SOCIAL ATTITUDE, SOCIAL BEHAVIOR, MOTIVATION

Social Attitude and Social Behavior

Social Attitude

Social attitude is an acquired tendency to evaluate social things in a specific way. It's characterized by positive or negative beliefs, feelings and behaviors towards a particular entity.

Types or Components

Social attitude has three main components: emotional, cognitive and behavioral. There are explicit and implicit attitudes. The emotional component is the feeling experienced during evaluation of a particular entity. The cognitive aspect implies thoughts and beliefs adopted towards the subject, while the behavioral component is the conduct that results from a social attitude. An individual is aware of his explicit altitude, and how it dictates his behaviors and beliefs. On the other hand, a person may not be conscious of his implicit attitude, although it still may influence his beliefs and behaviors.

People pick social attitudes from personal experiences or observation. Likewise, social roles and norms can dictate formation of attitudes. *Social roles* determine the behaviors an individual occupying a particular position or context in the society is expected to demonstrate, while *social norms* define the conduct that's acceptable to the society.

However, social attitude does not always lead to specific behavior. For example, someone may favor policies of a specific politician but fail to turn out to vote. Attitudes can be dropped the same way they're learned.

Social Behavior

Social behavior is behavior among two or more organisms, typically from the same species. Social behavior is exhibited by a wide range of organisms including microorganisms, slime moulds, social insects, social shrimp, naked mole-rats, and humans. Even though humans and animals share some aspects of social behavior, human social behavior is generally more complex.

Our social behavior arises from our social cognition. Especially when the unexpected occurs, we try to analyze why people act as they do. For example, Does her warmth and enthusiasm in relationships reflect really the romantic interest? Or is this the way she relates to every one? Does his absenteeism in the class really due to illness or laziness or due to stressful school environment?

Types

The different types of social behavior include emotional behavior, violent behavior, aggressive behavior, group action and prosocial behavior. Social behavior consists of conduct and actions exhibited by individuals within society. People's social behavior normally corresponds with acceptable actions within an individual's peer group, while most individuals strive to avoid the behavior society deems unacceptable.

- *Emotional behavior* is a form of social behavior that causes individuals to behave emotionally within groups and individually. This type of behavior expresses emotions such as excitement, fear, joy, anger, anxiety and sorrow.
- *Violent and aggressive behavior* commonly happens in crowds or groups. This occurs when certain individuals within a group act violently or aggressively, and others copy the behavior. The pressure to conform to the actions of the group normalizes the behavior. This type of behavior is common during instances of looting and rioting.
- *Prosocial behavior* is a social behavior that is viewed as altruistic. This type of behavior consists in helping others through selfless actions. For instance, prosocial behavior occurs when an individual helps another without expecting an action in return.
- *Group action* is a social behavior that occurs when people gather in large groups and attempt to change a particular aspect of society. Group action has a particular purpose, which influences the behavior in both positive and negative manner.

Differences between social behavior and social altitude are enlisted in Table 4.

TABLE 4: Difference between social behavior and social attitude

Social behavior	Social attitude
• Social behavior is behavior among two or more organisms, typically from the same species • Behavior relates to the actual expression of feelings, action or inaction orally or/and through body language • Social behavior includes emotional behavior, violent behavior, aggressive behavior, group action and prosocial behavior	• Social attitude is an acquired tendency to evaluate social things in a specific way • It's characterized by positive or negative beliefs, feelings and behaviors towards a particular entity • Social attitude has three main components: emotional, cognitive and behavioral • Attitude involves mind's predisposition to certain ideas, values, people, systems, institutions

How Social Behavior and Social Attitude are Inter-related?

An attitude is an evaluation of an object, person, act, etc. It can be explicit and implicit, and can be weak or strong, positive or negative. It can be changed but in the case of strong attitudes, this takes quite some effort and often leads to failure of efforts.

Behavior is, essentially, any output of the brain. Unfortunately, there is quite a big attitude-intention-behavior gap. It means attitudes do not always lead to concordant behaviors, and sometimes, people are not aware of their attitudes as well. Sometimes attitude and behaviour does not match each other. E.g., we may dislike a particular food and our attitude towards that food is very negative. But, when we go to a person's home and we are offered that food, we can not refuse, as it would be offending that person. We eat that food. Our behaviour is opposite to our attitude.

According to Dewey and Bentley (1949), a behavior is always to be taken transactionally: i.e., never as of the organism alone, any more than of the environment alone, but always as of the organic-environmental situation, with organisms and environmental objects taken as equally its aspect. This simply means that the behavior of a human being is to be taken into consideration considering many factors.

People hold complex relationships between attitudes and behavior that are further complicated by the social factors influencing both. Behaviors usually, but not always, reflect established beliefs and attitudes. For example, a student who believes strongly in parents may choose to strive hard in the school and work so that he can be the bread winner of the family by the time the parents are old. Ideally, positive attitudes manifest well-adjusted behaviors. However, in some cases, healthy attitudes may result in harmful behavior. For example, someone may remain in an abusive and potentially deadly domestic situation because they hold negative attitudes towards divorce.

Factors influencing Social Attitude and Social Behavior

Behavior can be influenced by a number of factors beyond attitude, including preconceptions about self and others, monetary factors, social influences (what peers and community members are saying and doing), and convenience. Someone may have strong convictions about improving the public school system in their town, but if it means a hefty increase to their property taxes, they may vote against any improvements due to the potential of monetary loss. Or, they may simply not vote at all because their polling place is too far from their home, or the weather is bad on election day.

Man as Social Creature

Along with our psychological make-up, our behavior is deeply influenced by social context. This is true both on a small scale, in terms of being affected by what others think and do, and on a large scale in terms of the norms and practices that dominate a society. Social psychologists believe that behavioral outcomes are determined by individuals, acting in the context of their social networks. Sociologists go further still, arguing that social norms and structures largely define our behavior, with little role for the individual. Proponents of 'practice theory', for example, argue that it is not individuals who should be the subject of inquiry, but shared practices such as watching TV, washing and cooking. Here are some of the social factors that influence people's behavior.

Commitment and Reciprocity

Commitment, especially public commitments which are monitored by others (such as in weight watchers), can have a strong bearing on our behavior. When someone has promised in front of others to do something, they are more likely to stick to it without reward or punishment.

We expect others to reciprocate good deeds, such as giving presents, doing favors or making sacrifices. This has implications for government's own actions – if it fails to display the behaviors, it is asking of the public this will go against people's desire for reciprocity and fairness.

Messenger

Whether people listen to information depends on who is speaking. Demographic and behavioral similarities between the messenger and their audience can improve persuasiveness. Peers (such as friends and family) can also be effective messengers, as they tend to be people we respect and trust. Evidence shows that when an expert delivers information, people are more likely to act on it.

Ego

People tend to behave in ways that make them feel good about themselves and that gains approval from others. Social marketers exploit this by trying to make desirable behaviors appear acceptable and pointing out the undesirable effects of certain behaviors, for example, highlighting the fact that smoking can cause yellow teeth and impotence.

Social Norms

Social norms "provide implicit guidelines on acceptable behavior". We perceive these norms either by watching what most people do ('descriptive norms') or by being told what to do ('injunctive norms'). Many studies have shown that people are strongly influenced by social norms. Telling people about existing social norm can help outliers come into line with the majority. For example, telling householders that they are using more energy than the average can help bring their use down.

Social Attitude, Social Behavior and Human Relationship

Personality develops in relation to social environment. Social environment consists of groups of other personalities and the methods of living, which they have evolved. The latter is known as ***culture***. From the psychology point of view, group life, including culture, furnishes the environment to which the human being must adjust himself if he has to survive. What the sociologists and anthropologists call culture patterns constitute the basis of ideas, attitudes, and habits of an individual. The individual does not grow up in a vacuum. He is doing all times reacting to a world around him, consisting of physical and organic objects, especially, of other human beings. It must have existed since the beginning of social life.

From the moment of birth, humans are social creatures. Indeed, without social interactions (the support of caregivers), no infant would survive. Even when we become capable of living independently, very few people seek to live in isolation. Instead, we generally welcome social interactions, and no study of behavior would be complete without considering these interactions.

Social influence can include direct influences, like group decision making, as well as indirect influences, like imagining how friends would react to a particular situation. Cognitive processes that we use in understanding ourselves and others, called social cognition, also plays a very important role. Stereotyping and attitude change are examples of social cognitive processes.

Motivation

Meaning

In modern days, psychologists and social scientists define motivation as a need or desire that energizes and directs behavior. In other words, motivation is defined as the desire and action towards goal-directed behavior. It gives the reason for people's actions, desires, and needs. Motivation can also be defined as one's direction to behavior or what causes a person to want to repeat behavior and vice versa. A motive is what prompts the person to act in a certain way, or at least develop an inclination for specific behavior.

Intrinsic Motivation (Fig. 2)

A person is intrinsically motivated if the desire for change comes from within the individual. The person may want to learn something because he or she is interested. Another person may want to accomplish a goal or task because it is something he or she feels competent at and enjoys doing.

Extrinsic Motivation (Fig. 2)

Extrinsic motivation, however, comes from outside the person. They are bribed to do something or they earn a prize or reward. Fear of punishment and coercion are also extrinsic motivators.

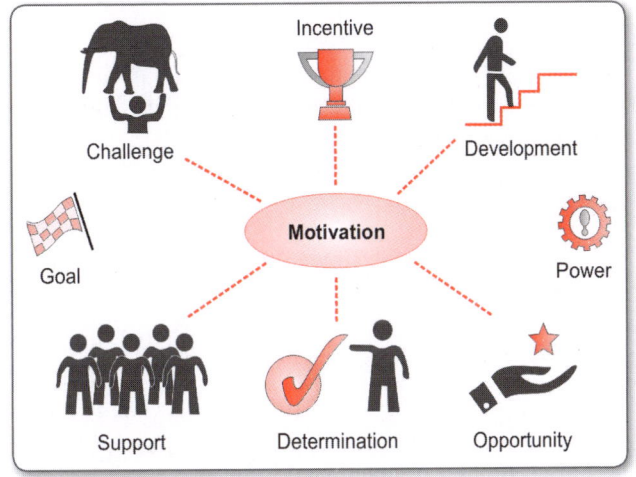

Fig. 2: Motivation can be intrinsic or extrinsic

Factors Influencing Motivation

Positive Influence and Negative Influences

- **Self-efficacy and competence perceptions**: First of all, the role of self-efficacy in the regulation of motivation should be defined. Perceptions of self-efficacy refer to individuals' beliefs about his or her ability to successfully accomplish tasks they are given and have been related to their successful engagement and persistence in tasks. The person's judgments about how likely he is to successfully accomplish tasks must be based on his perceptions of task requirements.
  When people are expected to do well, they tend to try hard, show persistence, and perform better. The individuals who believe they can and will do well are much more likely to be motivated in terms of effort, persistence, and behavior than individuals who believe they are not able to succeed.
- **Competition** is another important possibility. By setting a specific goal that can be achieved in a limited period of time, by one individual or by a group, can put the people's competition spirit to work.

Attributions and Control Beliefs

The basic construct refers to beliefs about the causes of success and failure, and how much perceived control one needs to affect outcomes or to control one's behavior. Individuals must believe that their efforts will lead to success. This assurance enables them to manage their activities and emotions.

Higher Level of Interest

High levels of both personal and situational interests are associated with more cognitive engagement, more learning, and higher levels of achievement. An individual's interest refers to the intrinsic pleasure he or she draws from completing the activity.

Environment

Environment plays a very important role in motivation of an individual. There is an old saying that in a positive environment, even a mediocre usually excels in all activities and even an excellent person can perform average in a negative environment.

Self Motivation for Attaining Life Goals

If you want something bad enough, you can achieve it. To reach your goals, you need to be motivated. But, self-motivation is not easy; it takes a lot of discipline and determination.

What is Self Motivation?

Self-motivation is having the drive and enthusiasm to achieve something without the supervision or influence of others. You take matters into your own hands, completing the tasks you're presented with. It's most certainly not a black and white concept; it's far from simple.

When you're more self-motivated, you feel more accomplished in reaching your goals. It's a great skill to have, as it can dramatically improve your quality of life. Once you understand the power of self-motivation, you can positively change many aspects of your life. It plays a huge role in career development, productivity and even job satisfaction.

Social scientists and psychologists believe that there are few practical steps to be a self motivated person (Fig. 3).

When it comes to self-motivation, there's a strong correlation between our goals and achievement. If you set goals, you will have something to work for. We all want to achieve things of value, this is what drives us and gives us self esteem. Our goals are crucial in terms of the direction we take, the way we spend our time, and the resources we use. When goals are set, it's easier to measure our progress. Keeping the goals defined and current is the best and most powerful way to keep yourself motivated.

If you put your priorities in check, there is no reason why you cannot achieve the life goals you dream of. If that was your dream since the age of 10, you could have reached your goals if you would have aligned your plan to action. If you are self-motivated and the goal is achievable, there is nothing that can stop you. Once you choose your goals, you can then create an action plan. How do you plan to reach those goals? You

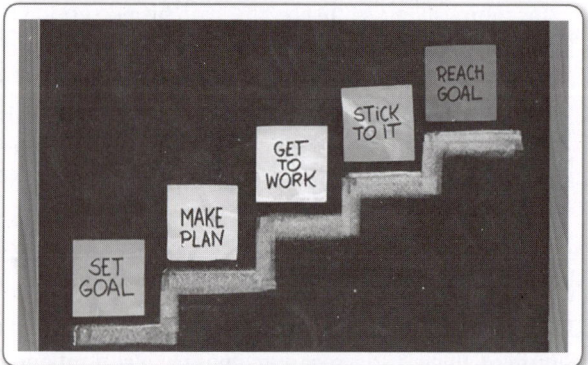

Fig. 3: Steps towards reaching the goals

want to be a nurse? Okay, start writing out your action plan. What education do you need? Who do you need to speak to? Are any apprenticeship programs available? Use the resources available to you. Don't look back and think 'I wish I did that.' You were able to achieve all along. If you were self-motivated, you would exhaust all resources. Self-motivation and hard work will allow you to reach any goal.

Make Your Goal Specific

This will allow you to know exactly what it is you're moving towards. For example: I want to publish a book in the next two years.

Make Your Goal Measurable

This helps in assessing the progress. In terms of publishing a book, break it down into deadlines. Next month you may approach various authors, getting advice. You will want to have your storyline completed, and the first chapter written. Once this is achieved, you can check it off. What's next? Move towards your next deadline. This will help you stay on track. It will also keep your motivation levels up.

Don't Make Your Goals Impossible

Make sure you can reach your goals. Each sub-goal may take a lot of effort, but you should know that they are possible. Millions of books have been published. This is something that is highly attainable. If you are weary of the publication process, which does not mean it's not attainable, you need to reach out and ask for help if needed.

Create Relevant Sub Goals

You will more than likely need to reach multiple sub-goals to reach your main objective. Make sure each goal is relevant to the final goal and to your life. The obvious sub-goals would be writing the content for your book. But, there are also other relevant goals to keep in mind. Do your researches, speak to experts in the field, and keep yourself motivated and determined. As long as you stay on course with your pre-planned goals, relevance will not be an issue.

Set Deadlines

You need to set deadlines and time frames for each goal. Once again, you need to be realistic, but you also need to push yourself. If you have a set date in mind to complete sub-goal one, you can maintain a high level of motivation without being overwhelmed. Once that sub-goal is achieved, you're one step closer.

Motivation and Human Needs

Maslow's (1943, 1954) hierarchy of needs is a motivational theory in psychology comprising a five tier model of human needs, often depicted as hierarchical levels within a pyramid. Maslow stated that "people are motivated to achieve certain needs and that some needs take precedence over others." Our most basic need is for physical survival, and this will be the first thing that motivates our behavior. Once that level is fulfilled the next level up is what motivates us, and so on.

The original hierarchy of needs five-stage model includes:

- **Biological and Physiological needs**: Air, food, drink, shelter, warmth, sex, sleep.
- **Safety needs**: Protection from anti-social elements, security, order, law, stability, freedom from fear.
- **Love and Belongingness needs**: friendship, intimacy, trust and acceptance, receiving and giving affection and love, affiliating, being part of a group (family, friends, work).
- **Esteem needs**: achievement, mastery, independence, status, dominance, prestige, self-respect, respect from others.
- **Self-Actualization needs**: realizing personal potential, self-fulfillment, seeking personal growth and peak experiences.

Maslow's Hierarchy of Human Needs (Latest 7 Needs model) (Fig. 4)

The Expanded Hierarchy of Needs

It is important to note that Maslow's (1943, 1954) five stage model has been expanded to include cognitive and aesthetic needs (Maslow, 1970a) and later transcendence needs (Maslow, 1970b).

Changes to the original five-stage model are highlighted and include a seven-stage model and a eight-stage model (Fig. 4), both developed during the 1960's and 1970s.

- **Biological and Physiological needs**: Air, food, drink, shelter, warmth, sex, sleep, etc.
- **Safety needs**: Protection from elements, security, order, law, stability, etc.

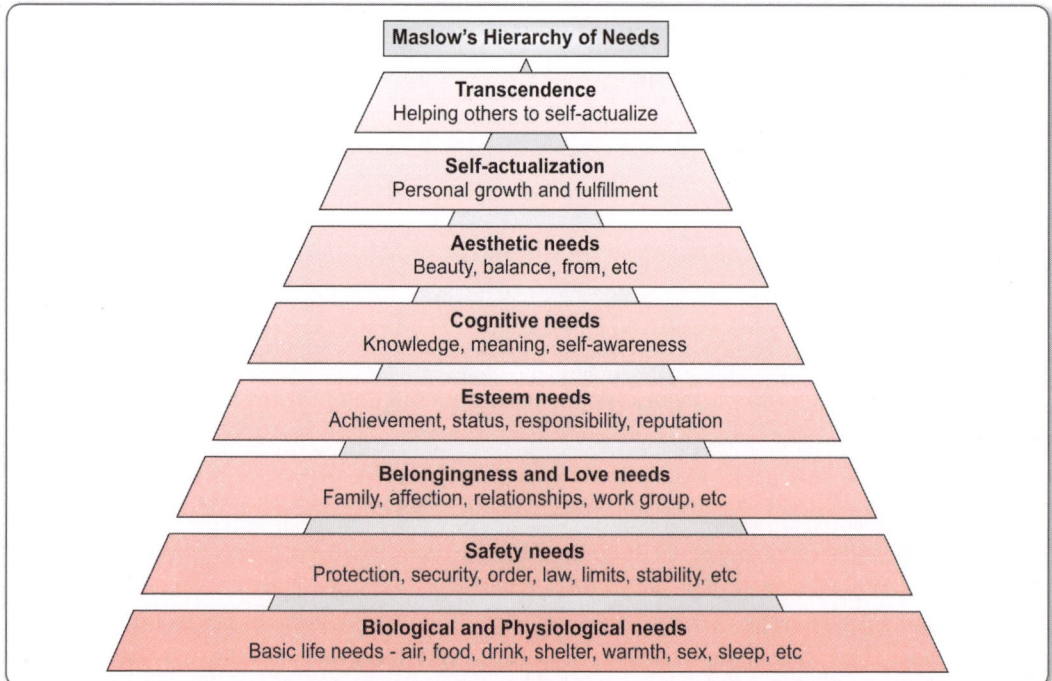

Fig. 4: Maslow's hierarchy of human needs (latest needs model)

- **Love and Belongingness needs**: Friendship, intimacy, trust and acceptance, receiving and giving affection and love, affiliating, being part of a group (family, friends, work).
- **Esteem needs**: Self-esteem, achievement, mastery, independence, status, dominance, prestige, managerial responsibility, etc.
- **Cognitive needs**: Knowledge and understanding, curiosity, exploration, need for meaning and predictability.
- **Aesthetic needs**: Appreciation and search for beauty, balance, form, etc.
- **Self-Actualization needs**: Realizing personal potential, self-fulfillment, seeking personal growth and peak experiences.
- **Transcendence needs**: Helping others to achieve self actualization.

INDIVIDUAL AND GROUPS

What is a 'Group'?

According to Harold H. Kelley and J.W. Thibaut, "A group refers to a collection of individuals, the members accept a common task, become interdependent in their performance, and interact with one another to promote its accomplishment". In other words, a group consists of two or more individuals, interacting with each other and interdependent, who have a stable relationship, a common goal, and perceive themselves to be a group. A group doesn't simply mean individuals possessing identical features. For example, a collection of students or musicians don't form a group. There are two principal types of group interaction, one exists when people are discussing ideas and is generally called a meeting, and the other exists when people perform task together and is called a team.

Types of Groups

Psychological Group

It may be defined as the one in which two or more persons, who are interdependent and each member's nature influences every other person. They share a common ideology and have common tasks. (For example, families, friendship circles, etc.)

Social Group

It may be defined as an integrated system of interrelated psychological groups formed to accomplish a defined function or objective. (For example, political party)

Formal Group

It refers to those, which are established under the legal or formal authority with the view to achieve a particular end result (For example, people making up the airline flight crew)

Informal Group

Informal groups are the ones that emerge naturally due to the response and common interests of the members of an organization who can easily identify with the goals or independent activities of the group.

Primary Group

The primary groups are characterized by small size, face to face interactions and intimacy among the members. Family groups are the example of primary group.

Secondary Group

The secondary groups are characterized by large size and individuals' identification with the values and beliefs prevailing in them rather than actual interactions (for example, occupational association and ethnic groups).

Membership Group

The membership group is the one to which an individual actually belongs.

Reference Group

The reference group is the one to which an individual would like to belong.

Command Group

The command groups are formed by subordinates reporting directly to the particular manager and are determined by the formal organizational chart (for example an assistant regional transport officer and his two transport supervisors form a command group).

Task Group

The task group is composed of people who work together to perform a task but involves a cross command relationship.

Interest Group

The interest group involves people who come together to accomplish a particular goal with which they are concerned (for example office employees).

Friendship Group

The friendship groups are formed by people having one or more common features.

Classification of Informal Groups

Many social psychologists classify the informal groups in different ways.

Mayo and Lombard Classification

- **Natural Groups**: It reveals no or too little internal structure
- **Family Groups**: These possess a core of regulars who exert marked influence on the behavior of the members.

- **Organized Groups**: These possess acknowledged leaders who set themselves dedicatedly with intelligence and skill to attain group integrity.

Sayles Classification

- **Apathetic Groups**: These groups possess consistently indifferent attitudes towards formal organization and are characterized by dispersed leadership, lack of cohesiveness, internal disunity and conflict.
- **Erratic Groups**: These groups fluctuate between antagonism and cooperation and are marked by the poorly controlled pressure tactics, behavior inconsistency, quick conversation to good relations with management, centralized and union formation activities.
- **Strategic Groups**: There is consistent antagonism, continuous pressures, high degree of internal unity and usually good production record in the long run.
- **Conservative Groups**: These groups are marked by the usual cooperation, limited pressures for highly specific objectives, moderate internal unity and self-assurance.

Dalton's Classification

- **Horizontal Groups**: These are associations of the worker, managers or any other member of equal ranks engaged in performing more or less similar works.
- **Vertical Groups**: These are composed of members from varied levels within a particular department, for example, workers, foreman, managers.
- **Mixed Groups**: These are the groups that are composed of members of varied ranks, departments and physical locations.

Group Formation through Social Relationship

United we stand, divided we fall. This is a famous proverb. From the prehistorical times, human beings started being in group for various purposes. People seek to join groups since the groups give the members stability and enhances their achievement capacity. Being a member of a group always gives a feeling of comfort and confidence. The main reasons propelling individuals to join groups are:

- **Sense of security**: The group enables the person in reducing the sense of insecurity and have a stronger feeling with few self doubts and more resistant treats when they are a part of the group.
- **Status**: The persons in a group can be easily recognized and a status is achieved by them
- **Develop self-esteem**: The groups can help a person develop a sense of "belongingness". This provides feelings of self-worth and develops confidence in its members.
- **Affiliation**: The groups can fulfill social needs. People enjoy the regular interaction that comes with the group membership.
- **Power**: The power is derived from the strength of closeness of the group members. Greater power is achieved when an individual is in group than being alone or individually.
- **Goal achievement**: The goal can be achieved more easily when a group effort is present as "UNITED WE STAND, DIVIDED WE FALL"

Stages of Forming a Group

Group development is a dynamic process, and probably never reaches a state of complete stability. There is strong evidence that groups pass through the standard sequence of the following stages:

- **Forming**: This is characterized by a great deal of uncertainty about group's purpose, structure and the leadership. The stage is completed when the members begin to think that they are a part of the group.
- **Storming**: The members accept the existence of the group but they are still resisting the constraints the group poses on them. There is a conflict as to who will control the group. When this stage completes, a relatively clear hierarchy exists in the group.
- **Norming**: In this, there is a close relationship between the members and the group demonstrates cohesiveness. There is a sense of group identity and this stage is completed when the group structure solidifies and the group has assimilated a common set of expectations defining the behavior.
- **Performing**: The structure at this point is fully functional and accepted. The group energy has moved from getting to know and understand each other to performing a task at hand. For permanent work groups, this is the last stage. But for temporary committees, team, task forces and similar groups, the adjourning stage is the last.
- **Adjourning**: The groups prepares to disband. The high task performance is no longer the required goal. The attention is towards wrapping up of activities and responses of the group members. The responses of the group members vary in this stage. Some are upbeat, basking in the group's accomplishments. Some are depressed over the loss of colleagues and friends made during the course.

Group Dynamics and Human Relations

Group dynamics refers to a system of behaviors and psychological processes occurring within a social group (intragroup dynamics), or between social groups (intergroup dynamics). The study of group dynamics can be useful in understanding decision-making behavior, tracking the spread of diseases in society, creating effective therapy techniques, and following the emergence and popularity of new ideas and technologies. Group dynamics are at the core of understanding racism and other forms of social prejudice and discrimination.

Group Dynamics refers to the study of forces operating within a group. Following are few of its salient features:

- Group Dynamics is concerned with group. Wherever a group exists the individuals interact and members are continuously changing and adjusting relationship with respect to each other.
- Changes keep on happening like introduction of the new members, changes in leadership, presence of old and new members and the rate of change – fast or slow. The groups may dissolve if the members are not enthusiastic about the goals.
- There may be rigidity or flexibility that influences a group dynamics. If the members get along well, there is smooth sailing for the group and if there is a conflict, it leads to problems
- The group organization is essential. It leads to greater group effectiveness, participation, cooperation and a constructive morale.

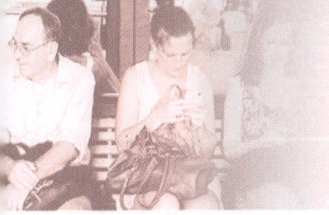

- Dynamic groups are always in continuous process of restructuring, adjusting and readjusting members to one another for the purpose of reducing the tensions, eliminating the conflicts and solving the problems, which its members have in common.

There are some principles for group dynamics which are as follows:

- The members of the group must have a strong sense of belongingness to the group.
- The more attractive a group member is to its members, the greater influence he/she would exercise on its members.
- The successful efforts to change individual sub parts of the group would result in confirming the norms of the group.
- Information relating to the need for change, plans for change and the consequences of the changes must be shared by the members of the group.
- The changes in one pact of the groups may produce stress in the other parts, which can be reduced only by eliminating the change or by bringing about readjustments in the related parts.
- The groups arise and function owing to common motives.
- The intergroup relations, group organization and member participation are essential for effectiveness of a group

Human relation is an area of management practice which is concerned with the integration of people into a work situation in a way that motivate them to work productively, cooperatively and with economic, psychological and social satisfaction.

Roles and Responsibilities of an Individual in a Group

Three types of roles are performed by members in a group. They are task roles, maintenance roles and hindering roles.

Task Roles

Task roles refer to the actions of individuals that help move the group by taking leadership roles.

Initiating

Initiating refers to proposing tasks or goals; defining a group problem; suggesting procedure or ideas for getting the task accomplished. It is done at the beginning of a meeting, when the meeting bogs down, or when the group needs direction or a new direction.

Information or Opinion Seeking

It includes requesting facts; seeking relevant information about a question or concern; asking for suggestions, ideas or opinions. It is done during problem solving, decision making, action planning and in group discussion.

Clarifying

Clarifying involves interpreting or reflecting ideas and suggestions; clearing up conclusions; indicating alternatives and issues before the group; giving examples and defining terms. It is performed at any time when the group discussion becomes too vague, too general or lacks focus or when a lot of information has been put out.

Summarizing

Summarizing is nothing but pulling together related ideas; restating suggestions after the group has discussed them; offering a decision or conclusion for the group to accept or reject. It is done at each transition of the meeting, when many different ideas or proposals are being considered, when the group gets off track and at the end of a meeting/ discussion.

Consensus Testing

It is the process of checking with the group to see how much agreement has been reached and how ready the group members are to consider a decision. It is conducted during problem solving, decision making and action planning.

Maintenance Roles

Maintenance roles refer to the actions of individuals that help preserve the relationships in a group.

Encouraging

It involves being friendly, warm, and responsive to others; accepting others and their contributions; regarding others by giving them an opportunity to contribute or be recognized. It is done regularly.

Harmonizing

It is nothing but attempting to reconcile disagreements; reducing tension, getting people to explore their differences. It is done when the group cannot reach consensus, when conflict of ideas, opinions or personality is preventing progress.

Expressing Group Feelings

It includes sensing feelings, mood, relationships within the group; sharing one's own feelings with other members. It is performed when the group is having trouble making a decision, when you sense a conflict in the group, as a check-in to see how the group is doing. The techniques used are verbalizing what you see as the feelings, mood, and tension in the group and openly acknowledging your own feelings about what is going on in the group.

Gate-keeping

It is helping to keep communication channels open: facilitating the participation of others, suggesting procedures that permit sharing remarks. It is done whenever you want to hear from the more silent members of the group and whenever you want to prevent a participant from dominating the discussion.

Compromising

It is used when your own ideas or status is involved in a conflict, offering a compromise which yields status; admitting error, modifying ideas in interest of group cohesion or growth. When the group is

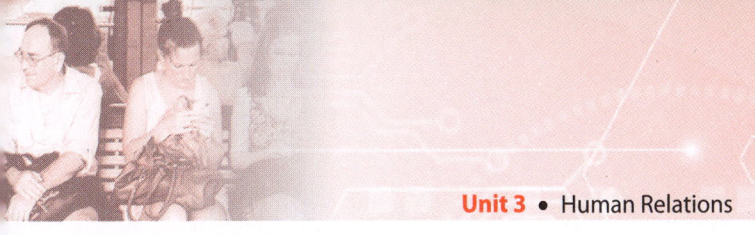

stuck, when trying to make a decision and there are opposing views, compromising will be of immense use.

Standard Setting and Testing

It includes checking whether the group is satisfied with its procedures and suggesting new procedures when necessary. It is performed when the group first meets together, whenever the norms that are developing prevent the group from functioning effectively.

We have discussed the two roles which are constructive in nature. But the remaining role is usually destructive in nature.

Hindering Roles

Hindering roles refer to actions of individuals that hinder the group's process and progress.

Dominating

The behavior shown is asserting authority or superiority to manipulate the group or certain members; interrupting contributions of others and controlling through use of flattery or patronization. The solution is to establish a procedure whereby each person contributes one idea to the discussion and then must wait until every other group member does the same before contributing again; interrupt the dominator, ask him/her to summarize the point quickly so that others can add their ideas, too.

Withdrawing

It is the process of removing self psychologically or physically from the group; not talking; answering questions only briefly. The solution is not to let conflicts remain unresolved; talk with the person privately to find out what is happening; direct questions to and solicit ideas from the avoider so this person stays involved.

Degrading

The behavior of putting down others' ideas and suggestions; deflating others' status; joking in a barbed or sarcastic way contribute to degrading. When your group first gets together, review your contract and ground rules with them, highlighting the rule that all ideas will be accepted; the first time someone criticizes another person, reinforce this rule.

Non-cooperation

The behavior is disagreeing and opposing ideas; resisting stubbornly the group's wishes for personally oriented reasons; using hidden agenda to thwart group progress. The solution is to incorporate statements in the original guidelines that deal with cooperation and interruptions, encourage this person to explain reasons behind his/her objection; look for any aspect of the position that supports the group's ideas so that this person moves from left to center field; refocus his/her participation as a recorder or process observer and ask the group to deal with this non-cooperative behavior.

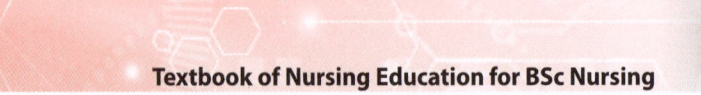
Side Conversations

The behavior includes whispering, giggling and having private side conversations with another person. The solution is to set guidelines and expectations at the beginning of the meeting, stop the meeting and ask those involved in the side conversation to share what they are talking about with the group, stop the meeting and comment that it is difficult for you to hear the other discussion or to concentrate on the topic at hand with side conversations occurring; privately talking with the distracters and discuss their expectations for the meeting's topics and empower others to confront the distracters with how these side conversations keep everyone from concentrating on the group's discussion.

Group Behavior and Communication

Successful working groups are marked by a range of different communication behaviors—actions people do with words and gestures, which they can practice and improve over time. Some of them are:

- **Listening**: Hear and make sense of what your colleagues are saying; use good, active non-verbal behaviors like looking at people when they speak, nodding your head when you agree with something, and sitting forward to show involvement.
- **Making clarifying statements**: Offer an explanation of a concept or issue which the group is trying to understand.
- **Deliberating and discussing**: Respond to other people, not simply pushing your agenda regardless of what anyone says; engage them by agreeing and extending what they say or by respectfully disagreeing with it and offering reasons.
- **Keeping the discussion on task**: If the conversation drifts, bring the group back onto task.
- **Eliciting viewpoints from others**: Ask people who haven't spoken what they think about an issue.
- **Offering feedback**: Give a colleague constructive comments on a project they did.
- **Mediating conflicts**: If there are disagreements and conflicts, try to find middle ground that satisfies everyone.

TEAM WORK

What is a Team?

A team refers to a group of people with a full set of complementary skills required to complete a task, job, or project. Team members: (1) operate with a high degree of interdependence, (2) share authority and responsibility for self-management, (3) are accountable for the collective performance, and (4) work toward a common goal and shared rewards(s). A team becomes more than just a collection of people when a strong sense of mutual commitment creates synergy, thus generating performance greater than the sum of the performance of its individual members.

In healthcare, teamwork is "a dynamic process involving two or more healthcare professionals with complementary background and skills, sharing common health goals and exercising concerted physical and mental effort in assessing, planning, or evaluating patient care"

Researchers have identified 10 teamwork processes that fall into three categories:
- Transition process (between periods of action)
  - Mission analysis

- ■ Goal specification
- ■ Strategy formulation
- ● Action process (when the team attempts to accomplish its goals and objectives)
  - ■ Monitoring progress toward goals
  - ■ Systems monitoring
  - ■ Team monitoring and backup behavior
  - ■ Coordination
- ● Interpersonal process (present in both action periods and transition periods)
  - ■ Conflict management
  - ■ Motivation and confidence building
  - ■ Affect management

What We Need to Build a Team? (7 Cs)

The researchers have identified several skills required to work effectively as a team and can be easily discussed under following headings

Communication

In any work team, communication must be clear and consistent. Members of the team need to remain open and actively seek diverse points of view to avoid falling into what group think. It's vital that each individual uses his or her voice and be heard. Because we all have different preferences in how we give and receive information, this can be challenging. Finding the right balance of cooperativeness and assertiveness is a skill, one that is applied differently in teams than it is in one-to-one interactions. Teams that are new or have been assembled for a specific project may need to accelerate the process of establishing clear communication. They may not have time to get acquainted and to work out style differences.

Collaboration

It requires time, planning and trust—three variables newly-formed teams may not have in abundance. To truly collaborate, team members need skills in problem-solving, negotiating and emotional intelligence. Unlike compromise (where all parties give up something), collaboration expands to be sure and every party's interests are fully met. As team members represent various interests, they may enter into the team with an agenda and, if so, will need willingness and ability to set it aside long enough to build something bigger.

Conflict Resolution

As a team skill, this one has two distinct parts. The first involves an ability to undermine the conflict and engage in healthy debate to bring more ideas and opinions into the discussion. The second is the ability to curtail unhealthy conflict and redirect those energies into a genuine collaboration. Neither of these skills is honed fully in routine settings. Working as a member of a team demands these skills, especially when the team is project-based and comprised of cross-functional representatives.

Cross-Functional Understanding

The old saying "seek first to understand and then to be understood" applies here. It's much easier though to judge and blame "the sales department" or "those engineers" or "penny pinchers in accounting." Developing broader view helps the team, especially if they are united around a common purpose for the team. Business acumen is also useful for any employee in any role -- that's why being a part of a cross-functional team is such a great opportunity.

Creativity and Innovation

Most teams are formed to solve something or to create something. Either way, team members will need to learn how to stretch beyond the status quo. In most roles, though, creativity and innovation are not a part of the day-to-day job. That's why these are considered to be qualities more often than they are thought of as skills. To be fully effective, a team needs to develop skills in innovating and creating. Even basic brainstorming has technique to it, but this is not widely known or used.

Change Management

Teams will likely be charged with implementing what they've devised. They will need to inspire others to get on board with the changes, and they'll need skills for overcoming resistance (the natural response to change). Since appointed team members are unlikely to be the direct supervisors of everyone involved in a change initiative, they'll also need skills of influence (vs. authority). These are all teachable skills, but teams seldom get the backing they need to be trained in these skills. When their change doesn't take hold, it appears the team failed to produce a good solution.

Coaching

Influencing others, resolving conflict, stretching to become more creative, leading change, adapting one's own communication style and collaborating cross-functionally—that's a tall order for a team. Perhaps the complexity of these first 6 C's is what prevents "the powers that be" from fully equipping teams. After all, it's much easier to simply assign the project and leave the team to its own devices.

The first 6 C's can all be acquired and practiced with team training. The seventh C is where these skills are mastered. When team members hold each other accountable for using these skills as they work together, coaching one another for continued development, that's where the magic happens. Think back to any successful team you worked with and this C—Coaching among peers—will be apparent. But it, too, is a skill and with a little training, team members can become much more effective.

Role of an Individual in a Team (Do's and Don'ts)

There are several roles an individual member has to perform, for the successful performance of the team. They are explained under Do's and Don'ts for the clear understanding.

Do's

- Be considerate. Stimulate others, by asking questions and making suggestions without pressuring them.

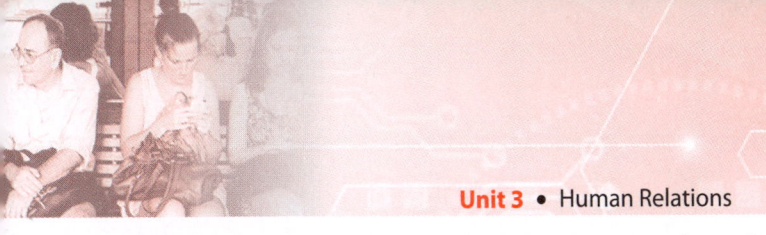

- Support the ideas of other people vocally. Silence may be understood as tacit approval or may be interpreted as apathy or disdain. When you like someone's idea, say so.
- Be aware of others' feelings. If feelings are getting in the way of the issues, address the feelings first and the issues second.
- Listen actively. Make sure that you understand the ideas of others. Paraphrase these ideas, as you understand them, in order to make sure you've got the message-and to help spur others on to refinements and new ideas.
- Invite criticism of your own ideas and work You can help to establish an open productive atmosphere by making it clear that you know your ideas are tentative and not necessarily perfect. Give permission to others to help you refine your ideas and writing.
- Accept that others are imperfect too. Particularly, be aware that communication breaks down in the best of groups. If someone misunderstands you, don't get exasperated or angry, and don't try to assign the blame for the breakdown in communication. Simply restate your idea.
- Feel free to disagree with the ideas of others and to critique the work of others but lay off the people. Don't identify peoples' names with ideas that you are criticizing.
- Remember that any non-obvious ideas initially appear strange, but that most of the best ideas are not immediately obvious.

Don'ts

- Don't continually play the expert role.
- Play a variety of roles.
- Don't pressure people unnecessarily.
- Don't punish people for their ideas.
- Don't continue an argument after it becomes personal-either for you or for your fellow group member.
- Don't give in too easily when your ideas are criticized. The excellence of the group is a product of constructive conflict.
- Don't fall prey to "groupthink" sacrificing high level thinking for the sake of group cohesiveness.

HUMAN RELATIONS IN CONTEXT OF NURSING

Nursing – A Humanistic Profession

Nursing is a humanistic profession. Nurses care and do the very best to save lives and if they can't, they provide dignity until the moment of death arrives. Nurses face ethical dilemmas daily—it is a calling. Nurses are the eyes and ears monitoring the patient's state of health and well being and must intervene appropriately when a patient's condition worsens. Florence Nightingale claimed that the essence of nursing rested on the nurse's capacity to provide humane, sensitive care to the sick, which she believed would allow healing. This approach is depicted through the well-known image of the lady with the lamp caring and healing the soldiers in the middle of the night.

Nursing takes place within an economic, social, and technological context that may influence the way nurses practice and the ways they interact with patients. Certain aspects of the healthcare environment are not congruent with a humanistic agenda in nursing. Some of the examples are:

- High technology in the form of computers, diagnostic equipment and pharmaceutical cures.
- Robots as analogs to nurses.

Self-concept, Self-image and Nursing

With the changing concept of health, it is necessary to promote positive relationships between a nurse and a patient and provide qualitative caring with the objective of providing high-quality medical service. To provide professional service based on advanced knowledge, experiences, and technology to meet such a demand, nurses need to establish a positive image as a professional and correctly perceive the attributes of caring, which has traditionally been considered essential to nursing. It is important to establish a positive professional self-concept in order to do their jobs effectively as a professional nurse in clinical area with healthcare professionals.

Although professional self-concept is an important factor to improve nursing profession in every aspect, the researchers in this area have explored it among nurses or determined its association with relevant variables. However, little research has been conducted on the association between caring perception and professional self-concept among several relevant factors. Caring is a central concept in expressing the originality of nursing as a profession. As a personal relationship between a nurse and a patient, caring is intellectual, developmental, and central to nursing practice.

It is a well known fact that the social image of a profession also largely contributes the self concept and self image of the members of that profession. It is been observed that the self concept and self image of nurses working in the western world are higher since nursing is one of top ranked professions in those countries. The other factors include the social security, remuneration and recognition from other members of health team.

Significance of Human Relations in Nursing Practice

Human relations refers to a systematic, developing body of knowledge devoted to explaining the behavior of individuals or people in the working organization or concern. Human relations are an integral process through which the individual's attitudes and work are combined or integrated. Purpose of human relations is to help in working more effectively with other people in organizations. It is a well known fact that nurses play a very significant role in connecting between patient and physician and among other healthcare professionals. The human relation skill is as important as other cognitive, psychomotor skills of rendering patient care. Human relations attempts to improve employee morale and motivation through an improved three way communications through employee involvement in the decision making processes. It emphasizes employee aspects of work rather than technical or economic aspects and tries to make employment and working smooth.

Nurse Client Communication

Patient-centered communication is a basic component of nursing and facilitates the development of a positive nurse-patient relationship which, along with other organizational factors, results in the delivery of quality nursing care. Nurses are frequently described in the literature as poor communicators; however, very few studies have examined patients' experiences of how nurses communicate.

Nurses largely affect society in the healthcare system by helping, supporting and caring for an individual, a whole family or even an entire community. While in the medical surroundings, the nurse becomes the primary contact for the patient in care and spends a lot of time with them. Before approaching a nursing care situation, a nurse needs to clear all judgments with respect to every individual, as there are many different religions, morals and personal beliefs in the world today. Therefore nurses need to develop the ability of quality communication skills, which helps to create great interpersonal relationship skills in nursing. Communication and interviewing are both skills needed to develop interpersonal relationships within the nursing environment. Communication skills are the first skills noticed in a person.

Nursing has many crucial elements, which are necessary to ensure a good quality of care. The nursing process is developed to encourage individualized care; this then achieves meeting all patient needs in and out of the hospital setting. Effective communication skills include the use of verbal and non-verbal language, vocabulary, listening and written record taking skills. The nursing interview and assessment process is a part of the nursing care plan, which is a crucial process to enable a nurse to assess a patient to full potential. These both help to develop a therapeutic interpersonal relationship, which is increasingly important for both the patient and their family. The relationship allows a patient to trust and feel comfortable with the people surrounding them while being cared for. These important nursing skills enable the highest quality of care for all patients in the nursing environment.

Nurse as a Member of Health Team

An interprofessional team is a group of people, who have certain common goals or objectives, which drives them to work together by setting aside individual goals. Inter professional team can be defined as "a dynamic process involving two or more healthcare professionals with complementary backgrounds and skills, sharing common health goals and exercising concerted physical and mental effort in assessing, planning, or evaluating patient care, accomplished through interdependent collaboration, open communication and shared decision-making, and generates value-added patient, organizational and staff outcomes". Freeth et al (2005) defined inter professional team work as "when two or more professional learn with, from and about each other to improve collaboration and the quality of care".

The roles played by nurses in the interprofessional teams are fast evolving. The importance of specialist skills for nurses is now recognized and new role have come up. A group of nurses called night practitioners literally run the hospitals at night. They are skilled to assist any department and are sometimes considered better than junior doctors too.

SUMMARY

Understanding self is very important aspect in development of an individual. The concepts of social behavior, motivation and social attitudes are very important concepts we need to understand to be effective healthcare professional. Nursing being a humanistic profession, the members of the profession need to have good human relations to be successful in the career. Team work is the key to the success in healthcare. Understanding group dynamics and principles of team work will help the members of any profession to be successful.

ASSESS YOURSELF

LONG ANSWER QUESTIONS

1. Describe the factors which play important roles in formation of human self.
2. Describe the expansion of human relations during the life-stages of growth and development.
3. Discuss the factors influencing Social Attitude and Social Behaviour.
4. Describe the stages of formation of a group.
5. What is the significance of human relations in nursing practice?
6. How understanding of group dynamics is helpful for a health care professional?
7. Explain Maslow's Hierarchy of Human Needs with suitable examples.

SHORT ANSWER QUESTIONS

1. What are the components of social attitude?
2. Explain the types of social behavior
3. Difference between social behavior and social attitude
4. How social behavior and social attitude are inter-related?
5. Discuss the factors influencing social attitude and social behavior.
6. What are the different types of group?
7. What are the stages of formation of a group?
8. Describe roles and responsibilities of an individual in a group
9. Define group dynamics?
10. Explain the significance of human relations in nursing practice
11. Explain the role of a nurse as a member of health team.
12. How understanding of group dynamics will be helpful for a healthcare professional?
13. What is the significance of human relations in nursing practice?

SHORT NOTES

1. Differences between positive and negative self-concept
2. Evolution of inner-self
3. Components of social attitude
4. Types of social behaviour
5. Difference between Social Behaviour & Social Attitude
6. Relationship between social attitude and social behavior
7. Different types of Group
8. Group dynamics
9. Role of nurse as a member of the Health Team
10. Significance of human relations in nursing practice

Contd...

MULTIPLE CHOICE QUESTIONS

1. **Types of social behavior are the following, EXCEPT –**
   A. Emotional behavior
   B. Group interaction
   C. Inaction
   D. Pro-social behavior

2. **A social factor which influences behavior is –**
   A. Environment
   B. Motivation
   C. Peer group
   D. Social norms

3. **Motivation is determined by –**
   A. Life challenges
   B. Life goals
   C. Determination
   D. All of the above

4. **Stages of forming a group**
   A. Storming
   B. Norming
   C. Performing
   D. Adjourning

5. **Effective communication requires all the following, EXCEPT –**
   A. Active participation
   B. Judgmental attitude
   C. Listening
   D. Open-mindedness

ANSWERS TO MCQS

1. (C)	2. (D)	3. (D)	4. (D)	5. (B)

BIBLIOGRAPHY

1. Hoffman, E. (1988). The right to be human: A biography of Abraham Maslow. Jeremy P. Tarcher, Inc.
2. Kenrick, D. T., Neuberg, S. L., Griskevicius, V., Becker, D. V., and Schaller, M. (2010). Goal-Driven Cognition and Functional Behavior The Fundamental-Motives Framework. Current Directions in Psychological Science, 19(1), 63-67.
3. Maslow, A. H. (1943). A Theory of Human Motivation. Psychological Review, 50(4), 370-96.
4. Maslow, A. H. (1954). Motivation and personality. New York: Harper and Row.
5. Maslow, A. H. (1962). Towards a psychology of being. Princeton: D. Van Nostrand Company.
6. Maslow, A. H. (1968). Toward a Psychology of Being. New York: D. Van Nostrand Company.
7. Maslow, A. H. (1970a). Motivation and personality. New York: Harper and Row.
8. Maslow, A. H. (1970b). Religions, values, and peak experiences. New York: Penguin. (Original work published 1964)
9. Wilson and Rosenfield. Managing Organizations. London: McGraw Hill Book Company. p. 9.
10. Jump up DuBrin, A J (2007). Human Relations Interpersonal Job-Oriented Skills (9 ed.). New Jersey: Pearson Prentice Hall. p. 2.

11. Jump up to: a b c Bruce, K and Nylan, C 2011, 'Elton Mayo and the Deification of Human Relations', Organization Studies, Vol 32, No 3, pp 383-405.

12. Jump up, Wren D and Greenwood R 1998, Management innovators: The people and ideas that have shaped modern business, Oxford University Press, New York.

13. Jump up, Bruce, Kyle. "Henry S. Dennison, Elton Mayo, and Human Relations historiography." Management and Organizational History 2006, 1: 177–199.

14. Jump up, Mcleod, M 1983, '"Architecture or Revolution": Taylorism, Technocracy, and Social Change', Art Journal, Vol. 43, No 2, pp 132-147.

15. Jump up, Taneja, S, Pryor, M G and Toombs, L A 2011, 'Frederick W. Taylor's Scientific Management Principles: Relevance and Validity', Journal of Applied Management and Entrepreneurship, Vol 16, No 3, pp 60-78.

16. Jump up, Taneja, S, Pryor, M G, Humpheries J H and Toombs, L A (2011). "Where Are the New Organization Theories? Evolution, Development and Theoretical Debate". International Journal of Management. 28 (3): 959–978.

17. Benne, K. and Sheats, P. (2010). Functional Roles of Group Members. Journal of Social Issues, 4(2), pp.41-49.

18. Mindtools.com. (2016). Benne and Sheats' Group Roles: Identifying Both Positive and Negative Group Behavior Roles. [online] Available at: https://www.mindtools.com/pages/article/newTMM_85.htm [Accessed 21 Jun. 2016].

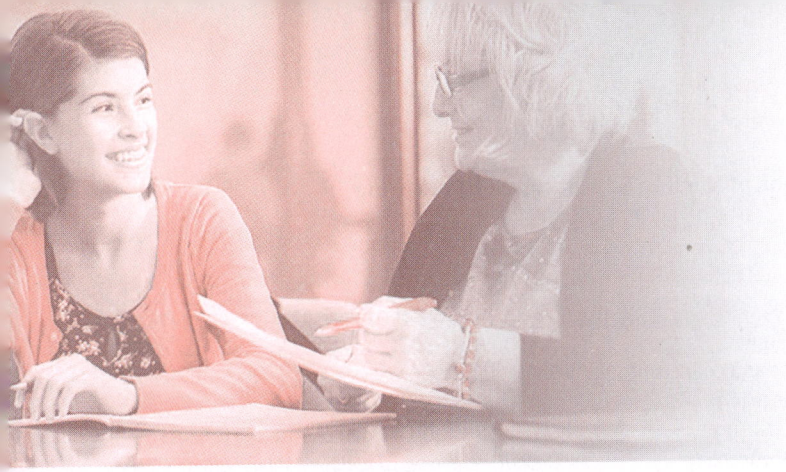
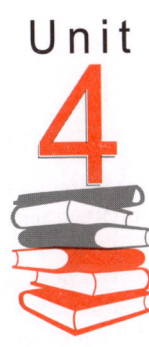

Unit 4

Guidance and Counseling

— *Mamtaz Begum*

CHAPTER OUTLINE

Concept of Guidance and Counseling
- Meaning of Guidance and Counseling
- Definition of Guidance and Counseling
- Difference Between Guidance and Counseling
- Comparison of Guidance and Counseling

Purpose, Scope and Need of Guidance and Counseling
- Purposes of Guidance and Counseling
- Scope of Guidance and Counseling
- Scope of Guidance and Counseling In Educational Organization
- Needs of Guidance and Counseling

Organization of Guidance and Counseling Services
- Principles of Guidance and Counseling
- Factors Upon Which Guidance and Counseling Depend
- Approaches of Counseling

Counseling Process
- Preparation of Counselor
- Role of Counselor

- Qualities of A Counselor
- Steps of Counseling

Uses of Tools In Counseling
- Standardized Test
- Types of Standardized Test
- Non Standardized Test
- Types of Non Standardized Test

Management of Crisis and Referral
- Definition of Crisis
- Characteristics of Crisis
- Types of Crisis
- Phases of Crisis Development
- Steps in Crisis Intervention
- Referral Service

Managing Disciplinary Problems
- Common Disciplinary Problems
- Managing Disciplinary Problems
- Teachers and Students Role
- Issues of Counseling in Nursing

📖 LEARNING OBJECTIVE

The learner will be able to

- Define guidance and counseling
- Differentiate guidance and counseling
- Recognize the purposes of guidance and counseling
- Discuss scope of guidance and counseling
- Identify needs of guidance and counseling
- List out principles of guidance and counseling
- Explain the influencing factors in guidance and counseling
- Distinguishes the role of counselee in changing approach of counseling
- Describe the qualities of a good counselor
- Discuss the role of counselor according to the need of counselee
- Enumerate the process of organising counseling service
- Classify the tools used in counseling process
- Describe the uses of various tool in counseling process
- Elaborate crisis management process
- Identify disciplinary problems
- Discover the issues of counseling in nursing

INTRODUCTION

Guidance and counseling is not a new practice; it is as old as society in human civilization. In human society, it was the role of older people to give advice and guidance to their next generation for sustaining with the changing environment. In a family, parents take the responsibility to shape the behavior of their children through information, advice, and role modelling. The inappropriate or socially unaccepted behavior of children is corrected with great patience and they also use some technique like scolding, praising, etc. These actions of parents are similar to the technique of counseling. In present days, we find guidance and counseling reaching many levels: parents guide and counsel their children, doctors and nurses do for their patients, lawyers do for their clients and teachers do for their students.

Guidance and Counseling as a discipline originated in America at the beginning of the 20th Century because of the society's emphasis on individual development. In 1908, Frank Parsons founded a Vocational Bureau in Boston and it was the beginning of vocational movement. Parsons concern and belief was that if individuals can understand their strengths and weaknesses, that knowledge can be used to choose vocational opportunities.

In India, the Gurukul system of education was teacher centered, where '*Guru*' had the supreme authority of taking decision for '*Sishya*'. Guru was very respectful and wise person in society. They had full control over their student and their word was valuable for students. The primary role of student was taking care of teacher and following his words. This kind of role and relationship indicates that Guru acted as his guide, adviser and great motivator. In the ancient Indian Universities like Nalanda and Taxila, the monks used to provide guidance to their students.

Guidance movement started in India at the beginning of 19th century. The first psychological laboratory was established in the year 1915 at Calcutta University and Batliboi Vocational Guidance Bureau, Bombay was established in the year 1941. A department of Psychological service and Research was established at Patna University in the year of 1945 and there was a provision for number of psychological tests and vocational guidance for students. In the 20th century, guidance and counseling become an integral part of student's overall development. Student's development occurs following a sequential process of orientation, adjustment and development. Each step in the process of development is dependent on guidance and counseling.

KEY TERMS IN GUIDANCE AND COUNSELING (FIG.1)

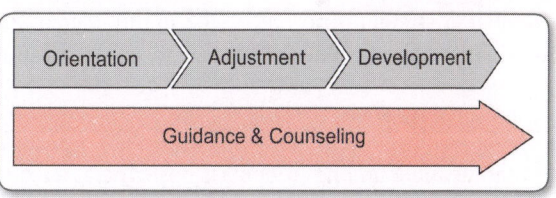

Orientation

The literal meaning of orientation is the adjustment or alignment of oneself or one's ideas to surroundings or circumstances. Here

Fig. 1: Key terms in guidance and counseling

orientation refers to introducing a student with his/her educational program, educational organization, educator, co-learners, and environment.

At the beginning of an educational program, the group of students are introduced with the following.

- **Educational Program**: It is the particular course in which students are interested in and are willing to continue in the present session. Educational program includes the combination of subjects and its placement with specified period, methods of teaching, uses of educational technology, mode of evaluation, activity of students, and the offering awards. Students are oriented thoroughly with the educational program through guidance and counseling and it helps them to justify the suitability of the program. Any wrong decision taken made by the student creates problem and maladjustment.
- **Educational Organization**: Students are introduced with the educational organization, its vision, mission, objectives, rules, regulation, infrastructure and facilities. Orienting with educational organization, students are enabled to recognize to what extent their desired need may be fulfilled. Inappropriate orientation or lack of student's recognition may create maladjustment.
- **Educator**: The group of educators involved in the teaching program are introduced with students, which facilitates adjustment.
- **Co-learners**: Students are also introduced with their co-learners with whom they need to interact more and are going to spend maximum their time. This learner group is dissimilar in many ways, therefore, it demands adjustment.
- **Environment**: It is the surrounding that includes living arrangement, food, drinking water, ventilation, sunshine, degree of noise and climate in which student has to survive. If the students are not guided with their immediate environment, problems may arise at any level.

Adjustment

After entering a teaching institution or educational organization, a student is oriented through guidance and counseling. Appropriate orientation helps students to decide whether to join the course or not. Once student joins a course, the next task is adjustment for which they need support in guidance and counseling. Adjustment is a kind of change that makes it possible for a person to do better or work better in a new situation. Adjustment is necessary to maximize the development of student. Without adjustment student may face problems at personal, interpersonal and extrapersonal level.

Personal

Students may not adjust because of some personal problem such as lack of intellectual ability, lack of interest, ill temperament, lack of motivation, value conflict, health status etc. For example, if a intelligent student is not interested in nursing course, he/she may develop many personal problems like psychosomatic illness, frequent absenteeism and failure.

Interpersonal

Maladjustment among students is observed as a result of some interpersonal causes such as mismatch of attitude, belief, and behavior with other co-learners or teachers. Sometimes, the differences of cultural practice, religious practice, food habit and language cause maladjustment and crisis between two or more students.

Extrapersonal

Maladjustment may occur as a result of extrapersonal causes. Extrapersonal causes are those, which are beyond the control of a person such as environmental pollution, natural calamities etc.

Development

Social Development

One of the main aims of education is the social development, which is supported through guidance and counseling. Appropriate social behavior—cooperation, healthy competition, harmony and fair play should be encouraged where as inappropriate social behavior like fighting, destroying equipments, ragging and substance abuse need to be discouraged and require repeated counseling for adaptive behavior. Important social values like respect for humanity, patience, toleration, etc. are exhibited to students as well as expected from students.

Intellectual Development

To develop intellectual capacity of students, various kinds of exposure, challenging tasks, and new information should be delivered in an attractive manner to the students. To identify difficulty, different type of tests are useful. Excellent performers should be encouraged and at the same time, poor performers should be counselled to identify the cause and to provide the required guidance.

Psychological/Emotional Development

Intellectual development is not only the aim of education but improving psychological health and emotional quotient is also desirable for a student's overall development. Some students join the nursing course with previous psychological or emotional problems due to genetic predisposition, family and societal causes, whereas some students develop psychological problems after joining the course. Any kind of psychological or emotional problems are to be identified as soon as possible and should be treated through guidance and counseling services. For example, development of psychosomatic illness like migraine and colitis are common among student. Students are also found with various levels of depression and anxiety, which requires treatment and referral services.

Moral Development

Inculcating moral values in students is very essential for making them productive and useful for the society. Absence of moral values like honesty, truthfulness, justice, goodness may cause behavioral problems like stealing, lying, quarreling, bullying, etc., which are corrected with appropriate counseling.

Spiritual Development

Spiritual development is the development of higher level of awareness or consciousness, which makes a person to realize the equal rights of all beings on the earth, to develop and to carry out their tasks, so the purpose of life is fulfilled. Lack of spirituality makes a person aimless and causes loss of potentiality. As awareness increases, pupil learns to assume his/her responsibility and achieve the educational objectives with less problems.

CONCEPT OF GUIDANCE AND COUNSELING

Meaning of Guidance and Counseling

Guidance is an integral part of education, without guidance it is difficult to achieve the basic goal of education. The basic goal of education is all round development of individual that includes physical, intellectual, social, emotional, moral and spiritual development. Guidance helps in achieving all aspects of development harmoniously. Guidance is the assistance given to individuals in making intelligent choices and adjustment.

Counseling is a scientific process of assistance extended by an expert in an individual situation to a person who requires it. Guidance and counseling are not synonymous terms. Guidance is relatively more comprehensive process, which includes counseling as one of the components. Counseling is a component of guidance, not all of it. Thus, all counseling is guidance but all guidance is not counseling.

Definitions of Guidance

Guidance is a process of helping individuals to maximize capacity for adjustment with intra, inter and extrapersonal environment.

- "Guidance is that aspect of educational program, which is concerned with helping the pupil to become adjusted to his present situation and plan his future in line with his interests, abilities and social needs."   **—Hamrin and Erikson**
- "Guidance is a process of helping every individual, through his own efforts to discover and develop his potentialities for his personal happiness and social usefulness."   **—Ruth Strang**
- "Guidance is an assistance made available by a competent counselor to an individual of any age to help him direct his own life, develop his own point of view, make his own decision and carry his own burden."   **—Crow and Crow**
- Guidance is an attempt to individualize education. Each pupil should be helped to develop himself in the maximum possible degree in all respects."   **—Kitson**

- "Guidance is understanding a person and making himself, so that he may bring about in himself and in his environment such change through which his proper development becomes possible."

  —Knapp
- "Guidance is a process which helps an individual to develop his personality fully and enables him to serve the society to the best of his capabilities and talents." **—Woodworth**
- "Guidance is a continuous process of helping the individual for development in the maximum of their capacity in the direction most beneficial to himself and to society." **—Stoops and Wahlquist**
- "Guidance is a process through which an individual is able to solve their problems and pursue a path suited to their abilities and aspirations." **—J.M Brewer**
- "Guidance is a process of dynamic interpersonal relationships designed to influence the attitudes and subsequent behavior of a person." **—Good**
- "Guidance is a service designed to help one individual or group of individuals in making necessary adjustment to environment whether that may be within the school or outside it". **—Proctor**
- "Effective education is guidance, and realistic guidance is self guidance." **—Carmicheal**
- "Guidance is the systematic professional process of helping the individual through education and interpretive procedures to gain a better understanding of his own characteristics and potentialities and to relate himself more satisfactorily to social requirements and opportunities in accord with social and moral values." **—Mathewson**
- "Guidance is a process of helping individuals through their own efforts to discover and develop their potentialities both for personal happiness and social usefulness." **—Labh Singh**

Definitions of Counseling

Counseling refers to an interactive process between two persons, in which one person helps the other person with an expertise knowledge and skill for the purpose of problem solving and capacity building.

- "Counseling is a series of direct contacts with the individual which aims to offer him assistance in changing his attitude and behaviors". **—Carl Rogers**
- "Counseling is essentially a process in which the counselor assists the counselee to make interpretations of facts relating to a choice, plan or adjustment which he needs to make".

  —Glenn F. Smith
- "Counseling is an interactive process that facilitates meaningful understanding of self and environment and results in the establishment and or clarification of goals and values for future behavior". **—Stone and Sherzes**
- "Counseling is a dynamic and purposeful relationship between two people, who approach a mutually defined problem with mutual consideration of each other to the end that the troubled one or less mature is aided to a self determined resolution of his problem". **—C.Gilbert Wrenn**
- "Counseling is an interactive process conjoining the counselee, who needs assistance and the counselor, who is trained and educated to give this assistance". **—Perez, 1965**
- Counseling is defined as a " process which takes place in a one to one relationship between an individual beset by problems with which he cannot cope alone and a professional worker whose training and experience have qualified him to help others reach solutions to various types of personal difficulties" **—Hahn and MacLean**

- "Counseling is a dynamic and purposeful relationship between the people in which procedures vary with the nature of the students' need, but in which there is always mutual participation by the counselor and the student with the focus upon self-classification and self-determination by the students." **—Wrenn (1951)**
- "Counseling is a purposeful reciprocal relationship between two people in which one a trained person helps the other to change himself or his environment." **—Shostorm and Brammer (1952)**
- "Counseling is a face-to-face relationship in which growth takes place in the counselor as well as the counselee." **—Ruth Strang**
- "Counseling is a form a interviewing in which the client is helped to understand himself more completely in order to correct an environment or adjustment difficulty." **—Wolberg (1954)**
- "Counseling is a mutual learning process involving two individuals one seeking help and the other a professionally trained person helping the first to orient and direct him towards a goal which leads to his maximum development and growth in his environment." **—Willy and Andrew**

Differences Between Guidance and Counseling

Guidance and counseling are not synonymous terms. Guidance is relatively more comprehensive than counseling. Counseling is a component of guidance, not all of it. Thus all counseling is guidance but all guidance is not counseling. The basic differences between guidance and counseling are:

- An advice or a relevant piece of information given by a superior, to resolve a problem or overcome from difficulty, is known as guidance. Counseling refers to a professional advice given by a counselor to an individual to help him in overcoming from personal or psychological problems.
- Guidance is preventive in nature, whereas counseling tends to be healing, curative or remedial.
- Guidance assists the person in choosing the best alternative. However, counseling helps in solving the problems by the person's own efforts.
- Guidance is a comprehensive process, that has an external approach. On the other hand, counseling focuses on in-depth and inward analysis of the problem, until client understands and overcomes from it completely.
- Guidance is given by a guide, who can be any person superior or an expert in a particular field but counseling is provided by counselor, who possesses high level of skills and has undergone professional training.
- In the process of guidance, level of privacy is less whereas in counseling complete secrecy is maintained.
- Guidance can be given to an individual or group of individuals at the same time, but counseling is always one to one.
- In the process of guidance, the guide may take the decision for the client. However, in counseling, the counselor empowers the client to take decisions on his own.

Guidance and counseling is comparable because both are used extensively in an educational organization for the general purpose of student's development. The differences between guidance and counseling are summarized in Table 1.

TABLE 1: Comparison of guidance and counseling

Basis for comparison	Guidance	Counseling
Meaning	Guidance refers to an advice or a relevant piece of information provided by a superior, for harmonious development of self	Counseling refers to a service provided by a professional counselor to enable the person in solving problems
Nature	Preventive	Remedial and curative
Approach	Comprehensive and extroverted	In-depth and introverted
Purpose	Assists in choosing the best alternative	It tends to change the behavior, through learning adaptive coping and solving problem by the individual itself
Provided by	Any person, superior or expert	A person who possesses high level of skill and professional training on counseling
Privacy	Less private	Confidential
Mode	One to one or many	One to one
Decision making	By the guide or client	By the client

PURPOSE, SCOPE AND NEED OF GUIDANCE AND COUNSELING

Purposes of Guidance and Counseling

As an integral part of education, guidance and counseling serve many purposes in development of students. The multiple purposes of guidance and counseling are as follows:

- **To establish a feeling of mutual understanding between student and teacher**: Mutual understanding is a necessary condition without which attainment of any objective is questionable. In a teaching learning environment, without student there is no existence of teacher, similarly without teacher, learning remains incomplete. So, the mutual understanding between teacher and student makes the presence meaningful for both.
- **To make a sense to recognize and use inner resources of an individual**: Self help is the best help and it is only possible when a student develops self awareness through guidance and counseling process.
- **To set goal that is best suitable for the individual**: Guidance and counseling is a helping process where assistance is provided to set goals that are suitable to individual.
- **To make plan that is practical and feasible**: To achieve educational objectives, appropriate planning is important. Teacher or the guidance provider helps students to plan their course of action considering their strengths and limitations.
- **To workout with present problem**: It is another important purpose of guidance and counseling. In the process of guidance and counseling, students learn to solve a problem efficiently.
- **To provide assistance in the process of development**: Every student has the potential for development with a varying rate, which is extended at optimal level through guidance and counseling services.
- **To develop capacity for self direction**: Guidance and counseling service not only helps a student to solve immediate problems but it enables the individual to develop his/her own capacity, which is necessary for self determination.

- **To encourage and develop special abilities and right attitudes among students**: Every individual has some attitude, which is based on their family and social background. All students may not have right attitude for learning new skills. Inappropriate attitude or negative attitude acts as a strong barrier and does not allow students to think differently. As a result, stereotype behavior becomes prominent. When students get engaged with the stereotype behavior, their hidden talent is not expressed. Through guidance and counseling service, students are encouraged to discover their special abilities and talent.
- **To provide necessary information**: Student receives information at various levels and amount through different media used in guidance and counseling services. Students receive information in the classrooms by the teachers in most formal way.

Scope of Guidance and Counseling

Guidance and counseling is a continuous process and may be required at any stage of life from childhood to adulthood and even during old age.

The unique nature of individuals makes them perceive the same event differently. As a result, they encounter varieties of problems at various levels in their day to day life, which demands guidance. Therefore, guidance is required for personal, social, emotional, and health problems as well for educational, vocational and professional problems. Guidance is a kind of service required for all groups of people including students, teachers, parents, professionals and general people.

Guidance and counseling are both generalized and specialized services. It is a generalized service, when a student is guided by his/her parent or teacher to improve his/her total performance in the school. It is a specialized service when a student is guided by a professional counselor to overcome his learning difficulty or to develop adaptive behavior while being anxious.

Guidance is a service provided to all group of students including poor performer to high performers.

Scope of Guidance and Counseling in Educational Organization

Diversity is common in an educational organization. It may or may not offer various educational programs but the learner and educator both come from different sections of society with varieties of needs and interests. To develop students in order to discover their full potential, guidance and counseling service is essential at every stage in an educational program. Throughout an educational program the guidance and counseling services are named as:

- **Preadmission service**: Preadmission service helps a student to understand their eligibility to a particular educational program and to choose the right course based on their interest, capability and available resources.
- **Admission service**: It is mainly concerned with selecting the right candidate for the right course, so that the student and the educational organization and society as a whole are benefitted. Admission service in a nursing college mainly comprises of a common entrance test and interview for selecting candidates with right level of intelligence and attitude.
- **Orientation service**: It is concerned with introducing the new group of students with the organization philosophy, vision, mission, rules, regulations, physical set up and faculty members. Orientation service also includes introduction to educational program and highlighting students and parent's role, informing available facilities and student welfare program and visiting the

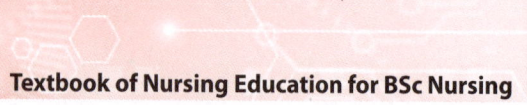

institute and surrounding area. It may last from a day to a week and is organized with the combined effort of guidance and counseling department of college and other faculty.

- **Student information service**: Information service is an essential part of guidance and counseling program. It involves collecting, maintaining, transforming and providing information to students as well as their adviser for making wise decision. Information may be categorized as personal, educational and social. Based on personal social information, students are enabled to make sense about their strengths, weaknesses and limitations and adviser also guides to inculcate the best set of qualities, moral values and develop philosophy of life. Educational information is useful for making the students about their progress, sources of knowledge, opportunity of higher study, etc. Adviser can utilize this information to diagnose student's individual problem, to help in adopting good learning habits.

- **Counseling service**: The counseling service involves helping the student to be aware about their role and responsibility considering individual limitation, to make choice wisely and to overcome difficulties in rational and easier way. Ultimately, it helps to strengthen the required qualities.

- **Placement service**: The placement service is considered as an important part of guidance and counseling because of globalization of nursing services. Through placement service, nursing students receive guidance for career opportunities and are able to analyze their career pathway. The nursing colleges of corporate world organize campus selection, conduct career conference and workshop to help nursing student for becoming global nurse, there by promoting their brand value.

- **Remedial service**: This section of guidance and counseling service is mainly concentrated to identify student's problems and provide remedial services for optimizing student's capacity. Minor identifiable problems are solved through guidance, where as major problems are solved through counseling service by professionals. Remedial services include teaching communication skills, social skills, time management skills and stress management skills, etc.

- **Follow up service**: Follow up services are concerned with identifying student's achievement in relation to their abilities, aptitudes and provided facilities. Follow up services are recommended not only for the present group of learners but also for the passed out students. Passed out students are assessed for adjustment with new job through telephonic interviews or questionnaire.

- **Research service**: Research as a part of guidance and counseling service is useful for evaluating the people who provide services and the process by which service is provided to students. Ultimately the guidance and counseling program could be modified based on needs of students and adopting newer approach.

- **Evaluation service**: It assesses and determines the effectiveness and efficiency of guidance and counseling program. Student satisfaction, percentage of passed out students, quality of student teacher relationship and placement in reputed organization are various indicators of guidance and counseling programs.

Needs of Guidance and Counseling

The need of guidance and counseling is realized by teachers and students. When it is realized by both the groups, it become more comprehensive and effective. Guidance and counseling service is needed at various level of development of students for a number of causes:

- To help in the total development of the student
- To enable students in making choice at various stages of educational career according to their interest and abilities
- To select, prepare and progress in an educational course or career
- To help the students in vocational development
- To develop best possible adjustment to the situations in school as well as in the homes
- To minimize the mismatching between education and employment and help in the efficient use of manpower
- To identify and motivate students from weaker sections of society
- To facilitate adjustment with the educational program and environment.
- To identify and help students who needs special help
- To resolve crisis through maximizing awareness and support
- To ensure the proper utilization of time spent outside the classrooms
- To increase the holding power of schools
- To make educational program successful
- To minimize the incidence of indiscipline

Developmental Need

Though the pattern of growth and development is similar among human beings but they grow and develop at different rates at different times due to their genetic inheritance and social heritage. To initiate optimal development and avoid gross deviation from standard, all students require various degrees of guidance and counseling services.

Health Needs

Nursing is a healthcare profession. As a healthcare professional, every nurse is trained in such a way that they should adopt all healthy behavior and practices. If nurse's behavior and practices are not healthy, they can't act as a role model for changing the behavior of clients. To develop healthy behavior and lifestyle practices, nursing students require appropriate guidance and counseling. Beside this, all student nurse should have a sound health, otherwise they can't actively participate in curricular and extracurricular activities. Student nurse is also guided to avoid occupational hazards like infection, needle stick injury, etc.

Social Need

Changing Family

Socialization starts from family and family is an ideal setting for bringing up children. Today this ideal setting, family has changed structurally and functionally. Increasing number of nuclear families or broken families, where children don't get the opportunity to share, to tolerate little frustration and to express anxiety has lead to development of many emotional and social problems. Anxiety, depression, and maladjustment are some common emotional and social problems among children and many major health problems can be prevented through guidance and counseling.

Changed Values

It is one of the deep rooted causes of many emotional and social problems, which influence the behavior of students, parents and teacher. Unrealistic expectations of parents and teachers creates more pressure on students and non achievement of those goal leads to frustration, depression, maladaptive behavior etc.

Urbanization

Since the time of industrial revolution, people have started to move from rural area to urban area and this trend is expected to continue in the new century. Population is increasing in the cities and the high cost of living is causing many social problems like poverty, homelessness, drug abuse, violence, crime, etc. Being a part of same society, students are not exempted from those social problems, for which they need guidance and counseling.

Industrialization

Advancement in technology and equipment is the result of rapid growth of industry. In the industrial world, the production, distribution and consumption of goods is increased, which demands specialization in education and occupation. To learn new skills and to adapt with changing environment, a student needs appropriate guidance and counseling service.

Cultural Diversity

Nursing profession is growing and maturing day by day and increasing number of students from different sections of society are interested to join this professional course. Students are diverse for their racial, ethnic, religious, language, food habits, socio-economic, and geographic background. Nurse educator needs to consider this diversity while preparing students to adjust and overcome maladjustment.

Globalization of Education

Globalization of nursing education is a trend, which demands to prepare student nurses in such a way that they serve mankind in any corner of the world.

Outcome-based Education

New pressure and demand is common in the educational organization as a result of challenges of outcome-based education. Now, educational program is evaluated by student's performance and placement, which a student can do after completion of a course. To achieve this target, new pressure and demand is placed on students and organization for which individual guidance and counseling is important.

ORGANIZATION OF GUIDANCE AND COUNSELING SERVICES

Principles of Guidance

Any guidance program should be based on the following eight principles, as stated by Hollis and Hollis. The principles are:

- **The dignity of the individual is supreme**: Human being is superior to any other animal on the planet and everybody has self respect and dignity that is not affected by color, caste, religion, social class or appearance. Any action of a person may be right or wrong but the dignity should never be neglected.

- **Every individual is different from each other**: There are some similar characteristics in a group of people as they belong to same ethnic group, speak a common language, or like to eat same food but they are different in many ways. Two identical people may not think, perceive or behave similarly because of their uniqueness. The quality and quantity of guidance required is totally dependent on the individual.

- **The primary concern of guidance is the social background of an individual**: Human being are social and as a member of any particular society, they develops similar attitude, follow same norms and practices that may be modified or changed when guidance is provided.

- **The personal perceptions and attitudes are the base on which an individual acts**: An individual's behavior is influenced by his/her attitude and perceptions, therefore the service provider needs to consider this for developing appropriate strategy.

- **The individual generally acts to enhance his perceived self**: Each person would like to inculcate the desired qualities, therefore the perceived self will be superior. The counselor and guide needs to understand how accurate is the perceived self so that required help and assistance can be provided.

- **The individual has the innate ability to learn and seek help for making choices that lead to self direction**: The autonomy or self determination is a fundamental right of an individual and that is protected by his/her deliberate action as learned naturally. An individual is allowed to be self directed with the supportive services of guidance and counseling program.

- **The individual needs a continuous guidance process from early childhood till old age**: Though the level of understanding is improved with age and experience, the complexity of life has also increased with the changing environment and diverse needs. Therefore, the service of guidance is also required continuously from early childhood till old age.

- **Competent and professional personnels can provide best form of personalized assistance and information to an individual**: A single individual or professional may not have all level of competence therefore he or she cannot give guidance to everybody. For example, an engineer does not have required competence for giving professional guidance to a surgeon.

Some Other Principle of Guidance

- **Holistic development of individual**: Guidance should aim in all round development of student. Academic achievement may be the primary objective of students but inappropriate health behavior, poor social and moral behavior is not desirable for any student. All aspects of development is interrelated so guidance is provided towards holistic development of individual.

- **Guidance is concerned with individual behavioral processes**: Every individual may not behave similarly in similar situation. After attaining a lecture session, a group of student may respond differently because of their listening behavior, level of understanding and previous knowledge. Therefore, the approach and technique of guidance or quantity and quality of guidance should be suitable for the individual student.

- **Guidance relies on cooperation, not on compulsion**: To provide effective guidance, cooperation is desirable both from the learner and guidance provider. Through cooperation, involvement is improved which leads to improvement in compliance also. The chances of mistakes are more with a compulsive act.
- **Guidance is a continuous and a sequential educational process**: An individual needs guidance throughout his lifetime, from childhood to old age. Therefore, it is a continuous process. There are some specific stages in every guidance process and it is aimed at changing behavior.

Principles of Counseling

The following principles should be followed during a counseling session.

- *Principle of self determination:* Human beings are basically self determining creatures, so it is the role of counselor to help in taking right decision but not taking decision for the client.
- *Principle of self understanding and self awareness*: A client should move towards a greater level of self-acceptance and self understanding without this behavioral change is not possible.
- *Principle of honesty:* A client should develop a greater level of honesty with respect to himself. Without this, self development is not possible.
- *Principle of need*: In counseling process, objectives should be based on the client's needs but not on the counselor's need.
- *Principle of Acceptance:* According to this principle, each client must be accepted as an individual irrespective of his/her feelings, thoughts and other characteristics.
- *Principle of permissiveness:* A conducive environment created by counselor is necessary, which allows ventilating the feelings of clients.
- *Principle of respect:* Providing due respect to an individual client is a basic condition for developing working relationship.
- *Principle of thinking with the individual:* Counseling emphasizes thinking with the individual. It is the role of the counselor to think about all the forces around the client to join client's thought process and to work collectively with the client regarding his problems.
- *Principle of learning:* Counseling is a process of learning, where the counselee learns some adaptive behavior and new techniques to solve problems. The counselor should enact the role of facilitator, by which process of learning become easy.
- *Principle of consistency with ideals of democracy:* All the fundamental rights of client should be protected during counseling process without violating the rights of others.

Factors upon Which Success of Guidance Depends

'Guidance is that aspect of educational program, which is concerned with helping the pupil to become adjusted to his present situation and plan his future in line with his interests, abilities and social needs' as defined by Hamrin and Erikson. Therefore, guidance is a kind of service provided to any individual based on his or her interests, abilities and needs.

The factors upon which success of guidance depends are as follows.

- **Recognizing the kind of help the individual learner requires**: In a teaching learning environment, student's needs are diverse and this increases because of their uniqueness. To meet the diverse needs of students, personalized assistance is required and to make it possible, the actual need should be identified and interpreted correctly.

- **Providing as much help as the learner needs at a given time**: The quality and quantity of guidance is never fixed for students and it is also true that extreme forms of guidance 'too much or too little' is dangerous. The quality and quantity of guidance must be determined in dealing with behavioral trends of students.

- **Strategic timing of help**: To serve the purpose of guidance and counseling, timing is very important. Organizing guidance and counseling service too early or too late is ineffective. The suitable time for educational guidance specially for deciding the choice of subjects is as early as 14–15 years after completion of secondary education and before entering for higher secondary course.

- **The amount and quality of the available resources**: The effectiveness of guidance and counseling service is not only dependent on the availability of resources but the amount and quality is also important. Among all other resources, the personnel who directly involves in guidance and counseling program can make a difference or greater impact through their instrumental or scientific attitude, instead of overenthusiastic, suspicious or indifferent attitude.

Approaches of Counseling

Based on the nature of counseling process and the role of the counselor, there are three approaches to counseling. These are directive, non directive and eclectic counseling (Fig. 2).

Directive Counseling

It is an approach of counseling where the counselor plays a dominant role. The counselor role is to direct the thinking of the counselee through using varieties of technique. The counselor may use the appropriate technique such as giving information, explaining, interpreting, advising etc.

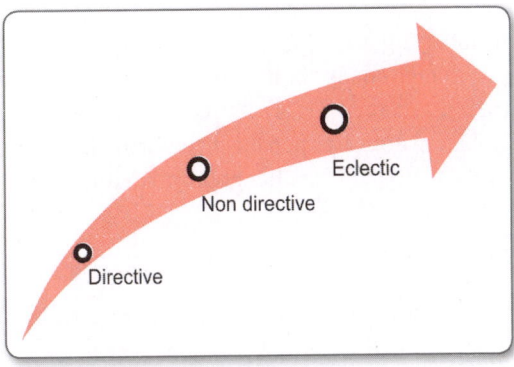

Fig. 2: Approaches of counseling

Non-Directive Counseling

It is also known as counselee centered approach where the counselee plays a predominant role. In this approach, the counselee is guided to use her/his inner resources to solve the problem.

Eclectic Counseling

In eclectic approach of counseling, strategy is formed according to client's level of knowledge, attitude and behavior. It is the combination of two or more approaches, which are developmental, preventive, and/or remedial in nature.

TWO BASIC COUNSELING APPROACHES :

- **The Dispensary Approach –**
  - Dispenser of cures
  - This is a Directive Approach – actively influencing or controlling the behavior of the counselee by changing his attitude or even the environment in which he lives.
  - Directive Counselor sees himself as the authority to advice, what he thinks as the best for the counselee.
  - Gives less attention for individual potential and abilities
  - Experienced counselor is sensitive to understand the circumstances, when to adopt this approach
- **The Bartender Approach – (Bartender = Drinking Partner)**
  - Non – directive approach
  - Counselee is offered companionship in his distress
  - Counselor is a helper, as he struggles with his difficulties, is with the counselee, but does not force his own views
  - Counselor respects the way the counselee sees his situation and tries to experience the way he is, putting himself in the counselee's shoes
  - Optimistic about the ability of the counselee to solve his own problem, this helps the counselee to have faith on himself to be responsibly independent.
  - The Counselor must have appropriate attitude and Interpersonal Skills

COUNSELING PROCESS

"Counseling is a purposeful reciprocal relationship between two people in which a trained person helps the other to change himself or his environment," as defined by Shostorm and Brammer (1952). It is very clear that counseling is a helping process where assistance is provided by a trained person for bringing change within the person or environment. To make the counseling process successful, counselor needs to prepare him/her appropriately for the situation, so that effective counseling services could be provided.

Preparation of Counselor

To provide effective counseling service, a counselor should prepare himself/herself. The preparation necessary in the area are given below (Fig. 3).

Educational Preparation

A counselor should have a Bachelor's or Master's degree in general education and the additional qualification as trained in counseling process.

Attitudes

Firstly, a counselor must possess an adaptive attitude towards life, so that he/she can prepare himself/herself as a professional counselor. Secondly, he/she should develop an experimental and scientific attitude, which enables to find the most useful and effective concept and techniques of guidance and counseling. The experimentally-minded counselor is neither misled by over enthusiasm nor inhibited or sidetracked by suspicion or distrust. The overenthusiastic person expects quick results and their judgement become emotional, so critical analysis is not possible. On the other hand, people who distrust others may reject good ideas and possibilities.

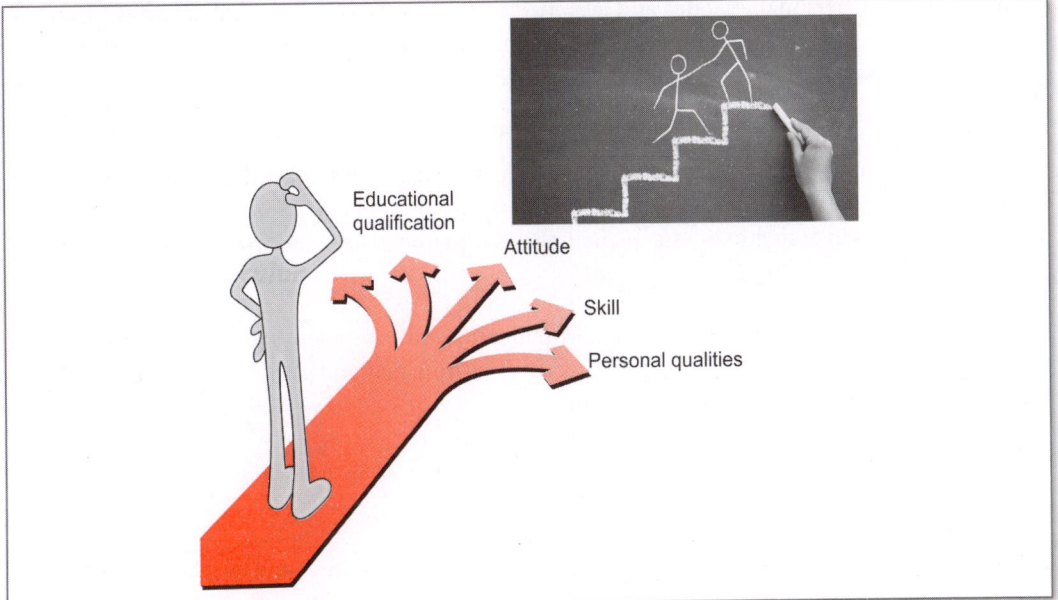

Fig. 3: Preparation of a counselor

Skills

To become a good counselor, some skills are essential to develop. The counselor should possess guidance and counseling skill as technical skill and some other skills including leadership, communication and skills in interpersonal relationship.

Personal Qualities

The counselor should present himself or herself attractively to the audience. This self presentation is exhibited through appearance, grooming, approach and communication. Some other important qualities which are necessary to inculcate that are-self awareness, high level of sensitivity, empathy, acceptance, patience, emotional stability, sincerity, and high sense of morality.

Qualities of a Counselor

To provide efficient and effective counseling service, a set of qualities are needed to be inculcated in a professional counselor. Each quality is very important for interdependent function in the process of counseling. A counselor should posses the following qualities.

Approachable

Counselor should be approachable, so that client can share his/her problems without hesitation. It is demonstrated through acknowledging client's presence, opinion and views and allowing to ventilate client's feelings.

Acceptance

Counselor should accept the client through conveying warmth, regard, concern, caring and non-judgemental attitude. The client should be accepted at any time, irrespective of his/her social background, caste, personal qualities and current situation. Professional counselors must be able to "start where the client is at." This phrase is used in counseling to describe the counselor's open minded and nonjudgmental attitude, thereby accepting the client in her current situation.

Empathy

Empathy is the ability to feel what another person is feeling. A professional counselor should be empathetic to client, thereby clients' feelings and thoughts are well understood. When the counselor understands clients in their most stressful and difficult situation, it helps to develop trust.

Genuineness

A good counselor should show genuine interest to identify and solve client's problem. Genuineness is interpreted through active listening, helping attitude, free from bias and providing correct information to the client. It helps in gaining faith from clients.

Communication Skills

A good counselor should have excellent communication skills that includes ability to listen and explain their ideas and thoughts clearly, considering entire environment, appropriate selection of channel, ability to recognize body language of client, congruency with spoken words and own body language etc.

Rapport-Building Skills

Counselors must possess a strong set of interpersonal skills for establishing rapport quickly with clients. Rapport building is possible through attentive listening, demonstrating concern and caring attitude to client. The counselor should avoid distraction by focusing client's problem and being non-judgemental. The counselor must give their undivided attention to clients and be able to cultivate trust and it is necessary to build rapport.

Problem-Solving Skills

A professional counselor should have problem solving skills thereby client's problem is identified timely and the client's strengths, weaknesses, support systems and coping abilities are also explored. With a good problem solving skill, a counselor is able to recognize negative thoughts and harmful behavior of client. After addressing the actual problem, all feasible solutions are identified and most suitable one is selected mutually.

Flexibility

Being flexible is one of the most important attributes of a professional counselor. Flexibility refers to the ability of adaptation with any situation. A professional counselor must be flexible so that the predetermined schedule or pathway may be changed according to the suitability and benefit of the counselee.

Self-Awareness

Self-awareness is the ability to recognize one's own desire, interest and attributes. A counselor must have the awareness about their professional competency so that the chances of mistake or wrong decision are minimized and also prevent from affecting the issues of counselee with that of counselor.

Multicultural Competency

Counselors must help people from all backgrounds. They should display multicultural competence and adopt a multicultural worldview that helps to relate and understand clients problems regardless of their race, ethnicity, religious or political beliefs or socioeconomic background.

Ten Do's and Don't's for the Counselor

Ten Do's	Ten Don'ts
1. Be natural and the way you are	1. Advice and be in hurry for a solution
2. Concentrate, but in relaxed manner	2. Question out of curiosity or uneasiness
3. Listen to the full message of the counselee	3. Moralize or intellectualize
4. Respond adequately, sincerely and creatively	4. Make the counselee depend on you
5. Communicate interest, warmth and understanding	5. Categorize or prejudice
6. Give prize or incentive (verbal)	6. Evaluate counselee's attitude or behavior
7. Deal with difficult situations in a sensitive and responsible manner	7. Talk too much or project yourself to impress
8. Use simple and direct language and stick to the main point	8. Encourage long narratives
9. Help to sort out and clarify the counselee's problem	9. Use technical terms
10. Help the counselee to take charge of himself	10. Write or make audio / video / photo record of the counseling process

Role of Counselor

Counselor may play the following roles.

Information Provider

Providing information to students and their parents is a part of guidance and counseling service. Verbal or written form of information is provided through lecture and discussion session and distributing leaflets, brochures and monograph. Information is provided in more comprehensive way through organizing career days, career weeks, career conferences, parent's day, etc.

Adviser

Giving advise is also very common in student guidance program. While expecting a desired behavior from student, advice is useful. To direct student's behavior in a particular way or shaping behavior in earlier stage, advice is recommended.

Educator

Counselor also act as educator as he teaches students regarding improvement of study habits and effective management of time and stress in a new environment to optimize their adaptive coping.

Planner

In the role of planner, counselor needs to identify available resources, actual and projected problems among learner, and objectives that have to be attained. The counselor also plans the actions against each objective, which has to be implemented by the group member of counseling committee.

Organizer

Organizing different guidance and counseling programs namely discussion session, counseling session, seminar, work shop and field visit is very important function in an organizer role.

Service Provider

Counselor provides services to the students, teacher, parents and society as a whole. They provide counseling services in terms of educational counseling, vocational counseling, career counseling, placement counselings etc.

Coordinator

A counselor role remains incomplete without coordination. In the role of coordinator, he/she has to coordinate with students, teachers, parents and members of guidance and counseling committee.

Researcher

A counselor need to perform the role of researcher because of the changing nature of teaching learning environment. To satisfy the diverse need of students with limited resources and to improve the quality of services, they must identify behavioral trends among students, most suitable techniques of counseling.

Counseling Process

Based on identified needs and nature of problem, the approach and type of counseling is decided but the basic steps are same. There are four steps of counseling process, which are interrelated to each other and the duration of each step may vary from client to client.

Step I: Establishing Relationship

In the first step of counseling process, the counselor and counselee are being introduced to each other. The initial task of this phase is building rapport, which advances towards development of trusting relationship. To develop a relationship of trust, the counselor and counselee should respect each other and maintain dignity. The counselor should ensure a comfortable physical environment, which facilitates uninterrupted interaction. Attentive listening, skill of observation and sensitivity of counselor is essential for establishing relationship.

Step II: Assessment

The second step of counseling process involves assessing counselee through obtaining relevant data and analyzing carefully. In this phase, the counselor creates a favorable environment so that client is expected to provide information in the area of personal, social, physical and psychological aspect. These multiple levels of information are used to state client's problems precisely. After assessing client's problem, diagnosis is made in relation to cause and observable behavior of client.

Step III: Goal Setting

Mutual goal setting is the main task in third step. It involves the agreement of counselor and counselee to identify goals that are reliable and achievable. While setting goals, the counselee's weaknesses and strengths are justified through critical evaluation of facts.

Step IV: Termination and Evaluation

This is the last step of counseling process, where problem is solved and counselee is enabled to handle similar problem independently. In this phase, both the counselor and counselee are aware about termination of relationship and feel comfortable

Students' Counseling Format

S. No.	Stages of counseling	Completeness		Reason -If 'No'	Remarks
		Yes	No		

I.	• Setting up the Relationship
	  ▪ Comfortable sitting arrangement
	  ▪ Ensuring privacy
	  ▪ Ensuring uninterrupted period of interactions
	  ▪ Relaxed attitude & environment
	  ▪ Gentle positive stroke to gain confidence				

II.	Unfolding the problem ▪ Listening to the feelings behind verbal words				
III.	Facilitating release of feelings ▪ Allowing outburst of emotions, unhindered				
IV.	**Encouraging expression of positive feelings** – (Opening JOHARI WINDOW)				
V.	Giving confidence to explore new ways				
VI.	Supporting in counselee's Self – Exploration and clarifying his doubts				
VII.	Assisting in analyzing all possible solutions				
VIII.	Helping in selecting a realistic Action Plan				
IX.	**Being available to him, when he takes action (if required) at a pre-set time** (Making decision)				
X.	Evaluation of the above counseling steps				

Source: Fr. Currie Joe, S.J. Barefoot Counsellor. Asian Trading Corporation, Bangalore, 1988, pa. 132

Future Plan of Action, with Date : _____

_____   _____

Signature of the Counselor   **Signature of the Counselee**

Uses of Tools in Counseling

Based on purpose, various tools are identified in a guidance and counseling program. The counselor may use multiple numbers of tools for a greater level of success. Tools are categorized into standardized and non standardized tests.

Standardized Tests

It is a measuring tool which measures a clearly defined set of behavior by following specific direction of administration and scoring system and provides accurate results.

Uses of Standardized Test

- To hold schools and educators accountability on student performance
- To determine the extent of learning standard is maintained
- To identify gap in student learning and academic progress
- To identify achievement gaps among different student groups
- To determine whether educational policies are working as intended
- To compare score of students within same schools and across schools.

Types of Standardized Test

IQ test

IQ, which stands for Intelligence Quotient, is a score of a person on a test that assesses intelligence. A person's IQ score is calculated by dividing a person's mental age (MA) by his/her chronological age (CA), and then multiplying by 100 (MA/CA × 100). Chronological age refers to a person's biological age. Mental age refers to the age, at which the person exhibits a particular level of performance on the test.

Definition

Intelligence tests are psychological tests that are designed to measure a variety of mental functions, such as reasoning, comprehension, and judgment.

Purpose

- To obtain an idea of the person's intellectual potential
- To recognize the deviation from standard
- To identify fitness for a particular teaching program or job
- To plan for educational counseling.

Types of IQ Test

There are four IQ tests which are most commonly used:
- Stanford-Binet Intelligence Scales (Table 2)
- Wechsler Adult Intelligence Scale (Table 3)
- Wechsler Intelligence Scale for Children
- Wechsler Primary and Preschool Scale of Intelligence

Description

To assess intelligence of a person, a variety of tasks are given. These tasks may include answering to a set of questions and solving mathematical problems. Some tasks may involve hand eye coordination and can also be bound to time. The raw score of an intelligence test is converted to standard score. The standard score is used to compare the individual's score to other people of same age.

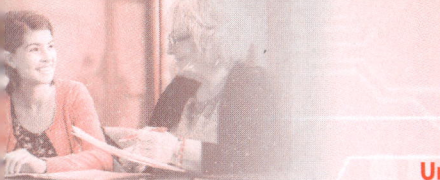

TABLE 2: **Stanford Binet Intelligence Scale**

Stanford Binet Intelligence Scale	
Genius	Over 140
Very Superior	120-139
Superior	110-119
Average	90-109
Dull	80-89
Borderline Deficiency	70-79
Moron	50-69
Imbecile	20-49

TABLE 3: **IQ range and its classification**

Terman's	Classification	Wechsler's	Classification
IQ Range	IQ Classification	IQ Range	IQ Classification
164 and Over	Genius or Near Genius	128 and Over	Very Superior
148 - 164	Very Superior Intelligence	120 - 127	Superior Intelligence
132 - 148	Superior Intelligence	111 - 119	Bright Normal Intelligence
113 - 132	Above Average Intelligence	91 - 110	Average Intelligence
84 -113	Normal/Average Intelligence	80 - 90	Dull Normal Intelligence
68 - 84	Dullness	66 - 89	Borderline Intelligence
52 - 68	Borderline Deficiency	65 and Below	Defective Intelligence
Below 52	Definite Feeble-Mindedness I		

Advantages

- It measures a wide variety of human behavior.
- It facilitates comparison among same age groups of individuals.
- It can predict academic achievement.
- It provides information about a person's mental strengths and weaknesses.
- It also suggests, at what extent an individual's potential matches with level of development and expectation.

Disadvantages

- Some intelligence tests produce a single score, which are a combination of different test score; thereby multidimensional aspect of intelligence is unexplained.
- It has a limitation to predict nonacademic intellectual ability of a person.
- Intelligence test scores are influenced by a variety of different experiences and behaviors; therefore, it should not be considered a perfect predictor of a person's achievement.

Achievement Tests

An achievement test is a test which measures the developed skill or knowledge of an individual. It is designed to measure an individual's level of knowledge in a particular area. In these types of tests, a series of task is presented to the person being evaluated and the responses are graded as per prescribed guidelines. The result is compared to a norm group. Norm group are the people who are in the same age group or grade level as that of the person being evaluated. Achievement test is backward looking because it measures how well students have learned and what they were expected to learn.

Uses of Achievement Test

- To measure the knowledge and skills of students
- To determine the academic progress that is learned over a period of time
- To identify the appropriate academic placement for a student
- To recognize suitable form of academic support.

Aptitude Tests

Aptitude test is a type of standardized test that evaluates the talent/ability/potential of individual in performing certain task, with no prior knowledge and/or training.

Aptitude test is used to assess verbal reasoning, numerical reasoning and logical reasoning, Work style and situational judgment of a person.

Uses of aptitude test

Placement Purpose

- Aptitude tests are widely used in educational organization for selection of students in academic and professional courses.
- Employer institution places the right candidate for right job.

Choosing Career

- Aptitude tests are useful to assist high school students in selection of academic courses such as Science, Arts and Commerce.

Prediction Purpose

- These are useful to make prediction about an individual's probable success in courses and careers.
- Aptitude test is used for measuring professional potential of a person. It helps to know at what extent a student is fit for the future occupation such as army, air force, business, law, medicine, etc.

Academic Improvement

- It assesses specific abilities of individual such as clerical speed or mechanical skill through Differential Aptitude Test (DAT)

Advantages

- It helps students to select educational program that can maximize career opportunity
- It guides student's decision, which involves investment of time and money.
- It facilitates the employer to select right candidates for a profession.
- An aptitude test can uncover someone's hidden abilities
- Employees get promotional opportunity based on aptitude test

Limitations

- Development and administration of aptitude test is not economic
- Aptitude test is quite stressful for the candidates
- Aptitude test is conducted in a created environment which is different than actual professional environment thereby predictive value of aptitude test is reduces.
- An aptitude test predicts probability, which is sometimes uncertain. As a result brilliant students sometimes fail to perform according to expectation and an average student is listed among the toppers.

Personality Test

A personality test is a standardized test designed to reveal some specific personality traits of an individual. In personality test, various aspects of personality such as temperament, emotional response, sociability, stability etc. are assessed.

Types of Personality Traits

Based on some characteristic features personality traits are classified as: Type A personality traits and Type B personality traits.

Type A personality Traits

People with type A personality traits are usually highly stressed, extremely ambitious and rigid in their attitude. They are very particular to time, over achiever, competitive, unable to relax and also have a high challenging spirit. They like to multitask and tend to be very impatient if something is not done within the planned time. They need to learn effective conflict management techniques and stress management skills. They should set realistic goals and consider everything making lifestyle changes.

Type B personality Traits

People with type B personality are calm and have an easy going attitude. They love fun in life and are relatively less competitive. They are able to relax and are not easily anxious or agitated. They take time to complete their task. They do not mind waiting in queues for getting their work done and do not get hyper if it takes too much time. They are also very tolerant and flexible and can change in order to adapt to changes.

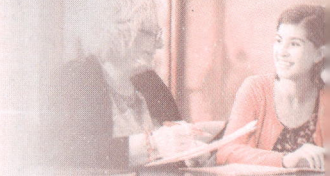

Purposes of Personality Test

- To recognize psychological makeup of a person
- To identify changes in personality
- To evaluate the effectiveness of therapy
- To diagnose psychological problems
- To select suitable candidates for a job

Uses of Personality Tests

- **Employment institution**: Personality test is used by the employer to select appropriate candidate
- **Health organization**: In health organizations, it is used specially in the department of Mental health and Forensic medicine. In medicine it is used for diagnostic, therapeutic and research purpose.
- **In the discipline of law**: To assess criminal psychology, lawyer uses personality test. It is also very important in cases where it is necessary to assess competency of parents in deciding child custody.

Types of Personality Tests

There are two basic types of personality tests: Self-report inventories and projective tests.
- **Self-report inventories:** It is a type of personality test where test-takers administer the test to the participant and based on their response, test score is interpreted. One of the most common self-report inventories is the Minnesota Multiphasic Personality Inventory or MMPI.
- **Projective tests**: It involves presenting a vague scene, object, or scenario to the respondents and then asking them to give their interpretation of the test item. Rorschach Inkblot Test is an example of projective test.

Advantages

- It is relatively easy to administer because it has some established norms.
- Among personality tests, self-inventories have much higher reliability and validity than projective tests.
- Many critical aspects of personality are tested, which is not possible to detect with any other test.
- In psychotherapy, setting projective tests allows therapists to gather a lot of information about a client within a short period of time

Limitations

- Some personality tests like self-report inventories have a limitation to detect accurate result because few people provide false answers to present self in a superior position or appear more socially acceptable and desirable.
- All people are not always good at accurately describing their own behavior, thereby overestimation or underestimation of personal characteristics leads to inaccuracy of test results.
- Some personality tests, especially self-report inventories, are time consuming
- In projective tests, different raters might provide entirely different viewpoints of the responses as the test result is highly qualitative.

Interest Test

Interests are acquired motivations. What an individual is willing to do is determined on the basis of his/her interests. Interest test is also known as career inventory or interest inventory. It is used to find a person's genuine interest in a job or course of education. If a student shows a genuine interest towards an educational program or vocational course then he/she is likely to perform better.

Uses of Interest Test

- To identify students interest in educational, social, recreational and vocational activities
- To diagnose students readiness for educational activities
- To plan the curriculum.

Nonstandardized Tests

Non-standardized tests are the various classroom tests that are developed by subject teachers for assessing learning outcomes of students after a specific unit of study. This type of class test is mainly used to identify student's level of understanding, motivation towards study, learning problems, acquired knowledge on selected topic, etc. Non-standardized tests cannot be used for comparing performance of two similar groups of students from different schools. Table 4 differentiates between standardized and nonstandardized tests.

Definition

A non-standardized test is one that allows evaluator to assess an individual's abilities or performances, but doesn't allow for a fair comparison between students of similar group.

Forms of Nonstandardized Test

Most frequently used non-standardized tests are the class test, portfolios, interviews, informal questioning, group discussions, oral tests, quizzes, exhibitions, projects etc. Class tests may involve written or viva test and written test includes: essay test, short answer type question, short note, multiple choice questions, etc.

In portfolios, a student performs his work over a period of time and teacher will evaluate it based on a scoring guideline. Here, students are also encouraged to reflect on their work, which enhances the learning process.

TABLE 4: Differences between standardized and nonstandardized test

Standardized tests	Nonstandardized tests
Uses Standardized test makes the teacher accountable for student's result, is used for fund allotment in schools and also used in making policy by administrator.	Non-standardized test is typically used for assessing students' performance on given instruction within a limited number of learners.
Measurability • Standardized tests are fairer that allows comparison among teachers or students. • Standardized tests cannot accurately assess some skills like creative writing.	• Non-standardized tests do not facilitate comparison among students or teachers. • Non standardized tests are more suitable for assessing some skills like creative writing.

Contd...

Standardized tests	Nonstandardized tests
Questions	
• In standardized tests, all students answer the same or very similar questions.	• Non-standardized tests can give different questions/assignments/tasks.
Grading	
• Test score grading is consistent and is not influenced by other conditions.	• Non-standardized tests may have varying conditions that influence how the tests are scored
Formality	
• Standardized tests are more formal in nature.	• Non-standardized tests are less formal and rely on situations, such as teacher's observations, student participation in classroom, etc.
Consistency	
• Standardized tests are controlled assessments that examine all students in a given geographic area evenly.	• It can't examine all students in a given geographic area evenly.

Interview Schedule

Interviews involve mainly verbal communication between two people, in which one person provides information to the other person. It is widely used in guidance and counseling program. The tool is used to gather information from various resources. Information is collected from the individual student or counselee as well as from parents, other family members, friends and class teachers. Interview provides an opportunity to understand the counselee better through observing non verbal mode of communication such as appearance, posture, gesture, etc. Structured and unstructured form of interview schedule is used in student guidance and counseling program. Structured interview is specific for situation and group of students and gives more valid and reliable data but the unstructured interview is also equally important for exploring an event or problem of students.

Observation

Observation as a method of data collection is very popular in guidance and counseling program. Observation may be participative or non participative and structured or un structured. Unstructured observation involves spontaneously observing and recording an event or behavior of counselee where the counselor needs minimal planning. Where as in structured observation, the counselor needs to plan, how the observation will be made, what to observe, and how to record, etc. Checklist and rating scales are commonly used tools in a structured observation. To observe class room behavior of students, a checklist may be used either in a single or multiple occasions by the counselor.

Rating Scale

Rating scale is a type of tool, which contains an ordered series of response category for a number of items which are constructed to measure a variable. Using rating scale, it is possible to measure student's satisfaction for their learning experience, quality of academic guidance received by them and frequency of indiscipline behavior observed in class room, etc.

Checklist

Checklist as a measuring tool is commonly used to observe whether some set of behavior is demonstrated or not by a person. It can also be used to find some list of characteristics is present or absent within a product. Checklist is also used by counselee as self report instrument when they are guided for adopting some learning behavior or quitting some maladoptive behavior like smoking.

Anecdotal Records

It is a type of tool in which important incidents are recorded based on factual data. In anecdotal record the description of incident is recorded immediately after the incident by the counselor. It gives information regarding student's attitude, habits, interest, adjustment, etc.

Questionnaire

Questionnaire is a form of self report, in which a person's written response is obtained. Using questionnaire, a counselor may gather information about knowledge, opinion, beliefs, and intentions of counselee on any particular topic. The information obtained through questionnaire is objective in nature because the question tends to have less depth. It has the limitation for clarification from counselee.

Cumulative Record

It is a comprehensive record of students, which indicates progress in academic, personal and social development in an orderly manner. Other than curricular activities, extracurricular activities also recorded in a cumulative record. It helps to find the consistency of student's progress on yearly basis; compare changes of attitude in the consecutive year and also between students. It helps the counselor to find the effectiveness of counseling program.

Sociometric Technique

Sociometric technique is used to measure an individual's social worth, values as viewed by his/her peers or social groups.

Record Analysis

An educational organization keeps various type of records of students from admission till course completion and even placement of students. These records are related to their personal and social information, health information, performance in curricular and extracurricular activities, interest, behavior, attitudes and so on. All these information are available from records and are useful for effective guidance and counseling program.

Informal Collection of Information

Everyday we interact with many people and continuously receive and provide information both in formal and informal way. Although the informal source is not valid and reliable like formal source, but sometimes it is useful. In a guidance and counseling program, the counselor collects information about counselee from class teacher, peer groups or friends without using any tool or formal interview.

SOCIOMETRY

Sociometry is a way of measuring relationships between people and it can discover, describe and evaluate social status and structure of people.

- **Sociometry is defined as "a method used for the discovery and manipulation of social configurations by measuring the attractions and repulsions between individuals in a group."** **—Franz**
- Sociometry is defined by as "the inquiry into the evolution and organization of groups and the position of individuals within them **—Jacob Moreno**

Sociometry is a way of measuring the degree of relatedness among people and it is useful in assessing behavior of a person in a group and determining the changes of behavior after receiving certain therapy.

Sociometric test is a method of examination, primarily used for obtaining data on social interaction among group members, nature of group structure and group function.

Uses

Health organization

- In health organizations, a counselor uses sociometry to recognize client's social development, problem of socialization, interpersonal relationships, etc.

Teaching Institutions

- By studying the choice of students through sociometry technique, the teacher can determine the nature and degree of social relationship that exist among the students.
- It is useful in identifying those students who are isolated, the ones who are not preferred by others.
- It is used to assign students in project work.
- It facilitates the appraisal of social adjustment among students.
- It is useful in assigning students in committees.

In Research

- It can be employed in a wide variety of research in the laboratory as well as in the field.
- In social science, medical science or business administration, sociometric test is used to identify, explore, and evaluate various aspect of human behavior, organizational behavior etc.

Business Organization

- It is useful to identify the people who are liked by many others and who can be a better leader of the group.
- Sociometric methods are used whenever human actions like choosing, influencing, dominating and communicating in group situations are involved.

Methods of Analysis of Sociometric Data

The methods of sociometric data analysis are described in (Fig. 4.)

Advantages

- Sociometric test is useful to present structure of social relations graphically
- It helps to understand lines of communication among people in a group
- It identifies degree of attraction or rejection experienced by group members
- It helps in finding out how the group processes work
- It helps in understanding the group dynamic in a class or unit of organization
- It helps a teacher to find which student would be congenial for a working group or companions for certain work.
- It is a simple and natural method of observation and data collection.
- It is easy to administer

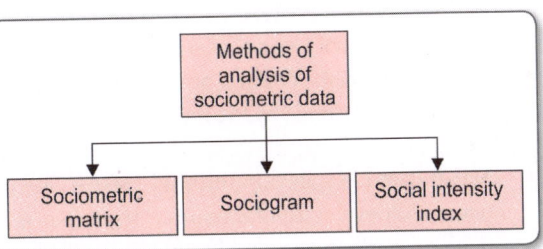

Fig. 4: Methods of analysis of sociometric data

Limitations

- Certain traits or qualities are very difficult to measure using sociometry and if at all they are measured, the measurement may not be accurate and free from subjectivity.
- **Some people may hide real relationship, which is not possible to measure using sociometry**
- **It is not economic in terms of money and time**
- **It is difficult to analyse.**

MANAGING OF CRISIS AND REFERRAL

Stressful situations are part of our life and we may experience it at any point of time in our day to day life. Whenever we face any stressful situation, we try to resolve it either using our own problem solving skills or taking help from others. When we fail to overcome any stressful situation or unable to minimize the level of stress, crisis arise that leads to disequilibrium. Stress is not uncommon for students. Nursing students also experience some level of stress and crisis.

Definition of Crisis

A sudden event occurs in one's life as a result of ineffective response to a stressor that disturbs homeostasis and is called crisis.

Characteristics of a Crisis

There are certain characteristics, on which the concept of crisis is developed. These are as follows:
- Crisis occurs in the life of all individuals at any point of time in their life.
- Crises are personal in nature. Same event may create crisis for one person but not for another.
- Crises are acute and not chronic.
- Crises are precipitated by specific identifiable stressors.
- Crisis has the potential for psychological growth and deterioration.

Types of Crises

There are mainly two types of crises: situational and maturational or developmental.

- **Situational crisis**: When a person loses psychological equilibrium in response to some life event and is not controlled by the individual. For example, loss of a loved one, witnessing a crime, illness etc.
- **Maturational or developmental crises**: The crises occurs in response to internal stressor and related to developmental issues is known as maturational or developmental crises. The common related issues are sexual identity, value conflict and capacity for emotional intimacy. Delayed or advanced sexual maturity both could be the reason of developmental crisis.

Phases of Crisis Development

According to Caplan (1946), four identifiable phases are there for crisis development, in which a person encounters stressors and progresses towards crisis.

Phase I: Exposure to a Precipitating Stressor

At the beginning of crisis developmental phase, the individual encounters one or more stressor. The person feels discomfort as anxiety increases and tends to minimize the anxiety level.

Phase II: Utilization of Previously Used Problem Solving Technique

In the second phase of crisis development, the individual becomes more anxious as the problem remains unsolved and a feeling of hopelessness and confusion is prominent. The person shows disorganization in his/her thoughts and activity. To minimize the anxiety levels, various problem solving techniques are used by the person that were previously used.

Phase III: Utilization of All Internal and External Resources to Resolve Problem

The individual may view the problem from different angle and find new problem solving technique. If the new problem solving technique becomes effective, higher level of skill is acquired. On the other hand, some person may overlook certain aspects of the problems and are unable to solve it. The second group of person does not gain anything instead, they lose their previous confidence and remain with similar or lower level of pre-morbid functioning.

Phase IV: Further Increase of Tension that Reaches to a Breaking Point

In this phase, the person is unable to solve the problem and the increasing levels of anxiety reaches to panic stage. The person can't think rationally and also shows impulsive behavior.

Steps in Crisis Intervention

Crisis intervention is a systematic process of solving immediate problem for the purpose of restoring previous levels of functioning and maintaining homeostasis. There are mainly four steps in crisis intervention that includes: assessment, planning, intervention and evaluation.

Step I: Assessment

It is the first step in crisis intervention, where the counselor's role is to develop a therapeutic relationship with the client and to collect information. For an effective crisis intervention, a counselor needs to explore the event to get relevant information, which has direct or indirect relation with crisis development and resolution. There are four identified factors, which have influence on development and resolution of crisis.

Precipitating Event or Stressor

Any factor which causes stress to an individual is known as stressor. Stressor may be internal or external and actual or potential. To recognize precipitating event or stressor, the counselor must know the problem or need of the client, the event that threatens those needs, and the onset of problem.

Client's Perception of the Event or Stressor

The client's perception of the event or stressor has a greater value for development and resolution of crisis. If any event is perceived incorrectly by a student, it can cause conflict, emotional isolation and mal-adjustment. Similarly overestimation about self preparation for examination may cause unexpected result and situational crisis.

Support System and Coping Resources

To find the support system and coping resources of client, a counselor needs to ask some basic questions that may be related to family type, relationship with each other, availability of support from friends or other strengths and weaknesses of client.

Client's Strength and Previously Used Coping Mechanism

The counselor must know the clients' strength that may be utilized in future for coping up in a better way. It is also important to know whether client had experienced similar problem before or not. If the client had previous experience of same crisis, then the technique of resolution and success is also important to know.

Assessment is the first step of counseling process, where counselor needs to assess the client thoroughly with the use of observation and interviewing. Generally after a crisis, client exhibits some behavioral changes along with alteration of emotion (Table 5).

Step II: Planning

It is the second step of crisis intervention where the counselor selects proposed action based on identified needs and problems. Mutual goal setting is the first task, which is done through analysis of previously collected data, considering clients strengths and weaknesses. The alternative solution for the problem is identified and evaluated for maximum benefit. The counselor also needs to think about the availability of resources.

TABLE 5: Behavior commonly exhibited after a crisis

Changes of behavior	Alteration of emotion	Physical manifestation
• Crying spell • Irritability • Overeating or under eating • Sleeplessness • Withdrawal • Substance abuse	• Anger • Apathy • Disbelief • Fear • Forgetfulness • Hopelessness • Helplessness • Sadness	• Backaches • Headaches • Fatigue • Numbness • Palpitation • Increased frequency of micturition

Step III: Implementation

It is the actual intervention for resolving crisis. In this step, the counselor may approach at various levels, using number of techniques that are suitable for the nature of crisis and affected person (Fig. 5).

Environmental Manipulation

It involves moderation of client's physical and inter-personal environment, which may remove the stressor or provide situational support. For example, a student who is in a crisis for maladjustment with other roommates can be shifted to another room.

General Support

It is a kind of support that is useful for every client irrespective of the nature of crisis. General support can be given by counselor through accepting the client, showing respect, dignity, empathy and demonstrating concern and caring attitude.

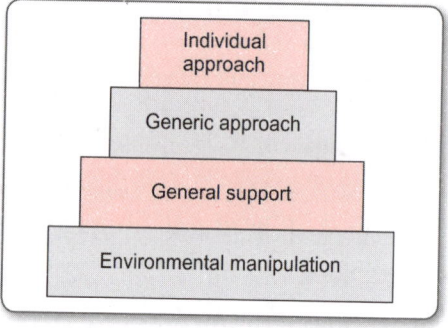

Fig. 5: Approaches of counseling

Generic Approach

The generic approach is suitable for a group of individuals who experience the same event and are in a phase of crisis or high risk for crisis. For example, generic approach is useful when a group of students witness accidental death and develop crisis.

Individual Approach

It is a client specific approach but not crisis specific. In this type of approach, the counselor must consider the characteristics of client, his strengths and weaknesses, support system, coping mechanisms etc. For example, individual approach is useful when a student has suicidal ideation after failure in examination.

Techniques

In the implementation phase of crisis intervention, various levels of approach are used by counselor. Similarly numbers of techniques are also used. Some of the commonly used techniques are: Catharsis, Clarification, Suggestion, Reinforcement of behavior, Support of defences, Raising self esteem and Exploration of solutions.

Catharsis

It is the release of feelings that takes place as the client talks about emotionally charged areas. It is used as a tension releasing measure but is never encouraged when an aggressive client tends to destroy things or likely to kill a person.

Clarification

It involves encouraging the client to express more clearly the relationship between certain events. It helps the client to understand the situation in a better way. For example, it is observed by the class teacher that, after the incident of fighting, you are not talking with anybody and not eating also.

Suggestion

Suggestion is a technique by which the counselor can influence a person to accept an idea or belief. It helps the client to think the event with a different point of view, which makes the client to feel less anxious and more optimistic. For example, "You may share it with your close friends or the person on whom you depend".

Reinforcement of Behavior

It is a technique of acknowledging an acceptable behavior of client.
For example, the student who is in a crisis because of her poor performance, one day responds well in the classroom. Teacher may appreciate it by "intelligent answer!"

Support of Defences

It is a technique used to encourage a healthy and adaptive defence.
For example, the student whose attendance was very poor and did not succeed in last term examination, but now coming regularly and showing more attentive response in classroom –is an adoptive defence that must be supported by teacher.

Raising Self Esteem

This technique is used to regain feelings of self-worth. During a crisis phase a client may have a feeling of hopelessness as the problem is not solved by him/her and need to take help from outside. The counselor's responsibility is enabling the client to handle the problem and overcome from crisis situation. For example, the student was in a crisis as a result of obtaining less marks in one test, the teacher can remind about the previous good performances.

Exploration of Solutions

It is a technique of searching an alternative form of immediate solution. To find an effective solution is the ultimate goal of crisis intervention. Using this technique, a counselor and client mutually explore a new way to resolve crisis. For example, a student is very upset due to her inadequate preparation before end term examination, she may go for group study with peers.

Step IV: Evaluation

Evaluation is the last step of crisis intervention, where the counselor needs to evaluate the effectiveness of crisis intervention. The effectiveness of crisis intervention is indicated through some positive outcome. Positive outcome of crisis intervention are stress reduction, regaining previous level of function, satisfying need and absence of maladaptive coping.

Follow up Service

After crisis intervention, client is reviewed in the follow up services. The client is assessed for successful crisis resolution, but if goal is not attained, then further session of counseling is require.

Referral Service

In an educational organization after providing available guidance and counseling services, if expected outcome is not observed, client may be referred for additional professional help. The client is also referred for higher level of services at any point of time during crisis intervention, if condition deteriorates or there is inadequacy of resources.

MANAGING DISCIPLINARY PROBLEMS

Common Disciplinary Problems

Indiscipline of students is not uncommon in any teaching organization. Though students are well informed about the rules and regulations of institution prior to admission, still they violate rules frequently. Commonly observed disciplinary problems are:
- Absenteeism
- Non-submission or late submission of assignment
- Indiscipline classroom behavior
- Strike
- Damaging or spoiling institutional property
- Ragging

Absenteeism

It is a common disciplinary problem observed among students. Though the Indian Nursing Council has prescribed rules on students' attendance for the clinical and non clinical subjects, the problem still exists. The students have the tendency to be absent more during the clinical days than nonclinical days. Some of the common causes of absenteeism are inappropriate preparation of assigned task, enjoying

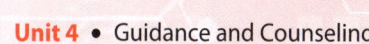

nonapproval holiday after a schedule holiday, lack of interest in particular subject and ultimately lack of motivation. This disciplinary problem could be managed by:

- Making aware about the requirement of attendance
- Establishing an appropriate monitoring system
- Identifying attendance rate of individual student
- Counseling of those student who are frequently absent
- Warning for incorrect behavior
- Taking disciplinary action as prescribed by discipline committee.

Non-submission or Late Submission of Assignment

Nursing students are expected to perform some curricular and extracurricular activities during their educational program as prescribed by the institution. One group of students fail to submit their assignment timely or do not complete it as a result of increased pending task. A number of causes may be related to this problem, which needs to identify and solve with a combined effort of student and teacher.

Student's Role

- Being aware about the curricular and extracurricular activity
- Preparing time table or schedule
- Following instruction in the theoretical and practical class
- Clarifying their doubt timely
- Seeking help or direction, if required
- Submitting assignment timely

Teacher's Role

- Appropriate assignment should be selected for students.
- Assignment should be relevant for the educational program.
- Assignment should be attractive and challenging for the students.
- Prior guidelines are necessary.
- Assignment should not be overloaded.
- Standard time should be allotted.
- Use of rewards and punishment should be done.
- Appropriate selection and use of disciplinary standards should be done.

Indiscipline Classroom Behavior

Classroom environment is disturbed by student's inappropriate behavior such as talking, sleeping, and watching mobile, while instructions are given by teachers. To promote appropriate classroom behavior, some necessary requirements are:

- Maintaining comfortable environments in the classroom such as temperature, ventilation, light, humidity, etc.

- Making aware about the rules and regulations of acceptable classroom behavior among students.
- Following prescribed disciplinary action while violation of discipline
- Avoiding discrimination while executing disciplinary action

Strike

Though strike is not very common among nursing students, but it is a serious disciplinary problem, which can be avoided through:
- Promoting better teacher student relationship
- Cultivating ethical and moral values
- Opportunity for effective parent, teacher and student interaction
- Adequate practice of curricular and extracurricular activities
- Active involvement of teachers in identifying student's problem
- Solving students problem.

Damaging or Spoiling Institutional Property

Loosing institutional property through intentional or unintentional act of students is increasing day by day. Damaging furniture, library books and equipments, audiovisual aids, etc. are very common incidents that are observed. The rate of incidents can be minimized through-
- Cultivation of ethical, moral and spiritual values
- Securing valuable goods and property
- Establishing strict disciplinary standards.

Ragging

The UGC's new regulation states ragging as " any conduct by any student or students, whether by words spoken or written, or by an act which has the effect of teasing, treating or handling with rudeness a fresher or any other student." All nursing colleges affiliated to INC have received a circular to set up anti-ragging mechanism.

ISSUES FACED FOR COUNSELING IN NURSING

Lack of Resources

To implement guidance and counseling program efficiently and effectively, adequate amount and quality of resources are important. To run a program smooth adequate amount of funds is not only essential but the other resources like man power, infrastructure, and adherence to time schedule are also equally important. The success of guidance and counseling program largely depends on the counselor, who should be competent to diagnose, predict, plan and provide cost effective service.

Lack of Interest and Positive Attitude of Counselor

The teaching faculty plays the additional role of counselor in most of the nursing schools and colleges instead of professional counselor. Lack of interest and positive attitude towards this additional role makes them demotivated. This demotivated faculty can't provide highest level of service.

Lack of Professionalism

In most of the nursing school and colleges, guidance and counseling services are provided by the teaching faculties who do not have required qualification. Many a times, they are not aware about their role and responsibility and are not accessible to students. They could not be able to provide services consistently because of workload.

Ethical and Moral Issues

It is a common and crucial issue of guidance and counseling services. Non compliance with ethical principle may result in ineffective services. Counselors have an ethical responsibility to recognize and protect the human rights that includes: right to self determination, right to privacy, right to confidentiality, right to fair treatment, and protection from discomfort and harm.

Lack of Awareness

Nursing students are not fully aware about the necessity and benefits of guidance and counseling service. Though the adequate level of guidance and counseling services is not available in every teaching organization, inappropriate uses of these services increase the magnitude of problems like stress, maladjustment, poor attitude towards profession, etc.

Lack of Compliance with Counseling Service

Noncompliance of nursing students with counseling intervention is a frequently observed issue in teaching organization. Student's shows nonadherence with guidance and counseling intervention because of incompetent counselor, lack of time, inconsistency of service and strong attitude, etc.

Common presenting issues for seeking counseling services among students are:

Depression and Anxiety

According to the report of American College Health Association, 45.6% of students had feeling of hopelessness, 30.7% were so depressed that it was difficult for them to function. A cross-sectional study of Ireland reported that 34% of nursing and midwifery students experienced depressive symptoms, 20% were poorly personally adjusted and 9% were poorly socially adjusted. In Taiwan, the prevalence of depressive symptoms among junior college nursing students was 32.6%. A cross-sectional survey conduct in a private nursing institute of Punjab, India reported that 73.03% nursing student experience anger followed by irritation (52.81%) very often over last 3 months. Other reported emotional problems were worry/anxiety (46.07%), loneliness (35.96%), etc. A correlational, cross-sectional study of Thailand reported that 50.1% Thai nursing students were depressed.

Academic Problems

A study of Taiwan reported that depressive symptoms were significantly related to grade point average, interest in nursing, interest in clinical placement, career planning after graduation etc. "Assignment and workload" as well as "teachers and nursing staff" were the highest sources of stress among nursing students in Saudi Arabia. The most frequent academic source of stress among Iranian nursing students was "increased class workload" (66.9%).

Psychosomatic Manifestations

A cross-sectional study of Punjab, India identified psychosomatic problems migraine headaches present among 49.44% of nursing students. Other problems as reported very often in were peptic ulcers (22.22%), constipation (23.60%) and loose motion (21.35%). Persistent psychosomatic complains are not a healthy behavior and have a risk of mental illness and behavioral problems.

SUMMARY

Guidance is a process of helping individual to maximize capacity for adjustment with intra-, inter- and extra-personal environment but counseling refers to an interactive process between two persons in which one person helps the other person with an expertise knowledge and skill for the purpose of problem solving and capacity building.

Guidance and counseling both ultimately serve the purpose of personal development. Scope of guidance and counseling is diverse, it may be required at any point of time in an individual's life from childhood to old age and for various kind of problems: personal, social, moral, spiritual, vocational and educational. In educational organization, guidance and counseling services are provided in various forms such as pre-admission service, admission service, orientation service, student information service, counseling service, placement service, remedial service, follow up service, research service and evaluation service.

Guidance and counseling is important to satisfy various personal and social needs of individual in a continuously changing environment. To provide an organized service of guidance and counseling, some basic principles are followed that include, principles of: dignity, individual difference, considering social background, personal perception and attitude, enhancing perceived self, continuity etc.

Success of guidance and counseling program depends upon four important factors that include: kind of help required for the client, level of help, availability of resources, quantity and quality of resources, and time orientation.

To get maximum benefit from guidance and counseling process, appropriate approach is selected. Counseling approaches are directive, nondirective and eclectic. Counselor may select the suitable approach for counseling but he/she has to play multiple roles such as information provider, adviser, educator, planner, organizer, service provider, researcher, etc. Efficient performance of counselor requires specific educational preparation, positive attitude, counseling skills and some personal qualities.

Guidance and counseling program is not a group of task but organized service that is provided by professional therefore it is important to consider the issues present which have greater impact. The issues present are related to counselor and counselee, which includes: lack of awareness among student, lack of resources, lack of interest and positive attitude of counselor, lack of compliance with counseling service, ethical and moral issues etc.

Counseling process involves five interrelated steps including: Establishing relationship, Assessment, Goal setting, Intervention and lastly Termination and evaluation. In each step of counseling process, a lot of interaction takes place between counselor and counselee with the use of some standardised and non standardized tools.

In every educational organization, some sort of disciplinary problems exist which need to be control through appropriate use of guidance and counseling services. Common disciplinary problems are absenteeism, non submission or late submission of assignment, indiscipline classroom behavior, strike, damaging or spoiling institutional property, ragging, etc.

Guidance and counseling service is not only essential to control and manage disciplinary problems, but it is also important for crisis intervention. Crisis is a sudden event that occurs in one's life as a result of ineffective response to a stressor that disturbs homeostasis. All types of crisis can be grouped as situational or maturational crisis but whatever the type, it has some phases of development. If crisis develops in one's life, it needs to be resolved as early as possible through a systematic process of intervention. Effective crisis intervention leads to restoration of previous functioning of client but ineffective intervention or deterioration at any stage demands referral service.

Assess Yourself

Long Answer Questions

1. Define the term counseling. Describe the characteristics of a good counselor. Write down the importance of counseling for a student lacking self confidence and self esteem.
2. Differentiate guidance and counseling. Discuss the approaches of counseling. Explain the steps of counseling process.
3. Discuss briefly about the scope of guidance and counseling.
4. Describe the types of counseling. Explain the factors on which success of guidance and counseling depends. To provide effective counseling service what kind of preparation is required for a counselor?
5. Discuss the common issues related to guidance and counseling program for nursing students.

Short Answer Questions

1. What is directive approach of guidance and counseling?
2. What are the basic differences between directive and non-directive counseling?
3. Why guidance and counseling service is require in an educational organization?
4. List the steps of counseling process.
5. What are the common disciplinary problems observed in educational organization?
6. What is crisis? What are the different types of crisis?
7. How do you recognize a client with crisis?
8. What are the levels of crisis intervention?
10. How guidance and counseling helps a student in preadmission service?

Contd...

SHORT NOTES

1. Scope of guidance and counseling
2. Needs of guidance and counseling
3. Principle of guidance and counseling
4. Phases of crisis development
5. Issues in guidance and counseling
6. Uses of non-standardised tool in guidance and counseling
7. Qualities of a counselor
8. Techniques of counseling
9. Role of counselor
10. Assessment in counseling process

MULTIPLE CHOICE QUESTIONS

1. In an educational organization, effective service of guidance and counseling is provided through organizing it:
   A. As early as possible
   B. As late as possible
   B. Timely
   D. As requested by student

2. To provide effective counseling service, the counselor should be:
   A. Over enthusiastic
   B. Suspicious
   C. Indifferent
   D. Instrumental

3. In directive counseling approach, the dominant role is played by:
   A. Counselee
   B. Counselor
   C. Parents of counselee
   D. Friends of counselee

4. In performing the role of coordinator, the counselor needs to coordinate with:
   A. Client and parent
   B. Client and teacher
   C. Client, parent and teacher
   D. All of them

5. Questionnaire is a form of self report in which a person's:
   A. Written response is obtained
   B. Verbal response is obtained
   C. Verbal and written response is obtained
   D. Body language is accepted

6. General support as an approach of counseling is used by counselor through:
   A. Accepting the client
   B. Refusing the client
   C. Criticizing the client
   D. Assigning task to the client

7. Intervention is the working phase of counseling process where the counselee and counselor are working towards:
   A. Problem identification
   B. Goal setting
   C. Achieving the goal
   D. Evaluating the performance

Contd...

8. **To predict fitness of student for an educational program, the appropriate test is:**
   A. Personality test
   B. Achievement test
   C. Aptitude test
   D. Intelligence test
9. **An achievement test is a test which measure the student's:**
   A. Developed skill or knowledge
   B. Social or political attitude
   C. Belief and values
   D. Personality and intellectuality
10. **A sudden event occurs in one's life as a result of ineffective response to a stressor that disturb homeostasis is referred as:**
    A. Stress
    B. Stressor
    C. Crisis
    D. Accident
11. **The technique of acknowledging an acceptable behavior of client is termed as:**
    A. Suggestive behavior
    B. Reinforcement of behavior
    C. Defensive behavior
    D. Supportive behavior

ANSWERS TO MCQS

1. (B)	2. (D)	3. (B)	4. (A)	5. (A)	6. (C)	7. (D)
8. (A)	9. (A)	10. (B)				

BIBLIOGRAPHY

1. Sharma RN, Sharma R. Guidance and Counseling in India. New Delhi: Atlantic Publishers and Distributors; 2004.
2. Kinra AK.Guidance and Counsellig. NewDelhi: Pearson Education; 2008.
3. Eiser A. The crisis on campus. APA 2011 Sep; 42(8). Available from: http://www.apa.org/monitor/2011/09/crisis-campus.aspx. Accessed August 4, 2016.
4. Horgan A, Sweeney J, Behan L, Mccarthy G. Depressive symptoms, college adjustment and peer support among undergraduate nursing and midwifery students. J Adv Nurs. 2016 Jul 19. doi: 10.1111/jan.13074.
5. Chen CJ, Chen YC, Sung HC, Hsieh TC, Lee MS, Chang CY et al. The prevalence and related factors of depressive symptoms among junior college nursing students: a cross-sectional study. J Psychiatr Ment Health Nurs. 2015 Oct;22(8):590-8.
6. Hamaideh SH, Al-Omari H, Al-Modallal H. Nursing students' perceived stress and coping behaviors in clinical training in Saudi Arabia. J Ment Health. 2016 Feb 5:1-7.
7. Kumar R. Psychosomatic complaints among nusing students-a cross sectional study from Punjab. DPJ. 2013 Oct; 16(2):343-49.
8. Neeraja KP. Textbook of Nursing Education. New Delhi: Jaypee; 2003.
9. SharmaSK, Sharma R. Communication and Education Technology in Nursing.. New Delhi: Elsevier:; 2012.

10. Rao SN, Hari MS. Guidance and Counseling. New Delhi: DPH; 2004.
11. Skinner CE. Educational psychology. 4thed. New Delhi: Prentice Hall of India PLtd; 2001.
12. Dandekar WN. Psychological Foundation of Education. Mumbai: Macmillan India Limited; 1976.
13. Sankarnarayanan B, Sindhu B. Learning and teaching nursing.4th ed. New Delhi: Jaypee; 2012.
14. Nayak AK. Guidance and counseling. New Delhi: APH Publishing corporation; 2007.
15. Townsend MC. Mental Health Nursing-concepts of care in evidence based practice. 7th ed. New Delhi: Jaypee; 2012.
16. Stuart GW, Laraia MT. Principles and practice of psychiatric nursing. 8th ed. StLouis: Mosbey; 2005.
17. Shrivastava KK. Principles of guidance and counseling. New Delhi: Kanishka publishers; 2003.
18. Kumar S. What are the Basic Principles and Characteristics of Counseling.[2]. Available at: http://www.publishyourarticles.net/knowledge-hub/education/what-are-the-basic-principles-and-characteristics-of-counseling/5379/. Accessed August 4, 2016.

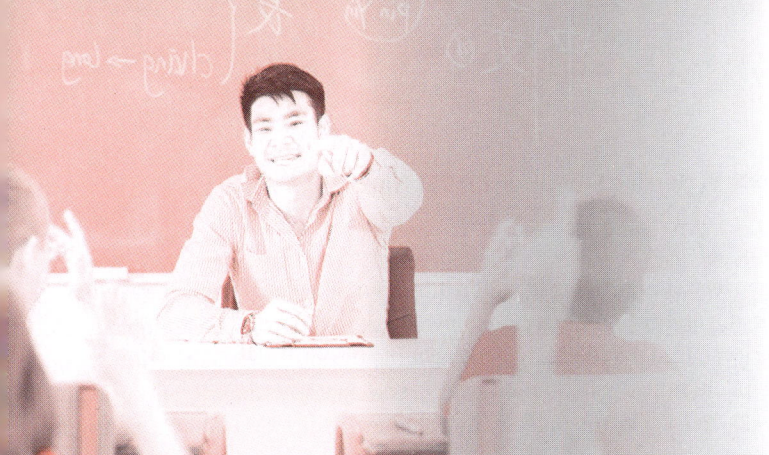

Principles of Education and Teaching Learning Process

— Anil Parashar

CHAPTER OUTLINE

Philosophy of Education
- Etymological Meaning of Philosophy
- Branches of Philosophy
- Essential Components of Philosophy of Education Statement

Schools of Education Philosophy
- Idealism
- Naturalism
- Pragmatism
- Realism

Aims of Education
- Social Aim
- Vocational Aim
- Cultural Aim
- Spiritual Aim

Functions of Education
- Towards Individual
- Towards Society
- Towards Nation

Nature and Characteristic of Learning
Maxims of Teaching
Formative Objective
- Smart

Bloom Taxonomy of Learning Domains
- Cognitive
- Affective
- Psychomotor

Lesson Planning
- Steps
- Types of Lesson Plan
- Approaches to Lesson Planning

LEARNING OBJECTIVE

The learner will be able to
- Etymological meaning of philosophy
- Identify the meaning of education
- Define the term of education
- Describe the philosophy of education
- Describe selected school of philosophies

- Identify the aims of education
- Explain the function of education
- Enlist the characteristic of learning
- Describe maxims of teaching
- Define objectives and enumerate the characteristic of objective

INTRODUCTION

Education is most important for every human being life. Education is that which transforms a person to live a better life and provide the ability to differentiate between right and wrong. Human beings is furnished with cultural, spiritual, moral and social aspects in life by education. Education plays a vital role in the personal growth of an individual and moreover, it enhances the confidence by giving us bulk of knowledge in many areas. Person learns in every moment every day. Education is strength of every person and enables him to solve any problem confronted by him in day to day living. Without education, a person is incomplete, thus education makes a person a right decision maker, responsible, dynamic, resourceful and enterprising citizen of strong moral good character. An individual develops like a flower and its fragrance spreads all over the environment by education. Education develops the individual in all fields, moreover, it contribute to the growth and development of society. Society also gets enriched the quality, heritage, culture, spiritual value, belief and moral ideals with the development of the individual.

Etymological Meaning of Education

The root of education is derived from Latin word "Educare "which means 'to bring up' or 'to raise'.
The word education originated from another term "Educere" which means 'to lead forth'.

Definition of Education

- By education I mean an all round drawing out of the best in child and man body, mind and spirit.
  —**Mahatma Gandhi**

- Education means enabling the mind to find out the ultimate truth which emancipates us from the bondage of the dust and give us the wealth, not of things but of inner light, not of power but of love, making this truth its own and gives expression to. —**Rabindra Nath Tagore**

- Education is the capacity to feel pleasure and pain at the right moment. It develops in the body and in the soul of the pupil, all the beauty and all the perfection of which he is capable of. —**Plato**

- Education is a natural harmonious and progressive development of man's innate powers
  —**Pestalozzi**

- Education is the development of good character. —**Herberts's**

- Education is the development in the individual of all perfection of which he is capable of. —**Kant**

- The aim of education is the development of valuable personality and spirituality, individuality.
  —**Ross**

- Education is the consciously controlled process whereby changes in behavior are produced in the person and through the person within the group. —**Brown**

PHILOSOPHY OF EDUCATION

The word 'Philosophy' comes from two Greek words – 'Philo' which means 'love' and 'Sophia' which means 'wisdom'. It is a love for wisdom.

- Education is gradual adjustment of the individual to the spiritual possession of the race. —**Buller**

- "Philosophy and Education are like the two side of the same coin: the one is implied by other; the former is the contemplative side of life, while latter is the active side" —**J.S. Ross**

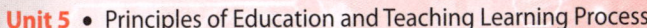

The main concepts and issue of education are reflected with the help of philosophy such as what is knowledge? what is the nature of learning? what is teaching?

Definition

- Philosophy is a persistent attempt to give insight in to the nature of the world and of ourselves by means of systematic reflection. **—R.W. Sellars**
- Philosophy like other studies aims primarily at knowledge. **—Bertrand Russell**
- Philosophy is unceasing efforts to discern the general truth that lies behind the particular facts, to discern also the reality that lies behind appearance. **—Raymont view**
- Philosophy is the science of knowledge. **—Fichte view**

Branches of Philosophy

- **Ethics**: It is also known as moral philosophy and a branch of philosophy that addresses questions about morality. It is related to the questions on morality and values and how they apply to various situations. Ethics seek the basis of morals and how they develop and how it should be followed.
- **Epistemology**: It deals with concept of knowledge, how we learn and what we can know? How do we have this knowledge? What do you know, really? And how did you arrive at it?
- **Logic**: It studies the rules of valid reasoning?
- **Metaphysics**: It is the study of the nature of reality and their relation such as god, person, thing, event, property, causation. The question typical of this branch is, hence: "What is there, really?"
- **Ontology**: It is the study of nature and existence. How might your view determine your classroom management?

Essential Components of a Philosophy of Education Statement

Philosophy of education statement is an integral component of teaching goal and how a teaching concept is transformed into real class room activities:
- Perception of teaching
- Perception of learning
- Teaching goals
- Executing philosophy of education statement
- Professional growth.

Perception of Teaching

It describes the meaning of teaching for teacher. Teaching process, and how you can facilitate those processes as an educator, issues such as motivating students, facilitating the learning process, how to challenge students academically and how to support their learning abilities should be addressed.

Perception of Learning

It describes what learning means to you and what exactly happens in learning. Use images to draw comparisons with known philosophies, you can directly relate what you think happens during a learning session based on your personal experience as an educator.

Teaching Goals

It describes goals for students and also list the various talents or skills that teacher expects from students to acquire through teaching. In addition to the goals that teacher have set for students, teacher should also provide the rationale behind these goals and how you will keep changing the goals to meet the growing learning needs of your students.

Executing Philosophy of Education Statement

The most important component of education philosophy statement is:
- Your elaboration of the different activities that you will implement to enable your students to achieve their goals.
- You have to illustrate how your perceptions of teaching and learning will be translated into real-time class assignments.

Professional Growth

In order to continue growing professionally,
- Teachers needs to set goals for themselves and also outline their ways to achieve these goals.
- The personal goals that you have set for yourself as an educator should thus be mentioned in your philosophy of education statement.

SCHOOLS OF EDUCATION PHILOSOPHY

Idealism

Idealism is derived from Plato's theory of ideas, according to which, the ultimate supremacy is of ideas. In idealism, ideas, feelings, and ideals are more important than material objects. According to idealism, the essential nature of man is spiritual, which is revealed in mental, religious and aesthetic areas.

Definition

- Idealism holds that ultimate reality is spiritualism. —**D.M. Dutta**
- Idealistic philosophy takes many and varied forms but the postulate underlying all this is that mind or spirit is the essential world, stuff, that the true reality is a mental character. —**J.S. Ross**

Idealism and Aims of Education

- Ensure the spiritual development
- Development of morality
- Self-realization of personality
- Development of intelligence and rationality: Adam defined education from the idealist point of view. According to him, there is a purpose in all objects and natural phenomenon. Man can understand the purpose as well as plan and organization.
- Preservation of cultural heritage. Make the child familiar with the enriched culture so that they are able to conserve, promote, and transmit it to the rising generation.

Fundamental Principles

- Focus –Universal mind
- Idealism believes man is a spiritual being
- Ideas are more important than objects
- Real knowledge is perceived in mind
- Principle of unity of diversity.

Idealism and Curriculum

- Idealistic curriculum is thought-oriented and gives importance to feeling and values. They believe that curriculum should be based on whole humanity and its experience.
- Literature, language, science, social studies and mathematics are included in the curriculum for intellectual development of the child.

Role of Teacher

- Teacher acts as a spiritual guide for the child.
- Teacher serves as a living model for the student.
- Teacher guide the child with love and affection that child achieve his full mental and spiritual development.
- Create a conducive environment and planned experience for child.

Idealism and Discipline

Idealists prefer the discipline on child. The main disciplinary factors are self-insight and self-analysis and self-discipline. This leads to inner discipline. The main task of education is the development of higher values of life through moral and religious education.

Method of Teaching

There is no specific method of teaching in idealism.

The following methods have been advocated by different idealists:
- Learning through reading
- Learning through lecture
- Learning through discussion
- Learning through imitation
- Learning through play way method and talk in group.

Naturalism

Naturalism is also known as materialism. According to naturalist, only nature is everything, nothing is before and beyond it. School environment should be completely free, flexible and without restriction. There should not be strict time table, etc. Nature will do all planning and processing. Development of child will be natural and normal. Naturalist do not believe in the spiritual development. They deny the existence of any such things as the supremacy of god, immorality of soul and the freedom of will. To them, there is nothing else than matter which is ultimate reality and the ultimate truth. Proponent of naturalism are Aristotle, Comte, Hobbes, Bacon, Darwin, Bernard Shaw and Samual Butler.

Definition of Naturalism

- Naturalism is a term loosely applied in educational theory to systems of training that are not dependent on schools and books but on the manipulation of the actual life of the educated.

  —**J.S Ross**
- Naturalism is a doctrine, which separates nature from god, subordinates spirit to matter and sets up unchangeable laws as supreme. —**Wards**
- Naturalism is not science but an assertion about science. More specifically, it is the assertion that scientific knowledge is final, leaving no room for extra–scientific or philosophical knowledge.

  —**R.B. Perry**
- Naturalism is a philosophical position adopted by those who approach philosophy from purely scientific point of view. —**Rusk**

Forms of Naturalism

- *Physical Naturalism*: It emphasises much more on physical science and accept that physical science is supreme. It studies the process of matter and phenomenon of the external world. It has no belief on morality, freedom of will and inner nature of human mind. It interprets the human activities and experience in terms of physical sciences.
- *Mechanical Naturalism*: Herbert Spencer is the main exponent of mechanical philosophy. According to him, universe is a machine which gets its form through matter and motion. Human being is considered as small part of this huge machine. Mechanical Naturalism has given rise to modern Psychology, which emphasizes the importance of conditional response and the effective principles of leaning by doing.
- *Biological Naturalism*: This form of naturalism based upon the Drawinian Theory of Evolution. Man is the supreme product of this process of evolution. This doctrine puts forward three principles to explain this philosophy:
  - Adaptation to environment
  - Struggle for existence
  - Survival of the fittest

Principles of Naturalism

- Man- as machine: The universe is a huge machine and man is consider a small machine
- Human being is the supreme creation of nature and considered as the supreme and superior most animal.
- Matter is the final reality. God, Soul, Mind, The Heaven and Hell, Freedom of will, Moral Value, Prayer, Wonders are illusion.
- Naturalist believes that all knowledge comes through senses.
- Law of nature controls all events and processes that occur in the world
- Provision of conducive environment
- Materialistic education: stress on the materialistic education then spiritual education.

- Material science is more essential, due to the rapid change of life, all inventions promote the comfort of human being.
- Man develops the society and fulfills his requirement. He adjusts and changes the environment according to his needs.

Aims of Education

- Self Preservation: It is important for human being to preserve and maintain the existence of life
- Human beings make a adjustment and harmony with his surrounding. Prepare the child for adjustment and ensure his health and happiness
- Autonomous development: According to T.P. Nunn, individual development should be free, fully autonomous and self acquired
- Struggle for existence: Children should be equipped physically and mentally to their environment and enable to survive in environment
- Man as a machine: The aim of education is to make the individual work effectively.
- Education should develop the child according to his inborn tendencies, interest, aptitudes and capacities.
- Attainment of social progress.

Naturalism and Curriculum

- Naturalists believe that there is no fixed curriculum.
- Curriculum must be child centered.
- Child can grow with fullest natural way with his inborn tendency, aptitude, interest and capacity.
- Every child is given the right to determine his own curriculum.
- According to Herbert Spencer, curriculum should contain physiology, biology, chemistry, arithmetic, home science and another scientific subjects as main subjects where as language, literature, art and other cultural subjects as subsidiary subjects.

Method of Teaching

Naturalists discard the traditional and bookish system of education. They have given freedom to the child for free expression, which leads to creative and innovative activities. They have given more stress on the following

- Direct Method
- Heuristic Method
- Learning by doing
- Play method, observation and excursion
- Learning through participation
- Other methods: Dalton method, kindergarten, montessari method

Role of Teacher

- Nature is the supreme teacher
- Teacher should not impose his authority

- Sympathy and affectionate towards child
- Sympathetic observer and guide
- As a gardner for the child
- Setter of the stage: According to Rusk, a teacher is a supplier of material, and opportunity and provides a conducive environment for the natural development of child.

Discipline

- Give full freedom to child to perform all activities which he likes
- No punishment should be given to child
- Discipline by natural consequences
- Favor of co-educational and residential school.

Demerits of Naturalism

- Do not give the importance on spiritual and moral aspects.
- Book system is totally rejected.
- Emphasis is given to science subject.
- Freedom to the child is given without restriction.
- Role of the teacher is limited.
- Discipline by natural consequences is harmful.
- Literature subject is totally neglect.

Pragmatism

This philosophy is known as the gift of American philosophy. It is also known as experimentalism due to the result oriented and experimental approach. It is a method of experimental inquiry extended in to all area of human experiences. Pragmatism uses all modern scientific method as the basis of philosophy. It is very closely connected with human life and human welfare. Pragmatism also known as humanistic philosophy of life. Scientific knowledge and scientific spirit are utilized to solve the human problem. Pragmatists emphasized empirical science. The chief proponders of pragmatism are CS Pearce, William James and Shiller John Dewey. Willam James defines pragmatism as "the attitude of looking away from first things".

Meaning of Pragmatism

The word pragmatism derived from the Greek word 'pragma', which means activity or to accomplish. Some scholars also believed that pragmatism has been derived from Geek word 'Pragmatikos', which means practicability or utility.

Definition

- Pragmatism offers us a theory of meaning, a theory of truth of knowledge and a theory of reality.

  —**James B. Prett**

- Pragmatism is a temper of mind, an attitude, it is also a theory of nature of ideas and truth and finally, it is a theory of reality.

  —**William James**

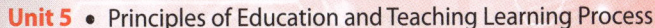

- Pragmatism is the doctrine that truth is practical efficacy of an idea.   **—William Durant**
- Pragmatism is an activity, engagement, encounter, based on the concept of practice, or workability of an idea or theory.   **—Arnold Reid**

Principle of Pragmatism

- *Changing nature of truth*: Pragmatism believes that truth is always not permanent. Sometimes a truth may be true to an individual with specific time and place whereas for others it's not. Truth related to certain things may be true for a person yesterday and may not be same for him in present or future. According to pragmatism, truth is always changing according to time, places and situations.
- *Faith in practice*: They believe in experience and experiment is the only criterion of truth. Value and life are determined by the human experience.
- *Emphasis on the principle of utility*: The things which are useful for human beings are true or right. According to Willian James "it is true because it is useful".
- *Significance of manpower*: Pragmatism has firmly been given importance of power of man. Man can create a conducive environment for his own development.
- *Importance of present and future*: Pragamatism do not stick to the past. Each individual has to solve the problems of his present and future life.
- *Emphasis on activity*: They have given more stress to activity. Human being is an active being and he learns all the aspect through activity, which also helps him to solve the problems.
- *Social value*: Man is a social animal and without society him existence is meaningless. They consider democracy, tolerance, responsibility and justice are the social value.
- *Importance of environment*: Growth of individual depends upon the interaction of the environment. Man always tries to adjust to the environment for growth.
- *Problems as a motivating factor*: Every person does the experiment to find out success of the problems in life. Problems are the main motivating factor to search the truth.
- *Flexibility*: Pragmatist believes that nothing is fixed and final in this world. Anything can be changed. Nothing is constant. Human life is also changing, whenever a human being finds a difficulty, he employs all his experience to find out the problem.

Aims of Education

- Personal and social development
- Reconstruction of experience
- All round development
- Activity and experience
- Adjustment
- Creation of value
- Motivating factor to solve the problem

Method of Teaching

They believe that every child is different from others, therefore, a fixed method of teaching cannot be used for all. Both the teacher and child formulate the teaching in such a way so that child can grow in a accurate way with practical work, and productive experiences.

Principles

- **Learning by doing**: Pragmatism has given more importance to experience and activity. Child can develop new ideas and clear concept through activity and experience. Learner develops the concept and necessary insight by his own efforts. Self experience makes the child more perfect than passive.
- **Integration**: It is the amalgamation of different subject leads the learning more effective. Subjects, which are closely related should bring as much as possible.
- Child should achieve some aims with or goal according to his interest, abilities and experiences. Pragmatism emphasizes self-learning with self-effort.

Role of Teacher

Teacher should play a role of a guide, open minded and friend to the children. He should understand the interest of child. He should select the educative experience to the learner. Teacher should create an environment of problem solving to the children. He should have the full understanding regarding the situation of changing society.

Discipline

Pragmatism do not believe any type of forced discipline. They strongly favor the social discipline. Play and work should go simultaneously, which gains the interest of the child while doing any work. Child develops self-confidence, co-operation, and self reliance. When a child develops all these qualities, he has a sense of social discipline.

Curriculum

The following principles are laid down by pragmatist

- **Principle of utility**: Only those subjects are included in the curriculum, which have the capacity to meet the present and future expectations. They suggest that geography, history and home science should be taught to girls
- **Principle of natural interest**: Only those activities are included in curriculum, in which a child has the interest. At the primary level, the curriculum should include reading, writing, counting art, natural sciences, craft work, etc.
- **Principles of experiences**: They are firm with the practical experience, curriculum should develop in such a way that child develop Innovative thinking, experience.
- **Principles of integration**: Child develop the natural interest and co relate the experience, when ever is integration of all subject in curriculum construction, Correlate the various unit will develop the firm concept and proper understanding in child.

Characteristics

- Education as life
- Education as growth

- Education as continued reconstruction of experience
- Education as a social process
- Education as a responsibility of the state.

Merits

- Importance of child
- Emphasis on activity
- Faith in applied life
- Social and democratic education
- Progressive and optimistic attitude
- Construction of project method.

Realism

Etymologically, realism means 'about a thing' or concerning some object. Realists believe that reality exists independent of the human mind. Realists believe that knowledge is acquired through senses is true.

Definition

- Realism is the refinement of our common acceptance of the world as being just what it appears to be. **—Butler's View**
- Realism means a belief or theory which looks upon the world as it seems to us to be a mere phenomenon. **—Swami Ram Tirth**
- The doctrine of realism asserts that there is real world of things behind and corresponding to the objects of our perception. **—J.S Ross.**

Principles

The following are principles of realism:

- **Observation and experiment**: Realists has given more stress on experiment and observation. Experiment can only be valid when it is tested and classified.
- **Phenomenal universe is true**: Realists believe the reality where as idealists believe spiritual aspect of universe.
- **Senses and knowledge**: Realism believes that human being is contact with external world through our senses leads knowledge which is true and real.
- **Importance of present life**: They firmly believe in present life unlike the idealist which is more supportive to spirituality Human behavior is based on the physical and material fact. They also emphasize the practical knowledge which helps the students to solve the present life problems.
- Main is the prime part of the material world, he obtain the knowledge through sense organ and mind.
- **Emphasis on reality**: Realist believe that reality is real, There is no place of imagination in realism at all. They believe the scientific method and experiment through which reality take place.

Forms

The following are the four forms of realism
- Humanistic realism
- Social realism
- Sense realism
- Neorelaism

Aims of Education

- Preparation of happy and successful life
- Development of physical and mental power of child
- Development of senses
- Maintain equilibrium between nature and social environment
- Value of vocational education
- Man is the prime concern in material world
- Grow a child in a real life.

Curriculum

Curriculum include subject which have real meaning in child life, he can learn and solve the problems of their life. The primary subjects that are very much essential in child life and child comes across in daily life such as nature, science and vocation have been included where as arts and geography are the secondary subjects. Mother–tongue is the foundation of development and vocation subject is needed for livelihood. Importance should be given more to experimental aspect.

Method of Teaching

- Gives more importance to experimental and observational method
- Avoid bookish knowledge
- Teaching based on the real life aspect
- Teach the child based on his capacity and strength
- Use of technology and scientific methods in studies
- Realist focuses on teaching their students with the scientific method of problem solving.

Role of Teacher

- Teacher is not given higher importance
- Good knowledge of the subject and need of the child
- Application of scientific principle at the time of teaching
- Teacher should involve the research and experimentation work
- Encourage the child to find out the new innovation and fact
- Teachers assess the children and provide a specific knowledge at a particular time.

Discipline

Moral and religious education have been given more priority. They emphasise self discipline with adjustment to external environment. In discipline, teacher's role is only to inspire and encourage the child sympathetically.

AIMS OF EDUCATION

In every walk of life, aims have unique importance. Without aims, the work, which we take up remain uninteresting and depressing. Indeed it makes the process lively. Aims give direction to activities. In the field of education, aims are very essential. In the word of John Dewey "an aim is a foreseen end that gives direction to an activity or motivates the behavior".

John Dewey suggested the criteria for aims:

- Good aims are related to real situation of life. They grow out of these situations and they can be achieved only under these situation.
- Good aims are flexible. These should be flexible enough to meet the demands of changing circumstances of life.
- A good aim represents a span of diverse activity. The real objective in pursuing an end is not the end itself but the course of activity itself which constitute the core of education.

Aims in Emerging Society

Individual aims and social aims are the most important aims of education. They are different to each other, individual aims give importance to free growth of individuality. Education helps the individual to develop each child in conformity with its special abilities. The success of life depends upon the development of this kind. It is believed that education must train and develop the individual in such a way so as to bring him up as a good citizen.

The individual aims of education have been emphasized by various thinkers:

- The naturalists like Rousseau believe that "the central aim of education is the autonomous development of the individual. Everything is good as it comes from the hands of the Author of Nature, but everything degenerates in the hands of man." God makes all things good, man meddles with them and they become evil. God creates everything good; man makes it evil. So individual should be given maximum freedom for its own development.
- Biologists believe that every individual is different from others. Every child has certain peculiar characteristics. Thompson says, "Education is for the individual". Individual should be the center of all educational efforts and activities.
- In present era, psychologists emphasize individual differences, every child is different from another with respect to his color, form, nature and mental abilities such as intelligence, thinking etc. The aim of education is to develop each child in conformity with its special abilities.
- According to progressive thinker, Sir Percy Nunn observes, "Nothing goods enter into the human world, except in and through the free activities of individual men and women and that educational practice must shape the individual. Education should give scope to develop the inborn potentialities through maximum freedom."

Social Aim

The followers believe that society or state is supreme or real. The state has complete control over the various parts of education the syllabus, teaching method, administration and organization of institute. The state will make the individual as it desires. It prepares the individual to play different roles in society.

Vocational Aim

Livelihood is important. Education must enable the students to stand on his own feet. Only living person has certain needs and requirements. An individual needs education in order to live. According to the recommendation of the Secondary Education Commission (1952–53), the aim of vocationalization of education is to improve the vocational efficiency of the students.

Cultural Aim

It is concerned with individual thought, good habits, social values and behavioral patterns. Education helps to protect the cultural heritage of the nation.

Spirituality Aim

Spiritual aims of education refer to those aims, through which national ideology and values are injected in the character of the present and future generations. In the absence of spiritual aim, one life is complete.

FUNCTIONS OF EDUCATION

Education is essential for every society and individual. Education helps the individual to develop the qualities, recognize the potentiality and towards society and nation

Function of Education towards Individual

Character Building

Psychologists believe that child character laid in the first few years of his life. It is developed by education mainly informal education. Education helps in development of moral character because child is not naturally capable with the power of distinguishing between the right and wrong. Socialization is an important factor for the moral development.

All Round Development

Physical, mental, social, emotional and spiritual development take place in child with the help of education.

Preparing for the Future

After completion of education, the child can earn its livelihood getting proper education, which has productivity.

Development of Personality

The informal development of personality takes place through his family, neighborhood and educationalist believe that development of personality of child is also one of the important objectives. Hence, the child may take various tasks, so that his personality develop. Games play an important part for personality development. The society plays important role for development of personality, i.e. communal life school, the forms of society control and traditions.

Helping for Adjustability

Education facilitates the child to adjust in environment.

Functions of Education towards Society

Encouragement of Social Welfare

Formal and informal education helps the child to think critically about the topic, which is presented to him. If he finds any mistake in it, he may think to solve the problems. In this manner, education is the basis for all social welfare program.

Development of Social and Moral Value

Education teaches the moral value and social value like cooperation, tolerance, sympathy, fellow feelings, love affection, respect towards elder, helping the poor and needy persons.

Providing Opportunity or Equality

Indian constitution says that equal should be treated equally under equal circumstances. Education teaches us to give equal opportunities in all aspects, irrespective of caste, creed, color, sex and religion.

Functions of Education towards Nation

Maintaining Communal Interest and Tradition

India is a country of many different cultural and linguistic groups. Education achieves this similarity through prescribed syllabi and various kinds of extracurricular program.

National Integration

India is a country of having diversities in respect of color, caste, language, diet, dress, habits and physical environment.

Educational integration leads to emotional integration. Education trains people for unity not for locality, for democracy and not for dictatorship.

Training for Leadership

A country can only grow, if it has an able leader in the field of a political, economical, cultural, artistic, social, moral and industrial. Education provides these leaders. This can be achieved by student's participation in various extracurricular activity.

Respect to all Religions

India is a secular state and it gives equal status to every citizen. There is no discrimination on the basis of religious beliefs.

PRINCIPLES OF EDUCATION

- Evolve independent and interdependent learning process for individual
- **Integration of knowledge:** students explore and adapt new ideas , thinking and demonstrating the value and means of relating what is known in one discipline to what is known in others. This will enhance the learning community.
- **Value:** Education nurture the whole individual with development of body mind and spirit, it also helps students thoughtfully shape their value and choices.
- **Skill and abilities:** Education prompt individual to express oneself effectively and creatively and to understand the world from various perspectives
- **Moral reflection and criticism:** Individual is abided and aware by the moral principles, and discuss moral issue openly and attentively, accept ambiguities and disagreements respectfully
- Develop supportive and productive environment that help the students to express themselves and promote active learning
- Find out the nature of problem ,analyze the problem and execute an appropriate solution
- Accept , and understand social change ,technology changes and individual development
- Decision based on the factual information rather than unrealistic opinion
- Access, organize, interpret, synthesize and apply information.

NATURE AND CHARACTERISTICS OF LEARNING

Learning is an important process of human behavior. Human beings constantly interact with the external environment and modify his behavior according to the environment to effectively deal with it. Learning always involves some experience direct or indirect and a continuous process. Everyday a new situation arises and an individual faces these situations in his own style.

Characteristics of Learning

Following are the important characteristic of learning:

- **Learning affects the change of behavior**: Learning bring the behavior change in the individual. It can be changed in verbal and non verbal communication and thinking process.
- **Learning is purposeful**: All type of learning has purpose. Individual also learns activity due to objective. He feels interested when there is an objective in activity.
- **Learning is experience and practice**: Experience makes the men perfect. These experiences provide new knowledge, skill and attitude.
- **Learning is adjustment**: Learning helps the individual to adjust with new situation. Individuals have various problems in his life and learning helps to solve the problems encountered by him.
- **Learning is intelligent**: Learning take place when there is meaningful and understandable processes occur which ensure longlasting learning.

- **Learning is a part of environment**: Learning can take place in conducive environment. It is in close relationship with environment.
- **Learning is growth**: Learning is a form of growth. Learning is a natural process and takes place at any time, child develops both physically and mentally through the learning experience.
- **Learning is both individual and social**: Child gets first learning experience from family, then society. These institutions have tremendous impact on child behavior pattern.

Nature of Learning

The main aims of education to bring a desired change in behavior. When child have changed behavior, it shows child has learnt. Learning can take place in response to felt needs. Learning is a complex process. Changes in behavior takes place when individual interact with particular situation, which carry on and affect the general behavior of individual to some degree. Changes in a form of acting, ways of expressing one's thought, attitude and feeling towards others are called leaning.

MAXIMS OF TEACHING

A teacher should be familiar with general maxims of teaching.

- *Proceed from known to the unknown*: It is always right that old knowledge serves a path from which, new knowledge can be introduced. Students have previous knowledge of the topic; teacher should utilize that partial knowledge before proceeding to new knowledge. While using the previous knowledge the teacher must see that it is perfect, definite and complete.
- *Proceed from simple to complex*: A teacher always introduces the simple material first, later followed by complex and difficult material. Simplicity and complexity should be determined by child's point of view.
- *Proceed from concrete to abstract*: It is important to teach a child with concrete material. The imagination is greatly aided by concrete material. Existing examples are to be given in order to prepare to learn abstract concepts.
- *Proceed from analysis to synthesis*: When things are separated into elements, they usually prove analysis, whereas in synthesis, different elements come together. For example if a teacher wants to explain about arthroscopy procedure to the students, then he explain joint structure emphasis on particular part (analyzing), and later explains about the procedure by combining all parts (synthesis).
- *Proceed from whole to part*: Whole theory is more meaningful then part. If a teacher wants to teach the students cardiovascular system, then present the whole system briefly and later teach in different parts.
- *Proceed from particular to general*: A teacher should always proceed from particular to general statement. The rule of grammar and science are based upon this principle.

Some others are as follows:

- Proceed from empirical to rational
- From psychological to logical
- From actual to representative.

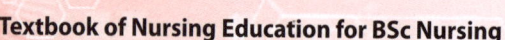

FORMULATING OBJECTIVES

Every organization has their own objective or desired state of affairs and allocates all the resources to achieve them. Objectives are the arrow that help the learner reach the target and well written objectives help to define the outcome of the activity. Objectives decide where we want to go and what we want to achieve and what is our destination. Objective is essential for successful implementation of any educational program. Evaluation can be made on the basis of objective. The differences between goals and objectives are given in Table 1.

Formulation of Objective; General and Specific

- **General Objective:** It is a description that a student's acquire with the aid of study unit. For ex : The students will be able to understand about the ....
- **Specific Objective:** There are four criteria for the formulation of specific objectives:
    - **Behavior:** How the student should be able to achieve the activity regarding subject matter, verbs is a tool to keep the student in a path that a teacher expect from students
    - **Content:** detail of substantive material, describe substantive material in most specific terms.
    - Condition of performance: it indicate the condition under which the students will performance, for ex : after attending the demonstration of oral care , students will be able to perform oral care correctly.
    - **Performance criteria:** it specifies the level of performance that a teacher accept for the successful attainment of objective

Definition

- An objective is a foreseen end that gives direction to an activity. **—John Dewey**
- Objectives are essential in all the key areas where performance and result directly contribute to the growth and survival of business. **—Peter F. Drucker**
- Objective is a term commonly used to indicate the end point of a management program.
  —Kontz and O'Donnell

TABLE 1: Differences between goals and objectives

Goals	Objective
Goals are long-term aims that you want to accomplish	Objectives are concrete attainments that can be achieved by following a certain number of steps
Goals may not be measurable	Objective can be measured
Goals are long-term	Objective usually mid to short-term
Goals are the wholes	Objective are the part of wholes
Ex.: I want to achieve success in the field of microbiology	Ex.: I want to complete this thesis on microbiology research by the end of this month

Characteristics of Objective

The following are the characteristic of objective:

Smart

It stands for "Specific, Measurable, Achievable, Realistic and Time-Bound."

Specific

It should be well defined, actual, detailed and able to render the detailed answer of everything, such as who, what, when, where, which and why.

Measurable

Frame concrete criteria is used for measuring the progress of an objective. Quality measurement uses the terms of amount, numbers and quantity, where as quality measurement explains in terms of accuracy, and standard guidelines.

Achievable

Make your goal attainable. Individuals enhance skill, knowledge, attitude and abilities to attain the objective. Plan a step wisely according to set of time frame to achieve the goal. Objective always motivates the person. Goals that may have seemed far away and out of reach eventually move closer and become attainable, not because your goals shrink, but because you grow and expand to match them.

Realistic

A goal can be both high and realistic. However, be sure that every goal represents substantial progress.

Time-oriented

A well defined timeline should be there to achieve the objective. It refers to the fact that an objective has end points and check points built into it. Deadlines are the action point for individual. Individual needs to be kept motivated when they have deadlines in their plan. Time is money! Make a tentative plan of everything you do.

Components of Writing Learning Objectives

According to Robert Mager, plan three components of writing learning objective:
- **Condition or Circumstances**: Objective is always formulated based on the condition under which the performance has to occur.
- **Performance**: Objective should write in such a way that learner must perform in a specific way to achieve the desired outcome.
- **Criterion**: It should be a performance-based criteria.

Bloom Taxonomy of Learning Domains

Bloom's Taxonomy was created in 1956 by the educational psychologist Dr Benjamin Bloom in order to promote higher forms of thinking in education, such as analyzing and evaluating. The Three Domains of Learning.

- **Cognitive**: Knowledge in terms of information or content
- **Affective**: Affections or emotional areas (attitude or self)
- **Psychomotor**: Manual or physical skills (skills).

Cognitive

The cognitive domain is knowledge and the development of intellectual skills. There are six major categories of cognitive areas starting from the simplest to the most complex. They are knowledge, comprehension, application, analysis, synthesis and evaluation (Fig. 1).

Affective

The term "affective" refers to affections and behavioral changes such as feeling, values and appreciation.

The five major categories are listed from the simplest behavior to the most complex as receiving, responding, valuing, organizing and conceptualizing and characterizing by value or value concept (Fig. 2).

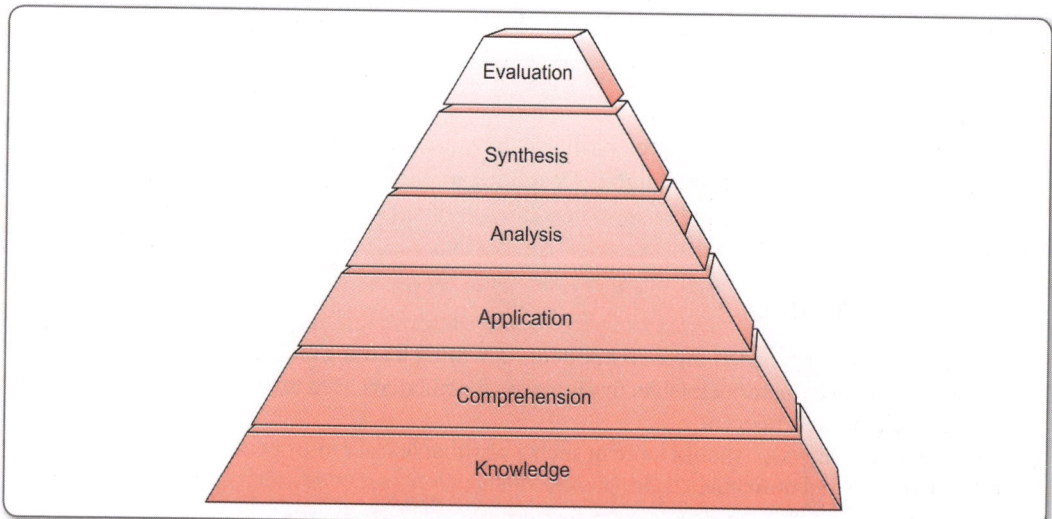

Fig. 1: Cognitive domain of learning

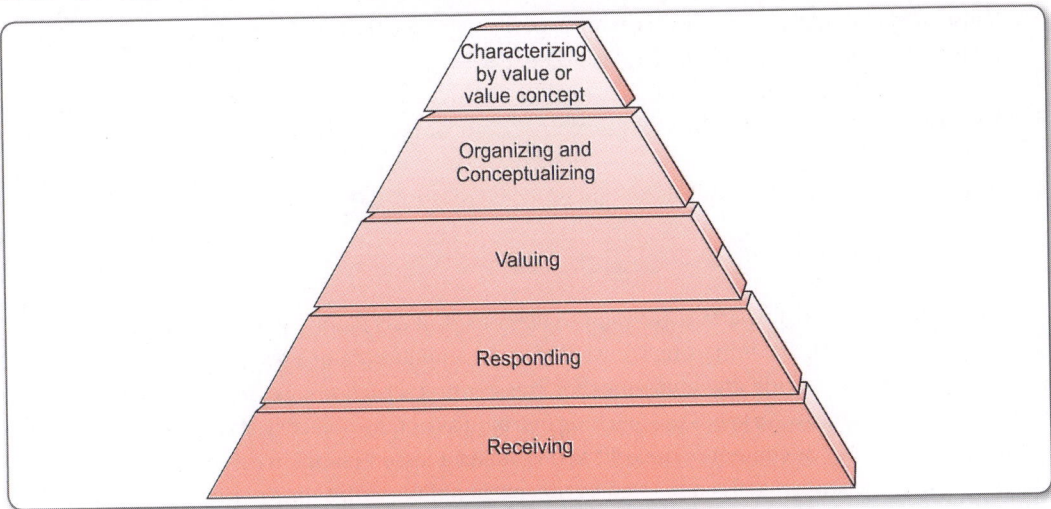

Fig. 2: Affective domain of learning

Psychomotor

The psychomotor domain (Simpson, 1972) includes physical movement, coordination, and use of the motor-skill areas. Development of these skills requires practice and are measured in terms of speed, precision, distance, procedures, or techniques in execution (Fig. 3).

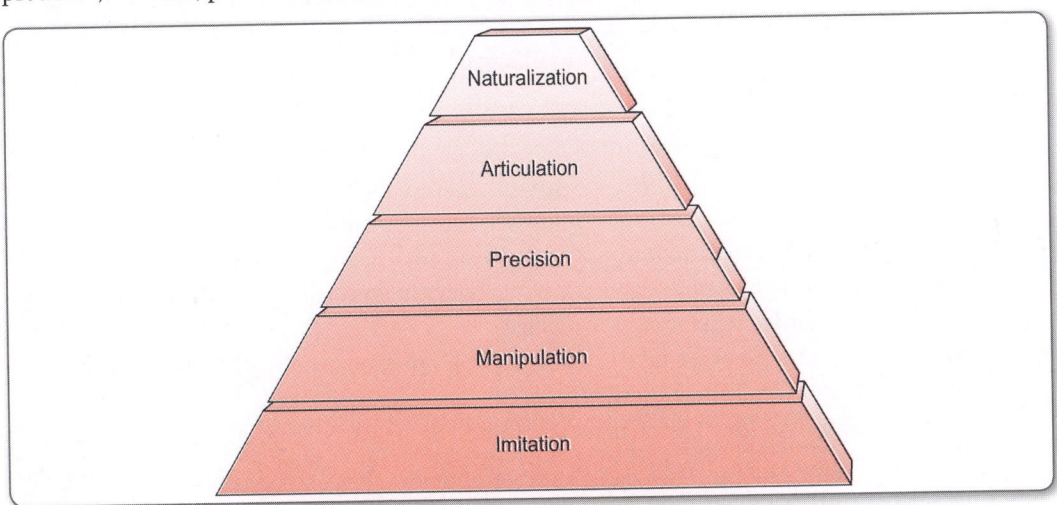

Fig. 3: Psychomotor domain of learning

Importance of Educational Objective for Nursing Students

- Educational objective described the desired behaviour that learner will exhibit and evaluate the outcome.
- It gives direction to the students for successful attainment of activity related to subject matter.

- It also helps the students to adapt lifelong experience and learning opportunities.
- Moreover objective helps to select appropriate teaching strategies and materials.
- Students will be determinant enough to explore the ideas and acquaint with condition.
- Student use critical thinking and all the learning outcome are assessed at the end of the learning situation.
- It helps the student to focus what they are expected to learn

LESSON PLANNING

It is a well known fact that whatever we want to execute, it needs planning, Lesson planning is also a planning of a teacher before imparting knowledge to the students about a particular topic. Theoretical knowledge does not provide any guidelines for classroom instructions. Lesson planning makes the teaching effective and always keeps the teaching in a path as per the objective. A teacher has to prepare the outline of the unit or content of the unit and is called a lesson plan. It is an insight, which will be given to students. Lesson plan is completed by the teacher along with a time period.

Definition

- Lesson planning is the title given to a statement of the achievement to be realized and the specific meaning by which these are to be attained as result of the activities engaged during the period.

  —NL Bossing
- All lesson planning involves defining the objectives, selecting and arranging the subject matter and determine the method and procedure. **—Binning and Binning**

Advantages of Lesson Planning

The following are the advantages while formulating the lesson planning:

- ***Provide systematic direction with a set period of time***: It provides a systematic and proper teaching and it will finish within a time framework.
- ***Suitable environment***: Objective will be prepared before delivering lecture. It also contain methods of teaching, teaching tactics, and teaching aids. It creates interest of pupils in the lesson and helps in creating an environment in the class teaching.
- ***Previous acquaintance***: Lesson plan is made of pupil's previous knowledge. Therefore, it will be simple for students to attain new knowledge.
- ***Teaching learning activities***: Lesson plan determines the activities for teacher and students, at the time of making lesson plan. Teachers formulate the activity, which will be performed in the class by the teacher and pupils.
- ***Audio–visual aids***: Teaching aid also helps the teacher to make the teaching effective. Teacher will determine the technique, strategies and aid that will be used by him in the class.
- ***Gives confidence during teaching***: It gives confidence to the teacher during teaching. Teacher is more familiar and clear to the topic during teaching.
- ***Discipline***: Lesson plan is teacher's homework. He explain in systematic manner and make the students busy in their work. This creates a excellent discipline in class.

- *Evaluation*: Lesson plan contains the evaluation. It give the feedback to the teacher about his teaching. Evaluation contains certain questions related to the topic. This helps the teacher to adopt different strategies of teaching, teaching aid, etc.
- *Time limitation*: Lesson plan provides the time for each steps of teaching, how much time a teacher can spend on a particular task and where to give more time.
- *Limitation of subject matter*: It has a limited subject matter, it avoids unnecessary material and he limits himself to only definite and limited aspects.

Principles of Lesson Planning

Clarity

The content is break down in sub stages, so that teaching will be more effective and interesting to pupils.

Knowledge

Teachers should know about the syllabus, activities, skills, subject and content

Variety

Teaching and learning should be interactive, so that there will be no boredom in teaching. Teaching and learning should contain a variety of activity. Classroom variety refers to different activities ranging from listening, speaking, reading, and writing. Classroom variety also refers to a wide range of materials to be used in class.

Coherence and Cohesiveness

In order to make a lesson plan, teacher should connect the activity with each other. Lesson plan appears as wholeness of harmoniousness. If activities are not connected in content and purpose, there will be no flow of classroom movement.

Flexibility

Flexibility is important in lesson plan and it comes while actual teaching. Teacher is free to change the content at time of teaching in order to make the students understand. Teacher is free to adopt the new teaching aid, language skills, and teaching strategies.

Steps of Lesson Planning

The following are the steps necessary for developing lesson plan

- *Clear objectives*: In order to make a lesson plan, the first step is to formulate the objectives. There will be general and specific objectives. No matter how entertaining your lesson may be, it will not impact if it does not contain the learning objective. When a objective is well defined, it creates interest of both learner and teacher. Objectives give a direction to the teacher to make a lesson plan effective.

- *Subject matter*: Content is much essential for effective or great lesson planning. It is important to organize all the things, which a teacher needs for perfect lesson planning. Content must be specific and related to the topic of the lesson plan.
- *Procedure*: Lesson planning procedure must include the activation of student's previous knowledge, teaching and learning activities and evaluation. In the method of lesson planning, there are general and specific objectives which are written before teaching. It depends upon the teacher to write teaching–learning activities, whether it is a lecture discussion, observation or participatory.
- *Evaluation*: Evaluation is a very necessary component in lesson planning. Teacher evaluates his/her lesson planning by asking questions to the students. How effective has been the lesson plan is determined by specific objectives.

Types of Lesson Plan

The following are the types of lesson planning:
- *Knowledge lesson plan*: This type of lesson plan contains the cognitive aspect of pupils. It enriches with the knowledge of various aspects of the particular topic.
- *Skill lesson plan*: These lessons are concerned with manual or other skills, which pupils will acquire by this lesson. Skills may be in writing, speaking, dancing, singing, gymnastic, handicraft, drawing etc. Student gets the benefit of skill training through skilled lesson. It not only benefits the students but also the society.
- *Appreciation lesson plan*: It is concerned with aesthetic or appreciation sense to students. These lessons appreciate students, so that they take interest in study. The lesson in music, art etc.
- *Activity lesson plan*: It is concerned with activity. The teacher assigns the task to the pupils and gives freedom to solve them. The student learns to perform collectively.

Approaches to Lesson Planning

For Lesson planning, various educationists have given different approaches for writing the lesson:
- Herbartian approach
- Dewey and Kilpattrick approach
- Morrison's approach
- American approach

Herbartian Approach

John Fredric Herbart was a great European educationist and philosopher of 19th century. He stressed that teaching should be planned actively, if we want to implement effectively. He applied the knowledge of psychology regarding the Learning process.

Based upon educational psychology, Herbart's educational ideology advocated the following four elements for a successful teaching.

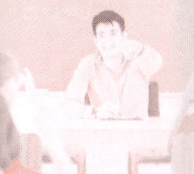

Interest

Whatever topic is presented to the students, they find the logic if the lesson plan has been made in a interesting way. Students pay the attention, when the topic is interesting. The teaching process should be interesting too.

Apperception

The entire knowledge is provided to the pupils from outside. Apperception of this external knowledge occurs in the unconscious mind of the pupils. By relating new knowledge to the previous knowledge of the pupils, their learning is simplified. Therefore, a teacher should proceed from known to unknown.

General Method

Learning activity occurs in a definite sequence. Therefore, the activities of the unit should be edited in a definite sequence.

Correlation

Knowledge is a single unit. All the subjects should be studied after correlating each other in the form of one unit.

Merits

- It is based on psychological appreciation.
- It is arranged in logical sequence.
- It uses the inductive and deductive methods.
- Previous knowledge can be correlated with new knowledge.
- New knowledge is acquired in new circumstances.

Demerits

- It is valuable in knowledge lesson.
- It has given same pace in all the subjects.
- Teacher has more active role than students.
- Teaching with different subjects makes it difficult for the students to understand.
- It does not considered the individual difference.

Morrison Unit Approach

Prof H.C Morrison gave this approach. In his book "The Practice of Teaching in Secondary Schools", he has emphasized unit method. Unit method is a more important approach:
- It is student-centered approach
- This approach considers the students needs and interests
- Unit is considered from the syllabus which can be divide in to unit and subunits

It has five steps
- Exploration
- Presentation
- Assimilation
- Explanation
- Recitation

Dewey and Kilpatrick Approach

Kilpatrick was the pupil of John Dewey. He was the former professor in education in Columbia. He was influenced by the pragmatism philosophy and believed that education should enter the real depth of life. The basic approach under Dewey and Kilpatrick is that the students can solve their life problem through this approach and acquaint with different types of experiences. Kilpatrick has mentioned seven steps in the project method:
- Creating the situation
- Selection of the project
- Purpose of the project
- Planning
- Execution
- Evaluation
- Reporting.

LESSON PLAN FORMAT FOR TEACHING

- Title of the course: _____
- Level of Student: _____
- Topic: _____
- Subject/ Unit: _____
- Duration: _____
- Date and Time: _____
- Class: _____
- Methods of teaching: _____
- Medium of Instruction (Language)- English/ Hindi: _____
- List of Teaching aids: _____
- Previous related knowledge of the students: _____
- Name of the student teacher: _____
- Name of the evaluator: _____
- **Objective**
  - **General objective:** The students will be able to understand about the
  - **Specific objective:** The students will be able to-

Contd...

Sl. No	Time	Specific objective	Content	Teaching strategies		Method of Evaluation
				Teaching- learning activities	Teaching aids	
1						
2						
3						

Summary: _____

_____

_____

Reference (in Vancouver Style)-:

1. _____

2. _____

3. _____

CLASSROOM MANAGEMENT

Effective classroom management is essential for teacher and learner. It includes all the aspects such as what is going on in the class and what the teacher has taught.

Definition

- Classroom management includes time management, student involvement, student engagement and class room communication. **—Farris**
- Classroom management consists of practices and procedures that a teacher uses to maintain the environment in which the instructions and learning can occur. **—Wong.H.K.**

Classroom Management Plan

- Clear rules and norms are set before planning the classroom management
- It is the agreement between the teacher and students to learn the content in the class without any interference and disturbance.
- Allow the students' input in classroom management, so that they are aware of violating the rules and regulation.
- Rules should be applicable to the pupils if they break the rules.
- The class teacher has insight to maintain and manage the students properly (Table 2).

TABLE 2: Difference between curriculum and syllabus

Syllabus	Curriculum
It is a specification of work	*Curriculum* as the '*Course of Actions,* course work, their content *and Experiences'* through which children become the adults, *for success in adult society.*
It covers the major areas of the subject - Sub areas of the subject	Overall goal of teaching –learning, deals with the entire set of the course
Syllabus is usually accessible to students	Curriculum is usually set out by the administration of an institute
Syllabus is descriptive in nature	Curriculum is prescriptive in nature

Essentials Points for Classroom Management

- *Understand your student*: Teacher should know each student as an individual. Build a teacher–students relationship with them based on trust and understanding. Teacher should show concern for every student. Talk informally with students before, during, and after class about their interests.
- *Establish a positive relationship*: Sometimes, students test the teacher. It is better to isolate the students who misbehave and not yourself. It is important to stay integrated with rest of the class. Teacher can change the student's behavior in the classroom. The teachers create a positive attitude for students toward the attainment of school goals. Teacher always provides the opportunity to express his concern about the academic work.
- *Praise is a powerful tool*: Praise can be used to transform a student's image and uplift the entire class. When praising students, it's important to be specific. Reinforcement is essential for a student to change their perception towards academic aspect. Clap and award are the positive reinforcements for students.
- *Create a safe learning environment*: An environment is important for student learning and motivation. The physical environment of the class such as proper lighting, room temperature, sitting arrangement, equipment and noise-free environment are some of the basic aspects which involves the students in classroom affairs.
- *Discipline*: If the teacher is more organized, there is more opportunity to focus on teaching and learning. This will help students respect the schedules. Make the obligatory rules of class and school, which are fair and consistent.
- *Be Patient*: The teacher should know how to respond to disruptive student behavior. Teacher should not take behavior personally and use positive self-talk.

SUMMARY

Education has one of its fundamental aspects the imparting of culture from generation to generation. Education encloses teaching and learning skill. It gives the firm foundation for the achievement of personal fulfilment. It also fosters individual development and prosperity Further it aim to acquaint the individual with knowledge, skill and attitude which enable them to lead a successful life. Society also enriches the quality, heritage, culture, spiritual value, belief and moral ideals with the development of individual

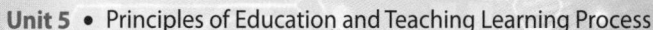

ASSESS YOURSELF

LONG ANSWER QUESTIONS

1. What is meant by teaching maxims? Write in detail.
2. What do you understand by realism? Discuss it.
3. What do you mean by education? Enumerate the aims of education and explain the social aim of education.
4. What are the different approaches to lesson planning? Discuss any one approach in detail.
5. Define lesson planning. Explain the principles of lesson planning.
6. What are the silent features of idealism as a philosophy of education?
7. Compare and contrast Realism and Pragmatism as philosophies of education.
8. Define Pragmatism. Explain the feature of pragmatism.
9. Define education. Explain the function of education in detail.

SHORT ANSWER QUESTIONS

1. Write a brief note on Herbartian approach.
2. Function of education towards individual.
3. Write about the essential components of a philosophy of education statement.
4. Write down the steps of lesson planning.
5. Enumerate the cognitive domain components.
6. Write down about Class room management.
7. Social aims of education.
8. What are the forms of naturalism.
9. What are the branches of philosophy.
10. SMART.

VERY SHORT ANSWER QUESTIONS

1. Define Education.
2. Write down the meaning of Philosophy.
3. What is Epistemology?
4. What was the main contribution of Plato?
5. What are the merits of pragmatism?
6. Enumerate the cognitive components of Bloom Taxonomy.
7. Enumerate the steps of Morrison's unit approach.
8. Enumerate the psychomotor components of Bloom Taxonomy.
9. Define classroom management.
10. Enumerate the essential points for class room management.

Contd...

MULTIPLE CHOICE QUESTIONS

1. By education, I mean an all round drawing out of the best in child and man body –mind and spirit – who said this?
   A. Swami Vivekananda
   B. Bertrand Russell
   C. John Dewey
   D. Mahatma Gandhi

2. The branch of philosophy, which deals with concept of knowledge is:
   A. Metaphysics
   B. Epistemology
   C. Logic
   D. Ethics

3. Which philosophy focuses on the experience:
   A. Existentialism
   B. Pragmatism
   C. Idealism
   D. Realism

4. Which Philosophy is known to Materialism:
   A. Naturalism
   B. Pragmatism
   C. Realism
   D. Idealism

5. What is most important in lesson plan:
   A. Teacher
   B. Content
   C. Student
   D. Home work

6. Appreciation lesson plan focusses on:
   A. Aesthetic sense to students
   B. Performance of students
   C. Activity of students
   D. Knowledge of students

7. Which method of lesson planning lays more emphasis on unit method:
   A. Herbartian lesson plan
   B. Morricon's approach
   C. Blooms approach
   D. Dewey and Kilpatrick approach

8. The following are the characteristics of objective, except:
   A. Specific
   B. Measurable
   C. Active
   D. Realistic
   E. Time Bound

9. Following are the major categories in cognitive domain except:
   A. Knowledge
   B. Comprehension
   C. Application
   D. Analysis
   E. Organization
   F. Evaluation

10. According to Bloom Taxonomy, precision is categorized under:
   A. Cognitive domain
   B. Affective
   C. Psychomotor domain
   D. Sensorial domain

ANSWERS TO MCQs

| **1.** (D) | **2.** (B) | **3.** (B) | **4.** (A) | **5.** (C) | **6.** (A) | **7.** (B) |
| **8.** (C) | **9.** (C) | **10.** (C) | | | | |

BIBLIOGRAPHY

1. Sharma BL. Maheshwari BK. Teaching of Social Science. Meerut: R.Lal Book Depot; 2013
2. Saxena Swaroop NR, Chaturvedi Shikha. Teacher in Emerging Indian Society. Meerut R.Lal Book Depot; 2011.
3. Rather AR. Theory and principle of education. New Delhi: Discovery publishing house; 2007.
4. Chandra SS, Sharma kumar Rajendra. Principles of Education. New Delhi: Atlantic publishers and distributers; 2004.
5. Bhattacharya Srinibas. Philosophical foundation of Education. New Delhi: Atlanic publisher and distributors.
6. Singh YK. Guidance and Career Counselling. New Delhi: APH Publishing; 2010.
7. Bloom Benzamin S, Taxonomy of Education Objective. N.Y: David Mckay Company, Inc; 1956.
8. Agarwal JC. Theory and Principles of Education. New Delhi: Vikas Publications;1996.

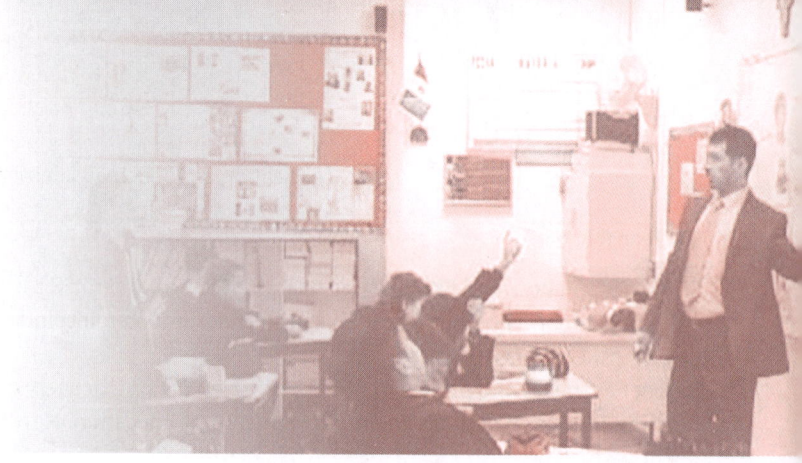

Unit 6

Methods of Teaching

— Nancy Fernandes Pereira

📖LEARNING OBJECTIVE

After the completion of the chapter, the learner will be able to –

- Define teaching
- State the principles of teaching
- Describe the features of good teaching
- Enumerate various methods of classroom teaching
- Discuss the importance of various classroom methods of teaching
- Recognize the advantages and limitations of various classroom methods of teaching

- Compare different classroom methods of teaching
- Identify the appropriate methods of classroom teaching during class presentation
- List out different clinical methods of teaching
- State the purposes of clinical teaching method
- Describe each clinical method
- Distinguish the limitations of each clinical teaching method

INTRODUCTION

A set of human behavior is infinite. Similarly, a set of teaching behavior, which is a subset of human behavior, is also infinite. For every element belonging to the set of human behavior, there exists a corresponding element in the set of teaching behaviors. This suggests that these two sets are equivalent. However, it is important to know, what is the distinguishing characteristic between these two sets of behavior. The distinguishing characteristic here is *intention*. Teaching behavior is intentional; it's basic intention is that somebody learns something.

Intentions can be as simple as knowing the name of the object and as complex as development of the character of the student. The complexity of the teaching behavior varies directly according to the complexity of intentions.

The heritage of teaching is as rich and old as the heritage of human race. Since the time of Socrates, Plato, and Aristotle, the people working in different fields have been trying to describe teaching learning process. However, there is a long standing controversy whether teaching is an art or a science. If teaching is an art, then it has to be developed like any other art. On the contrary, if it is not an art, then the skills of teaching should be developed among those who want to become teacher. In teaching, the teacher has to use his/her creative and intuitive skills at the same time while using his/her skills of teaching. If one teaches the same subject, requires to constantly improvise to move from what is routine in the expression of learning material that does not depend on fixed structures like formulas, rules and algorithms.

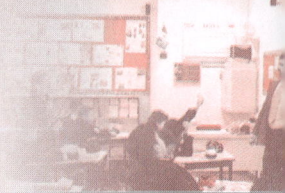

DEFINITION OF TEACHING

Many philosophers, developmental psychologists, learning theorists have put forth a number of definitions of teaching. Teaching is the arrangement of situations, which lead to desirable bonds and makes them satisfying'. —**Thorndlike**

- 'Teaching is the means where by society trains the young in a selected environment as quickly as possible to adjust themselves to the world in which they live' —**Yoakam and Simpson.**

Therefore, one can state that teaching is neither providing the knowledge required by students nor advising regarding a specific learning content, it involves integrated knowledge and skills passed on to students for enhancing the academic growth and ability to use this knowledge in life. It can also be summed as an interaction between student, subject and the mentor to bring out a new learning experience. Teaching involves providing useful information, stimulation and direction of learning to the student as being employed in modern times. It is helping the student to make effective adjustments and guiding the student's activity and training of their emotions. It's a process by which the mentor molds his/her prodigy's character through any of the following ways: intellectually, socially, emotionally, and physically, to mention a few, by using effectively communicating to them his/her ideas on the subject.

Teaching may be done formally or informally. It can be a one way method as in yesteryears, where the guru taught and students absorbed without questioning. It can be a two-way method where teacher teaches and students interact in the class with the teacher, clarifying, questioning, and debating so forth. In today's twenty-first century, teaching uses multi-way method i.e. students are not exclusively dependent on teacher; they have access to not just textbooks but multimedia as well. Hence, learning is constantly taking place. This poses a challenge for the teacher to make teaching effective and interesting in the classroom.

Teaching is influenced by teacher's own ability, mastery of the subject, environment created in the class, goals of society, available material and the training he/she has received. It's important that the teacher takes into account the student's needs, interests and goals. Although in nursing, a teacher has to follow the prescribed syllabus, he/she has to ensure its utility in the field in the students will work later. While teaching, teacher has to remember that it should be student-centric irrespective of the adopted which method of teaching. As and when required a teacher also has to ensure. Although the focus of the content.

PRINCIPLES OF GOOD TEACHING

In the teaching learning process, the role of teacher and learner is important and at the same time, the context, learning objectives, teaching medium, learning outcome are also very important.

Keeping this in mind, the principles of teaching are follows:

- In teaching learning process, teacher must recognize the individual difference in the students.
- Teaching must be learner-centered.
- Teacher should understand the interest of students and use effective methods, thus, creating the interest of the students and maintaining it.
- Teacher should be critical but should encourage the students by recognizing, appreciation and approval for their performance.
- A teacher should provide a challenging to the learner and should be able to create a situation through which the student learns effectively.

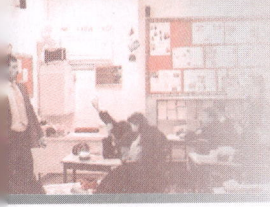

- Teacher should create an inquiring environment for the students, which will stimulate imagination, and facilitate and promote learning.
- Teacher should conform to the aims of nursing education by planning the learning experience, carrying it out effectively and evaluating at the end of the experience to ensure that the desired learning experience was delivered.
- Good teaching should help in the all round development of the students.
- Good teaching should incorporate various methods depending on the subject, situation and the needs of learning.
- Good teaching should not seek perfection in a single method.

FEATURES OF GOOD TEACHING

- Good teaching involves essential skills to guide learner.
- It is planned carefully.
- It is co-operative and suggestive to the students.
- It is democratic in nature.
- It is stimulating in nature.
- Although it takes the student's previous experience in account, yet it is progressive in nature.
- It is both diagnostic and remedial.
- In other words, good teaching liberates the mind of the learner.

Therefore, good teaching should follow the **maxims of teaching:** moving from what a student knows to what is unknown to him/her; teaching what is simple first and then moving to complex content; definite to indefinite; concrete to abstract; particular to general using both deductive and inductive thinking process; and keeping in mind the psychology of the learner.

There are a **number of methods** that the teacher can employ in the **classroom** to teach: Lecture method, discussion, seminars, discussion, role play, project, assignments, symposium, field trips, exhibition, computed-based/assisted learning, micro teaching, problem-based learning (PBL), simulations programmed instruction, and self-instructional modules (SIM).

The teacher can use demonstration in the classroom as well as in the clinical area. In the **clinical area,** teaching method that can include clinical teaching, nursing rounds, clinical reports, patient-based case study, bedside clinics, process recording and nursing conferences.

The teacher has to use various teaching techniques and methods while giving instructions; a lot of which is verbal structuring in the classroom to introduce new concepts, principles, generalization, procedures, etc. This is done most often in the colleges even today through lectures.

LECTURE METHOD

Lecture method is the oldest method used for attaining the objectives laid for teaching a specific topic and education as a whole. To ensure effective lectures, one must be aware of the style of lecturing, skill of teaching method and organization of teaching content. Lecturing style is highly individualistic but there are certain styles discussed by theorists.

Oral Lecture

In this method, the teacher depends largely on their verbal ability and communication skills. Though the teacher may structure the lecture properly, it may not be sorted as per the objectives written for the lecture. Sometimes they fail to mention the objective of the class to the students. The teacher does not use any visual presentation like black/white board, overhead projector, diagrams or power point presentation, which may be considered as negative aspect of the lecture. This method is usually used by the teacher of humanities and social science.

Exemplary Lecture

In this style of lecture, the teacher is against reading the lecture and resists providing a detailed content on the topics to the students. They confidently organize the lecture in a logical flow and support it with visuals, depicting the process or steps involved in the topic. The teacher ensures by repeating key points and summarizes points appropriately. They expect students to go back and read further on the topic. This method is mostly used by biomedical science teachers.

Information Providing Lecture

Teachers using this style act as newscaster in their classroom. They structure their class well but have an inclination to reproduce from their lecture notes. This aspect may affect their presentation of lecture, even if visuals are used and teacher is very certain and self-reliant. He/she gives complete content in their lecture, leaving very little for the student to explore. This style is mostly found to be used by teachers from the science and engineering.

Amorphous Lecture

This style of lecture is the most negative style of teaching in lecture method. The teachers using this style have no set objectives and do not prepare their lesson adequately. As a result, their presentation is deficit of impact as compared to other styles of lecture. This style may be used by teachers from the science and engineering.

Self Doubters

The teachers using this style would have problem in identifying and organizing their lecture content. While teaching, they stay away from the lecture notes prepared by them. As a result of adopting this style, the teacher has a feeling of dissatisfaction because of not attaining the set of objectives. This style may be adopted by the teachers in most of the fields.

STEPS IN LECTURE METHOD (FIG. 1)

Experience is not the only factor determining the style of lecturing. While senior teachers may be slightly different in their style than juniors, the former are likely to use illustrations in a more outstanding manner during the lecture. To make lecture method more effective, the teacher has to keep the following things in mind:

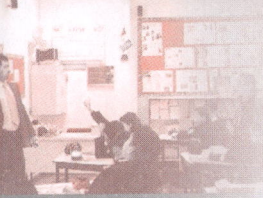

Set Induction

Set induction is also referred to as introduction. It influences the outcome of teaching. Its function is to focus the student's attention, use some previous knowledge to build upon, to provide structure or framework for the lesson and to advance or to give meaning to new concepts or principles. While the teacher observes the classroom, he/she prepares a suitable physical/emotional environment, asks questions based on previous knowledge, arouses curiosity of the students and creates dissonance in the classroom.

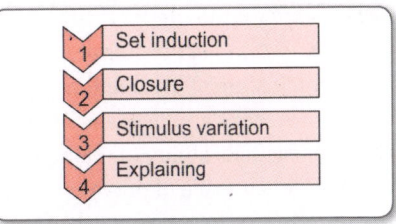

Fig. 1: Steps adopted for effective lecture

Closure

It complements set induction/introduction. It draws attention to the end of a specific learning sequence or of an entire lesson by focusing on what has been learned. Effective closures or conclusions reinforce what has been learned by reviewing the key points of a lesson and relating to other material the students have already learnt in the class. The function of the closure is to help the students in retaining the important points presented in the class and to introduce activities for future learning. Here, the teacher summarizes in the light of the objectives, links with similar situations, future learning and reviews with different aspects.

Stimulus Variation

It refers to the process of teaching or teacher liveliness. Variation in teaching can occur in different ways i.e. in the pattern and level of interaction between teacher and student; between students, for example, debate introduced in the lecture; and variation in the media and material instruction, for example, teacher can provide handouts or videos and build lesson around it or change the teaching style.

The purpose of introducing stimulus variability is to arouse and sustain student's attention to relevant aspects of teaching and learning. It provides opportunity for stimulating curiosity and motivation and helps in building positive attitude towards the subject, the teacher and the institution. It caters to the sensory preferences and facilitates learning. It promotes learning by involving students in a variety of attractive and purposeful experiences at varied cognitive levels. The teacher needs to use gestures, verbal focusers, change the pattern of speech, use audiovisual aids and change the interaction pattern.

Explaining

It is described as a systematically organized verbal process aimed at establishing understanding in an arbitrary manner that does not depend on a particular content or particular teacher. The success of explanation is indicated by the degree of understanding demonstrated by the students.

The function of explaining is to establish cause-effect relationship and to link different aspects of the subject matter i.e. events, objects or action etc. The factors that contribute to the effectiveness of explanations are the continuity of thought i.e. the flow of sequence and the fluency, simplicity in use of vocabulary, avoiding grammatical complexity and explicitness of content.

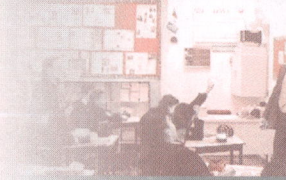

A clear explanation depends upon:

- Identification of the components to be related, for example, objects, events, processes, etc
- Identification of the relationship between the components that is casual, justified, interpreting
- The teacher's ability to speak with clarity, fluently and using appropriate vocabulary in the class
- The teacher's ability to maintain continuity of thought in relation to the content that has a logical flow, follows rule of providing examples wherever needed, make interlinked statements and avoid unnecessary repetition.

QUALITIES OF A GOOD LECTURE

The length of lecture should not be too long or too short and in both cases, holding students' attention is very important. The qualities of a good lecture are described below:

- It should address one topic or concept.
- It should simplify technical terms.
- It should include well acquainted examples and representations.
- There should be a natural flow while explaining technical content.
- A good lecture should use case illustrations from clinical area.
- It should be based on available facts/reality.
- It should be used in various innovative ways.

Activities to be used in Classroom to Enrich Teaching

There are a number of activities that a teacher can incorporate to make the lecture interactive and integrated. This helps in engaging the students actively and facilitates better interaction between student and teacher and it also helps to vitalize the learning process by providing a change in pace.

The activities that can be integrated are as follows:

- Questioning
- Pros and cons grid
- Debate
- Guided analysis
- Case study
- Buzz group
- Brain storming
- Quick test
- Non evaluator quiz

Questioning

It is the simplest form of interactive teaching tool. It can make students active and gauge their level of interest, if they are able to comprehend.

Teacher's Role

- Develop key questions before class as one should not depend for questions to occur on the spot.

- Decide when to ask. Put forth questions which students will be able to respond to. It is preferable to use open-ended questions rather than close-ended questions like answering in yes or no.
- Prepare questions covering a range of difficulty level. It's good to have some questions which rely on general knowledge to encourage the students to answer and participate actively.
- Questions with more than one concept should be asked to assess student's ability to link analyses before responding.
- One question at a time should be put forth to avoid confusion i.e., avoid firing one question after another.

Function of Question in Class

Discussion is enhanced when appropriate questions are posed in the class room. Questions asked in the early part of the class serve to stimulate and gauge level of students' knowledge or previous learning; in the middle of the class to prevent boredom and sustain enthusiasm; and at the end to conclude key points and build base for next lecture/class.

Pros and Cons Grid

This technique, when used in class, encourages critical thinking and also develops analytical skills among students, i.e. helps them to think out of the box for solutions or strategies. This essential skill is needed for students to deal in the clinical area. Students can evaluate the positive and negative aspects of procedures, techniques, actions etc.

Teacher's Role

Divide the students into small groups. Instruct the students with the number of pros and cons each group/ individual should develop. Allow them 5–10 minutes for discussion, i.e. give them time to think. The teacher or a student may be nominated to put the pros and cons list by students on the chalk board. Teacher can compare the points that are repeated to indicate their importance.

Function of Pros and Cons Grid in Class

It stimulates discussion, used to evaluate course material/nursing intervention and discuss strategies in nursing management class.

Debate

Using debate, different points of view can be expressed by a large group without disturbing the decorum of the class. Teacher can jointly or independently plan the debate before hand or it can emerge spontaneously from lecture point.

Teacher's Role

Teacher should describe the background, context and objective of the debate. Set ground rules for the discussion and group the students according to their point of view or according to their seating. Assign a point for agreement or ask which group is going to be for and against. Invite one of the students to start

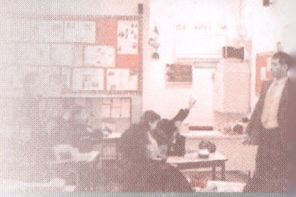

by stating their point and then continuing the debate from the other group. The teacher can appoint a moderator or moderate himself/herself. The teacher should remember that it may start slowly but gets picked at the point when students get comfortable and are encouraged to participate. The teacher should not express judgment at any point as it may embarrass the students but may ask questions to provoke new ideas. Debate should not be stretched beyond 10–15 minutes.

Function of Debate in Class

It is used to build ideas, encourage thinking critically and encourage healthy competition.

Guided Analysis

It can be incorporated when the students are on a field trip or observing a procedure under the guidance of teacher. Time required to conduct a session is about 30–50 minutes.

Teacher's Role

- Identify a text content, news/journal article, a procedure or a research abstract/methodology as an exercise to practice.
- Distribute the copy of the selected exercise among students, it may be performed as a group or an individual activity.
- Do the analysis of the selected activity before the students, so that it helps them to understand the steps to draw conclusions, which may be supported by putting points or developing flow charts on the board, using additional reference material to finalize conclusion.
- Provide opportunity and adequate time ranging from 5–10 minutes to critically analyze the selected content independently and facilitate analyzing ability under the guidance of the teacher.
- Choose team leaders among the group to present their report and provide feedback to each group.

Function of Guided Analysis in Class

This activity can form the basis of the class or session to be covered for that hour. The activity may be started after a brief lecture on the type of document/procedure, objectives of the exercise and area to focus on the document/procedure that will be analyzed in class.

Case Study

This method was first adopted by faculty of law and business schools. The care provided by the students to the patient can be analyzed, as well as unusual conditions observed in patients can be studied through case study method. Similarly, teachers who teach different subjects can modify and use this technique as per the need. It facilitates application of theoretical content beyond the class room and assures its utility in practical area. The required time is about 20 –50 minutes.

Teacher's Role

- Identify content which can be used as study material for case study, like case narrations, classic case studies or videos of cases. For example, when taking class of management, one can get video of a case dealing with problems related to collective bargaining, or news article on staff nurses-ethics in patient care etc

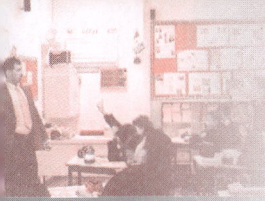

- Provide students with guideline to aid analyzing
- Encourage students to note down their findings either in group or independently
- Examine the arguments raised by student on the case
- Provide guidelines and encourage students to comply
- Avoid giving your point of view.
- Be an observer and speak only when you need to get students back on track
- At the end of the discussion, help the students to link it to the course content and theoretical concepts.

Function of Case Study in Class

Case study can be used as an example to simplify course content or build the lecture around it so that one can keep referring back to it.

Buzz Groups

It is another method that can be incorporated in class. When a lecture span is of 2–3 hour duration, students need to be stimulated through questioning or issue can be posed to get a different view point. Since everyone interacts at once, a noise is generated which energizes the participants. When they feel there is nothing more, no new idea or view is generated. For this activity, students/participants can be formed in group of two or four but not more than seven so that everyone has opportunity to share their view. A representative from a group reports to all in the class.

Purposes

- To encourage creative thinking
- To encourage innovative ideas
- To allow expressing one's view point/idea
- To generate a large reservoir of information.

Teacher's Role

- Select that topic from the lesson about which students have some background information and assign it to the students.
- Split the students into a group of 5–8 students depending on the size of the class.
- Ask the group to select a team or group leader to note the points and present at the end of discussion.

Advantages

- Buzz groups help students to develop new ideas.
- It allows assessing the temperament of the audience/participants by monitoring their interaction.
- It gives opportunity to students to assess their learning.
- It improves confidence to implement theoretical learning in clinical practice.

Limitations

- Teacher may be unfamiliar of its use in the class.
- Time required is more if it is not properly planned.

- A group leader to lead each buzz group is needed else there will be a chaos.
- More time is required to rearrange the seating in the class.

Brain Storming

This activity is taken up to generate new ideas and get quick reactions. This facilitates elicitation of unusual concepts. The group interaction revolves around coming up with something, which no one had thought before. All ideas that are generated get equal weightage and none are discarded. It encourages and stimulates even the timid students to speak up and contribute.

Teacher's Role

- Teacher should motivate students to freely express their ideas even if it does not seem important.
- A representative or teacher herself can list points on the chalk board/chart as they are generated. Later teacher along with the students may assess the feasibility of the points/idea/concept/steps of procedure etc.
- All the similar points are grouped and arranged under subheadings so that the most appropriate may be chosen.
- The activity should be planned for a stipulated time period so that it prevents losing track of time and diversion from the main theme.

Function of Brain Storming in Class

- To generate new concepts, ideas within short time using the experience of the participants and their thinking process
- Unlike a buzz session, a brainstorming session can work well with a large group and usually takes less time.

Advantages

- Many ideas and concepts can be quickly generated in short time.
- It is also useful in encouraging weak students for participation.

Limitations

It is time consuming and needs skill to organize and facilitate.

Quick Test

The quick test is short written activity in class that requires just 3–5 minutes. It helps to know if the students have understood or have clarity of the topic that is covered in the class. It also helps to know if the students are able to answer/respond. It also provides information without making the students aware that they are being assessed on the topic taught in the class. It also helps in reviewing the class quickly that assures the teacher whether the students have understood the content or not.

Teacher's Role

- Give a hint for the test such as "what was the most important clinical feature of this condition?" or "what were the main features covered in this lecture?"

- Give few minutes to the students before noting down their response. Then give few more minutes to pen down as many points as possible.
- Since there is no grading, students may not be asked to put their names that facilitates in expressing their views.
- Objective questions for example, fill in the blanks, match the following, define the terms, etc. may be corrected by exchanging the sheets among them in the class for quick assessment and the answer key may be given to the students.

Functions of Quick Test in the Class

- Quick test can be given either at the beginning of the class as review or end of the class to assess what is learned. This motivates and builds students' confidence.
- It also assures whether the students have understood or grasped the content.
- The quick test findings can be used to base the next lecture or session.
- It provides the opportunity to clarify and answer queries, which in turn builds faith and trust that teacher is capable of satisfying/clarifying their doubt and makes the next class interactive.

Non Evaluator Quiz

A non-evaluator quiz motivates participants to be attentive and focused during the session without making them uncomfortable or feeling challenged. It also provides data without students becoming aware that they are being evaluated. It does not require much time; allotted time could be 5–10 minutes.

Teacher's Role

- Prepare a list of questions, which will generate one word answer or quick response on a sheet of paper/display using overhead projector.
- Students may write their response or answer orally.
- In case they are writing, they need not write their names as there is no grading. This will allow them to write without hesitation.
- If sheets are collected, feedback can be given in the next session.
- Use variation when using non evaluators quiz.
- It can be assessed in class itself where students correct each other's responses based on the answer key read by the teacher.
- The students may be divided into two teams and each team will respond to questions in turn. If a group does not answer the question, it is to be passed to the next group giving opportunity to score a point. This will encourage competition. However, the disadvantage is that the timid or quiet students may not participate as students who are vocal may dominate.

Function of Nonevaluator Quiz in the Class

It helps to assess the knowledge of the students before initiating a lecture or at the end of the class, if they have understood the topic and summarization has to be done.

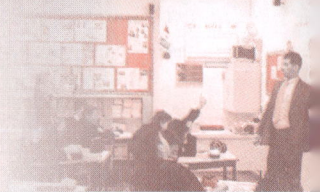

Advantage

- It motivates student to answer and helps in evaluating the learning done in the class.
- It also helps the teacher to evaluate the effectiveness of the content taught.

SEMINARS

It is a short intensive course study, where specialists come together to discuss/consult a selected topic or technique. There may be several or one keynote speaker in each seminar. All the speakers are experts in their own field or topic.

Classification

- Mini seminar at class room level
- Seminar at departmental/institutional level
- National seminar at national level
- International seminar at International level

Seminar as a Method of Teaching

It is a discussion method of teaching where an informal group of 10–15 (not more than 25–30 participants) learners participate to solve problems following scientific approach and analyze or learn a topic, for example, a seminar on neonatal resuscitation/IV line management, etc.

It is an organized, guided discussion with a focus on the discovery of new relationship by the participating individuals. It differs from intellectual initiative. The students play an active role in seminar.

Purposes

- To provide opportunity in participating in discussion methods that involves scientific analysis
- To allow students to do considerable library research prior to the seminar
- To promote critical thinking and problem solving skill
- To promote team spirit and cooperativeness
- To develops communication skills.

Characteristics

- Seminar is a type of group discussion methods.
- In a classroom level of seminar, the group generally consists of 10–15 participants.
- Persons involved in the seminar are called as Organizer, Chairperson, speakers and participants.
- An ideal seminar should last for 1–2 hours.

How to Conduct a Student Seminar?

- The topic is initially presented by the presenter followed by group discussion.
- The leader should keep the discussion within limits so the focus of discussion can be maintained, Care should be taken to avoid stereotypes.

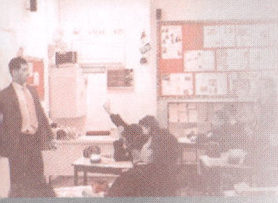

- In student seminars, students present their data in an informal way under the leadership of the teacher, followed by a teacher-monitored discussion. In higher group of learners, the student leader appointed may function as a monitor.
- All members take part in discussion in an informal but orderly manner.
- The student chairman should be skilled in encouraging the timid participants.
- A student secretary may record the problems that come up and the solutions given to them, or make note of points of discussion.

Steps in Organizing a Seminar

- Define the purpose of the seminar.
- Relate the topic of seminar and discussion to the main concept or the objectives.
- Direct and focus the discussion on the topic.
- Help students to express their ideas and keep the discussion at a high level of interest so that they attentively listen to those who contribute the ideas.
- Plan comments and questions that relate to the subject and also guide and direct the discussion.
- Set time limitations for each person's contribution.
- Guard against monopoly of the discussion by any member of the seminar.
- Plan for summary at intervals during the discussion and also before concluding a session, correlate concepts that are expressed for the purpose of discussion.
- Have the discussion recorded by a student as a recording secretary or by tape recording. This allows to review the content or to make notes.
- Plan for teacher and student self-evaluation of the progress made towards the immediate objectives.

Role of a Teacher

- Select the topic that can be handled by students.
- Give reasonable time for preparation of the topic.
- Remain in the background in the seminar, but sit where the whole group can be seen.
- Help in the initial stages if the student doesn't know how to proceed.
- Be sure that essential points are not overlooked and gross inadequacies are corrected (preferably by the other members of the class if they cannot, then teacher should add or correct).
- Make sure that all members have a share/chance to participate in the discussion and that irrelevant discussion is avoided.

Advantages

- Students get involved in the learning process when seminar method is used.
- A properly conducted seminar has potentials to teach students to analyze the content and searches for relevant content to be included for the presentation.
- Individual student and the group as a whole try to gather content for the seminar.
- Exchange of facts and ideas occurs to crystallize group opinion.
- The problem solving skills of the students are sharpened by participation as they learn to plan and organize the seminar.
- The students develop critical thinking skills as they participate in the seminar.

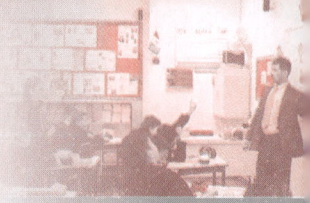

- A seminar helps in self-learning and promotes independent thinking.
- It develops ability to see own problems that increase because of personal difficulties and can be compared with those of the group.
- Skillfully directed seminar promotes group spirit and cooperation.

Limitations

- Seminar is a time consuming process.
- It cannot be applied to freshers or to a new subject.
- Timid or weak students may initially feel nervous or find it difficult to deal or present the topic.
- Students lacking the power of vocabulary or language mastery may find it difficult to express themselves.
- If subject knowledge is poor, unnecessary discussions arise.

SYMPOSIUM

Symposium is an interesting method of teaching by which concepts and topics can be discussed. It also helps the participants and experts to clarify their own ideas and thoughts and drawing conclusions regarding a particular issue or a topic.

Meaning of Symposium

Symposium is coming together of likeminded individuals from the same faculty/field with the purpose of sharing views on a selected topic, where in some present the views and others form the audience. Symposium is a discussion method where exchange of ideas, concept and strategies occur on a topic/area of interest. Symposium is a series of speeches on single aspect of a topic.

Purposes

- To recognize and comprehend various dimensions of a given topic or subject
- To refine skills of decision making and provide solutions/strategies to issues
- To be sensitive to the problems faced by patients due to disease
- To sensitize students/participants on a topic/disease/culture and emotions
- To facilitate the participants to form protocol related to the issue/condition
- To investigate a problem from several points of view
- To boost students' abilities to speak in the group
- To encourage the students to study independently.

Characteristics

- Symposium helps to comprehend a topic or problem.
- The audience is allowed to take a stand related to the issue or a problem.
- This method is used in higher classes for specific theme or a problem.
- It develops a feeling of cooperation and adjustment.
- Symposium technique helps in achieving the objectives of synthesis and evaluation.
- It provides different views on the topic of the symposium.

Principles

- The speeches may be persuasive, argumentative and informative.
- Presentation is objective and accurate.
- This method always includes a summary at conclusion.
- Every speaker presents their content uninterrupted.
- The convener introduces the theme and may also give the key note address.
- All the presenters are seated facing the audience with the convener in the middle or at one side.
- The seating arrangement can be done according to the content being presented. if it is 'for' and 'against' an issue, presenters may be seated on two sides of the stage and the convener center stage.

Guidelines

- The convener of the session introduces the subtheme and highlight key points.
- Each speaker is allocated 15–20 minutes.
- Each speaker would present their conviction, reasoning or contention, sharing new data or drawing out feelings.
- After completion of presentation by each speaker, the session is open to the audience so they can clarify or add to the issue/topic.

Advantages

- Symposium can be used to address a large group or class.
- This method can be frequently used to present broad topics for discussion during conventions and organization of meetings.
- In symposium, the principle of organizing is high as the speeches are planned beforehand.
- It gives a deeper insight into a topic.
- It directs the students for continuous independent study.
- This method can be used in ethics or topics that can generate different opinion.

Limitations

- Symposium does not provide adequate opportunity for all the students to participate actively.
- It has limited audience participation.
- The speech is limited to 10–20 minutes.
- Question and Answer session is limited to 3–4 minutes.
- It has possibility of overlapping of subjects.
- The speakers have the liberty to prepare and present the content where in the chairperson cannot restrain them from expressing on the theme. They can present any aspect of the theme or problem.
- There is a possibility of repetition of content. As each presenter may present subtheme that overlaps with other speakers, which is sometimes difficult to comprehend for the listeners.
- If the subthemes are not presented simultaneously, then the listeners are not able to understand the theme correctly.
- The listeners remain passive in the symposium because they are not given an opportunity to seek clarification and question in between the symposium.

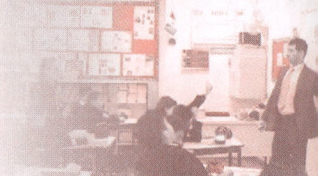

DISCUSSION

Discussion involves interaction between two or more individuals. In the classroom, it includes the facilitator and learner who interact in a discussion. In this method of teaching, an individual listens and speaks, which make it a proactive learning process than the traditional lecture method. The process fosters sharing of learned experiences, concepts and attitude by involving students/participants, which may bring about a positive change. It can be used to build a lesson on the basis of what is known to the students and also to deduce if they have learned.

Types of Discussion

It is of two types: Group discussion and Panel discussion.

Uses of Discussion Method

When students have some information on a selected topic, a broad outline can be developed before starting a lesson. For example, in maintaining body mechanics while transferring patient, many of the steps can be elicited by students through a discussion. The learners contribute from their real life experience. It also helps to demystify issues, ideas and concepts, if point of difference also arises in the process. Being a proactive process, discussion stimulates better learning among students as compared to a passive method adopted by lecture.

Uses of Discussion for Application

It helps to make learning more permanent and encourages application of what is learned in clinical practice. The teacher can help to connect and correlate concepts to clinical practice. After completing a teaching session, a teacher can pose a question or make a statement that can stimulate discussion.

Uses of Discussion to Obtain Feedback

Based on the contribution of the students, it is evaluated that to what extent learning has occurred and content is comprehended. Discussion method can be adopted in combination of other teaching methods to enhance learning experience. This also provides feedback to the teacher to improve her own skills of teaching and motivate to use variation in teaching.

How to Conduct a Discussion?

It can be incorporated by the teacher in the class, where she may lead or get a student to lead.

- Co-relate appropriate case story/anecdote to make discussion factual.
- Integrate similar situations and solutions.
- Contribute ideas or personal opinions.
- Share/add one's view point based on one's own learning.

Irrespective of who leads the discussion, it should be within the framework of the goal of the lesson/topic. It's the onus of the teacher to ensure the goal of the lesson is met and students do not stray from the topic. The facilitator has to ensure that the decorum is maintained so that insignificant discussion is avoided.

PANEL DISCUSSION

In this method of teaching, a topic is divided into four or five students who function as panelist; one of the students plays the role of moderator. The moderator introduces the topic and invites the panel members to present their point of view. The moderator may put questions to stimulate discussions among the panelist. Before closure of discussion, opportunity is given to students in the audience to put question or to present their view point. If the audience does not participate, the moderator has to put questions to the audience to stimulate discussion. When the session comes to an end, the moderator concludes and presents the key points or highlights of important aspects of the discussion.

The role of the teacher is to plan the topic to be assigned for panel discussion, allocate time frame for preparation and conduct the panel discussion. Teacher ensures the panelists sit in a semicircle fashion with moderator in the center. Teacher ensures that the group rehearses before the presentation so that each member is aware of the content that the other will present. Sometimes, the teacher may assume the role of moderator, if panel discussion is held for the first time in class or select a bright and mature student with ability to control the group.

Advantages

- Emphasizes on learning instead of teaching
- Facilitates participation by everyone in the class
- Encourages reflective thinking and self-expression
- Inculcates respect for others point of view or idea
- Spirit of tolerance is inculcated
- Learning is made interesting and provides opportunity for assimilation of content.

Limitations

- Panel discussion method is not appropriate for all the topics.
- It can be used only for students who have some basic knowledge of the topic.
- Some of the students may feel shy or reluctant to take part, while others may try to dominate in a group discussion.
- In panel discussion, the audience may feel nothing to contribute and remain as passive participants.
- There are chances when the group or panelist may deviate from the topic.
- If there are differences in the group or among the panelists, it may result in disagreement.

PROJECT METHOD

It is one of the modern methods of teaching based on the philosophy of pragmatism. Activities are given on a selected theme/concept. Based on it, students have to complete an assignment, which provide real life experience to students and they need to participate actively.

Definition

Projects are activities carried out by the students with a purpose to master a skill, technique or to sensitize them in a natural environment.

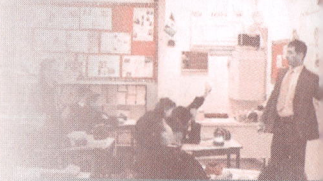

Project is the means through which students are exposed to real life situation issues/problems and encourage developing strategies independently or as a team, simultaneously learning to share and corporate.

It is a voluntary undertaking, which involves constructive effort or thought and eventuates into objective results.

According to Kilpatric, "a project is a whole-hearted purposeful activity proceeding in a social environment."

Characteristics

- It has some definite attainable goal.
- It is an activity done outside the class room.
- It is performed in a real situation, thereby giving a real experience.
- It is directed and planned by the students.
- It is practical in nature and the emphasis on a single concrete achievement.
- It promotes inquiring attitude, so as to reach a feasible solution.
- The project has to be done by the student themselves, which motivates them to think creatively.
- Students in the process of completing their project develop a scientific temperament.
- It provides learning experience, which comes from doing by one self.
- It helps student to work in team, and also to be resourceful.

Types of Project

Individual and Group Project

- **Individual project:** Individual project is solely done by a student, so that he may acquire the required experience to meet the needs of the goal or learning. This student is solely responsible to plan and execute the complete project.
- **Group projects:** These are the projects dealt by number of individuals with different skills or interests to develop strategies for solving a problem or issue. As a result, students learn to work together/function as a team with individuals of different personality and maintain team spirit.

  The project is planned and executed by a group of students. The project is divided into subparts that are assigned to each member of the group. On completing their part, the project is assembled.

Simple and Complex Project

- **Simple projects:** These are short projects with single theme that permits students to explore its different facets. They require less time to complete and yet gain a deep insight on a selected aspect. For example, in a project on growth and development, specific age group is divided into groups in class. Each group focuses on one specific age. This allows in-depth learning.
- **Complex projects:** Complex projects are those that have two or more aspects and require more time and technical skills and different dimensions/faculties are involved. Students learn to appreciate contribution of various subject experts, who have contributed to a device, or structure. For example, "Taj Mahal" as a project for architecture student –its history, structure, water system, aesthetic sense; similarly, for nursing students, a project on ventilator: understanding the principles involved, impact on the lungs, psychology of relatives, biomechanics involved etc.

According to Kilpatrick, there are four types of projects:

- **Constructive project:** It involves tasks that require students to recreate a device or make a working model or yet device a modified version of the original equipment/instrument. It may include preparing a model like water purification plant, model of infection control at ICU, isolation unit, nurses' station for ICU, etc.
- **Aesthetic project:** It is based on developing a sense of valuing a piece of work/art by involving students so that they recreate a musical composition, a design, articles, identifying medicinal plants, water purification mechanism, etc.
- **Problematic project:** It is to enhance student's analytical skill where they can identify or come up with strategies to resolve the situation/issues or hindrances. These are project for intellectual development through critical and creative thinking such as solving some patient problems, modification of procedure based on availability of articles.
- **Drill project:** It enhances and improves the manual dexterity, presentation skills, where the student is expected to repeat the same skill to achieve perfection and speed in carrying out a task. In this type of project, main aim of learning is acquisition of some ability/skill, for example, making a fracture bed, CPR, setting up of labor room or steps of delivery.

Criteria for Selecting Project

- The learning activity must be problematic in nature.
- The activity should have academic weightage.
- It should not be time consuming, inexpensive and material should be easily accessible.
- It should be difficult yet stimulating and should give a sense of satisfaction.
- It should not be the only method employed to complete a syllabus.
- Project should be selected according to the student's interest.

Role of the Teacher

The teacher has to play some role while selecting project as method of teaching, which include the following:

- Should act as a mentor
- Motivates students to work as a team
- Prevents students from getting dejected because of error
- Ensures each student must finish the task
- Encourages taking leadership role to complete the task
- Gives useful tips in case the students face hindrance or thought block
- Conducive environment should be created for free expression of ideas
- Monitor the task to ensure its pace is on schedule and fulfilling the objective
- Assign task as per their level of knowledge and capacity to achieve
- Should be motivated and proactive
- Should create an attitude of sharing within and between the groups
- Equality should be maintained among students while implementing the project
- Should have adequate knowledge and awareness of project completion

Steps Involved in Project Method

- **Step I – Identify the reason:** Identifying the reason of selecting a particular topic as project is the first step from which objectives are determined. The project should not appear as a punishment or an assignment merely to keep them busy but have learning value.

- **Step II – Identify the issue:** In the second step, project related issues are clarified such as to what extent teacher's supervision is required to complete the assignment, funding, time constraint etc. Teacher can entice/attract them to this methodology for learning but the final decision should be of student as learning should be student-centered.

- **Step III – Planning:** The teacher helps the student to work out the sequence of the project and its requirements, but the idea and concepts should come from students and the teacher's role is merely of a mentor.

- **Step IV – Execution:** In this stage, students implement their laid out plan following sequence after the required data and equipment/articles have been assembled. Teacher has to ensure that they do not deviate or lag behind the planned schedule also check, if they are following the plan made to complete the project.

- **Step V – Assessment:** Assessment of the project should not be done only by the teacher but it should be assessed by peers also. Firstly, assessment includes the objectives of the project and secondly, every step of the project needs to be assessed.

- **Step VI – Reporting and Recording:** It is the final step in the project, where the individual student or group is responsible to report about all activities of project. The report may be submitted in written format as per the guidelines including project plan, implementation, completion, and experiences of difficulties/hindrances faced. The contribution of every team member should be acknowledged and list of resources tapped can be included. The documentation can become a reference for future projects. It may be submitted as a booklet on its completion or the projects are displayed for teachers and other students to understand and learn.

Advantages of Project Method

- Gives the students a free rein to express themselves
- Sustains the interest and enhances ability of the students
- Identifies individual potential
- Develops creative and analytical thinking
- Contributes to all-round development of the student
- Provides opportunity to students to introspect their work
- Builds confidence to plan and execute with the best of their ability and maintaining the standard
- Project method is student-centered rather than being only subject or teacher-centered
- Student's learning need and desire to explore are met
- Develops a temperament of critical thinking
- Provides adequate opportunity to develop coordination of their physical skill and creative skill
- Supports holistic development of the student
- Contributes to learning and improving group dynamics and developing sense of togetherness, endurance while collaborating with others
- There is permanence of acquired knowledge, which will be retained for long time as students have acquired it themselves
- It helps to widen their perception and understanding
- Stimulates students to deal with issues and difficulties in a positive way and getting the best out of the situation
- It helps in developing social norms and social values among the learners.

Limitations

- The word project may be misunderstood.
- The project cannot be planned for all subjects.
- Project cannot cover all subject matter; it only cover the selected portion.
- Irrelevant aspects may be assigned as a project.
- Project as a method of teaching is time consuming.
- It is expensive.
- Required resources may not always be accessible.
- Repetition of matter may occur in two or more projects if poorly planned.
- It requires a competent teacher who guides students.
- Through this method students learn by doing and learning is limited to that activity.
- Sometimes the project may be assigned for course completion instead of challenging and need based topic that may result in non-attainment of learning objectives.

ROLE PLAY

Role play is enactment of a scenario where individuals would react to different situations. It can be used to sensitize student in different situations, which helps to develop empathy. While performing role play, it provides opportunity to sensitize to fact and life situation. It is widely accepted method of teaching in number of disciplines like nursing, medicine, management, etc., i.e. for counseling patients or relatives, conflict management, etc.

Uses

- To catch attention of audience before a session
- To introduce a difficult topic
- To understand complicated situations
- Through role play information is disseminated in an interesting way
- To link different dimensions of the subject matter under a broad frame
- To rehearse before actually getting in to a situation
- To develop skills in leadership and social interactions
- To practice selected behavior in a real life situation without the stress of making mistakes
- To improve on interviewing techniques
- To explore complex issues and deal with potential conflicts during meetings.

Teacher's Role

- Create scenario from clinical experience or by writing a story/script from scratch.
- Clarify objective of using a role-play to teach a selected topic.
- Provide a brief of the setting, in which the act is occurring.
- Assign students to the part that they have to play/enact.
- Involve students in taking part as role player, observer, reporter etc. rather than being passive observers.

- Give time for students to get in to the character they have to play.
- Keep the role play short, not more than 5–10 minutes, if used for introducing a topic.

Advantages

- Helps to stimulate and build interest at the beginning of teaching session
- Builds enthusiasm among students
- Improves the students' ability to disseminate information to a large audience through visual presentation
- Teaches to appreciate different situations
- Motivates students to think out of the box
- Helps to integrate different aspects
- Helps to realize sensitive issues
- Provides a chance to clarify personal issues that have been encountered
- Provides opportunity to get in to the skin of the character and comprehend the depth and breadth of the scenario/issue.

Limitations

- Role plays require active participation of the learner; being a passive observer does not helps in attainment of educational objectives.
- To perform effective role play, it needs time to rehearse.
- Students may not feel comfortable in playing all types of character.
- At the times of role play, it may arouse disturbing feeling because of negative role.

TUTORIAL METHOD

It is a method of teaching where a student is directly mentored by the teacher through tuition or coaching. Tutorial teaching method is a follow up study of lectures, highly individualized and remedial in nature. The principle of teaching, individual difference is followed while selecting this method. This method is often adopted when teaching Anatomy, handling instruments used in Operation Theater or in obstetrics nursing. This method is also used for improvement of weak students. Once the teacher finishes teaching a topic or demonstrating tutorials, they need to be planned for ensuring skills are learned or content are mastered.

Types of Tutorial Classes

- **Supervision tutorials:** This type of tutorials is selected for students with above average intelligence.
- Teacher assigns a problem to the student and he/she is asked to present a paper on the problem. Audience may put questions and the student has to answer them. When he is in a difficulty to satisfy the queries of the audience, the teacher helps by giving appropriate and satisfactory answers to the listeners.
- **Group tutorials:** This type of tutorials are arranged for students with average or low level of intelligence. Those students, who have not understood the subject matter after attaining the scheduled class, are grouped together. Teacher provides them remedial teaching and thus, helps to make the lecture clear and legible.

- **Practical tutorials:** This type of remedial class is used to teach practical subjects, specially when students have difficulty to develop certain skills. These tutorials can be organized after lecture and are practical in the subjects like nursing foundation, obstetrics, etc. These tutorials are basically employed to achieve psychomotor objectives.

Uses

- To ensure the student has learned correctly and is able to deal with complex content.
- To simplify content and facilitate learning.
- To develop psychomotor skills perfectly.

Advantages

- Student gets undivided attention of teacher.
- It gives opportunity to learn under individualized coaching.
- Through individualized teaching, a teacher gains the faith of students that motivates them.
- It facilitates to diagnose individual student's problem.
- Proactive participation is stimulated and promotes safety.

Limitations

- Requires high competence in teacher to teach skills.
- More number of teachers are required, as they need to work with small groups of students.
- It is not economic in terms of time and money.
- Increased number of students makes it difficult to solve the problems of each student.
- Even in tutorial groups, equal opportunities are not provided to all the students.
- There are some students who dominate the tutorial group.

FIELD TRIP

It is a method of teaching that facilitates to gather direct experience away from classroom through observing places, objects and procedure. It breaks monotony of classroom or changes routine pattern and facilitates learning in natural setting. A field trip can be arranged to teach Hospital Management regarding the functions of administrator. In some subjects like community health nursing, anatomy, physiology, nursing education and nursing administration, learning is enhanced by field trip. For anatomy, a field trip can be organized by visiting anatomy lab or to see postmortem at the mortuary of the hospital. In the subject of nutrition, food hygiene or the preparation of a particular item is shown through visiting the central kitchen or department dietetics.

Purposes of Field Trip

- To make a connection between practical and theory.
- To supplement classroom instructions.
- Can be used as an introduction to a unit or a culminating actively.
- To provide an authentic learning experience.

- To facilitate in gathering experience through all five senses: observing, touching, hearing, smelling and tasting.
- To retain learning as students learn using different methodology.

Types of Field Trip

There are two types of field trips, Physical and Virtual.

Physical Field Trip

Physical field trip refers to visiting an outdoor for attaining certain educational objectives. It may include visiting education centers, hospitals, science centers, museums, zoos, fire stations, agricultural operations, natural resource operations etc.

Virtual Field Trip

It is a kind of field trip, in which learners do need not to move physically from one place to another but they visit a website and explore their interest area. Example: http://www.uen.org/utahlink/tours/- the website will allow you to visit and explore by subject various educational learning field trips, create your own field trip or visit other virtual field trips that are located across the web.

Teacher's Role

- Developing a plan at the beginning of academic year
- Reviewing past experience, difficulties encountered and unexpected holidays
- Prior to the field trip, obtain the required permission, instruct students on dress code, articles to be carried, decorum to be maintained and the academic background for the field visit
- Prepare and communicate the objectives to students and the institution
- Provide guidelines to students with a list of questions or checklist that should be their focus so the trip becomes effective
- After the field visit, as soon as possible debriefing is very important.

Advantages

- Students are energized by the excitement of experiencing unknown.
- It facilitates socialization.
- It provides opportunity to learn in an unstructured way.
- Student learning can be interest-driven, not teacher and curriculum-driven.
- Learning becomes more holistic and integrated.
- Learning is enriched and reinforced with multimedia experience.

Limitations

- If the number of students is increased, the trip becomes a socializing event and fails to attain actual learning objectives.

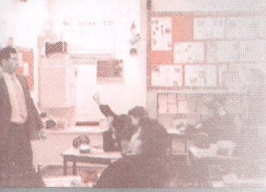

- Inadequate supervision may lead to indiscipline among students.
- While moving to new places, students might get lost from the group.

PROGRAMED INSTRUCTIONS

It is an autocratic method of teaching where response of the learner is strictly controlled by the programer. It is a method of self-study for acquiring factual knowledge. The main focus is to bring desirable change in the cognitive domain of the learner's behavior. In this method of teaching, principle of operant conditions is followed. In programmed instruction, selected content is analyzed and broken into smaller elements and each element is independent and complete in itself. The subject matter is taught step by step and immediate confirmation of correct response provides reinforcement to the learner and encourages moving forward for the next step. Wrong responses require feedback. Physical presence of the teacher is not necessary. He may come to give instructions regarding the program. Students are left for learning at their own pace.

Types of Programed Instructions

There are three types of this teaching strategy
- **Linear Programing:** Linear programming is used to teach all subjects. In this type of programed teaching strategy, progressive chain elements are presented and the last step is mastery level when students complete the learning. It is based on five fundamental principles: Small steps, Active responding, Immediate confirmation, Self-pace and Student testing.
- **Branched Programing:** It is generally used in mechanical fields.
- **Mathematics:** Retrogressive chain of elements is presented where first step is the master level and last step is the simplest element.

Uses

- It is useful for the students who cannot attend regular classes.
- It helps students to catch up with the rest of the class when they have joined the course late and missed classes due to illness.
- It is used to review and update learner's knowledge.
- It helps learner to become familiar with newer equipment and procedures initiated in the clinical area.
- It provides opportunity to students to bridge the gap between theory and practice.

Advantages

- There is no fixed time for study, therefore, students may learn at their own pace.
- In this method, students attain educational objectives through learning by doing, therefore, knowledge retention is longer.
- Immediate confirmation of the results provides reinforcement to the learners.
- Students develop mastery over the content as they receive feedback to wrong answer.
- It provides opportunity to study on the job.

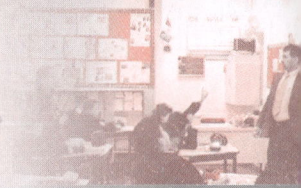

Limitations

- It is costly as a trained person is required to design the program.
- It requires longer time to prepare, if covered portion is increased.
- Only cognitive objectives can be achieved by using this method of teaching.
- There is no scope of students' creativity, as their responses are highly structured.
- In absence of the teacher, students may spoil the disciplinary tone of the class.
- It is not applicable for all levels of learners, i.e., primary level of education.

ASSIGNMENT METHOD

It is a method of teaching, which allows students to acquire academic competency independently without offering contact hours for completion of a given task. Assignment may be given at individual level or group level. It is generally used for students of higher classes and is not appropriate for primary standards. Students are instructed to prepare the content in written form. It enables student in organization of knowledge, assimilation of fact and preparation for examination.

Types of Assignment

There are four types of assignment that include Preparatory assignment, Study assignment, Revisional assignment and Remedial assignment.

- **Preparatory assignment:** This type of assignment is given on a topic that is planned to be discussed on next class; therefore, students are well prepared, become more attentive and interactive too.
- **Study assignment:** Students are assigned to complete a written task on a specific topic, chapter, problem or issue. Each student has a varying degree of interest, IQ and motivation; therefore, it allows expressing their abilities.
- **Revisional assignment:** This type of assignment is given to assess a student's understanding on a topic that is taught before. It also helps to check the retention of knowledge and allow practicing more.
- **Remedial assignment:** It is given to overcome weakness on particular topic or area where student's result was not satisfactory before. It helps students to clear their misunderstanding.

Purpose of Study Assignments

- To equip students to understand a topic before attending a class.
- To encourage student's participation/interaction in classroom that helps to attain learning objectives.
- To acquire integration of students' abilities.
- To provide opportunity for revising study material completed in classroom.
- To enrich study content.

Advantages

- In this method,, students have to carry out the tasks in their own time.
- Increases coverage of study material.

- Reduces classroom time.
- Students gives adequate attention to the topic assigned.

Limitations

- Inappropriate selection of assignment does not help to attain learning objectives.
- It produces inappropriate standards of results as all students are not equally motivated.
- Its evaluation is time consuming for teacher.
- Demotivated students are less benefitted.

WORKSHOPS

The term workshop has been drawn from engineering. According to this, workshop refers to an area where a group of persons work together to complete tasks with their hands to produce something. There are different training workshops like the railway workshop, roadway workshop, etc. Similarly in education, workshops are organized to develop skills in question paper setting and writing of lesson plans. In nursing, there are workshops in research methodology, on CPR, and mastering different skills where knowledge is provided with hands on skill.

Workshop is defined as coming together of a group of individuals of 10–25 with an intention to deal with similar areas of interest or problems to refine their skill through intense work out and practice.

Purposes of Workshop

- To solve problems encountered in teaching and learning
- To improve patient care
- To understand a critical issue
- To develop skills in performing task independently
- To determine strategies
- To use different medium and approaches of teaching.

Objectives of Workshop

- The workshop is organized to achieve the following objectives:
- To solve the problem that is encountered by a professional nurse
- To determine teaching strategies for any particular context of teaching learning
- To train nursing professionals with advanced technology/procedure/tools etc.
- To design a framework for professional practice in particular area
- To justify present nursing practice in selected area.

People involve in Workshop and their Role

To conduct a workshop, a number of people are involved. They are the organizer, convener, expert/resource person/speaker and participants. In every role, there are some specific tasks and responsibilities.

- **Organizer:** A workshop can be organized by a group of nursing students or learner/teaching faculty/nurses working at a clinical area etc. They have active role in all the three stages of workshop namely planning, implementation and evaluation.

- **Convener:** Convener is one of the organizers who takes the leading role throughout the workshop. The convener is responsible to finalize the appropriate theme, opening the theme, coordinating with other member of organizing committee and looking after overall formalities.
- **Experts or Resource persons:** Experts or resource persons are the ones who deliver speech in the respective area as decided by the organizing committee or organizer. Along with speech they also provide hands on training to the participants.
- The participant: Participants are the center of attraction in a workshop. Based on their learning, need and background, the theoretical and practical component of teaching is selected. Their interest and participation ensures the success of the workshop.

Stages of Workshop

Planning Stage

In the first step of planning, an appropriate theme is finalized. Secondly, it is evaluated for its practicability, availability of resource persons and participants. Duration of workshop also needs to be planned; whether it would be 2 days or more depending on the theme and content to be covered. It may last even 10 days also. Fixing the date, day, and venue for hosting the workshop is also important. Organizer needs to make arrangement for lodging and boarding of its participants, speakers and delegates. Organizers will also make preparation of schedule for the session and duration per session. A plan has to be made for providing hands on experience for the participants.

Implementation Stage

In this stage of workshop, organizer starts to work according to the given responsibility. Organizers look after hall arrangement. Accommodation committee is responsible to book the hall where it is planned. Other necessary arrangements are done to accommodate participants and resource persons. Members of invitation committee are responsible to invite participants, resource persons and delegates. Members of refreshment committee are responsible to arrange food. People in registration committee do the registration of each participant and speaker. Members of scientific committee are involved in organizing session of workshop, preparation of souvenir, workshop report and certificates etc.

Evaluation Stage

Workshop is evaluated by the participants, organizer and delegates. Evaluation can be done through input, process and output format. Input evaluation refers to evaluating different types of resources (venue, teaching content, audio-visual aids, resource persons and food) in terms of quality and quantity; Process evaluation refers how the workshop was conducted and output evaluation refers to evaluating the outcome in terms of acquiring knowledge.

Teacher's Role

- To evaluate student's plan for its feasibility
- To supervise students during organization phase
- To solve problems, if problems arise

- To involve all student actively in their allocated task
- To evaluate students' performance and giving feedback.

Advantages

- It facilitates to develop higher cognitive and psychomotor skills.
- It helps in developing professional efficiency.
- It is useful to impart knowledge in a structured environment.
- It can help to develop individual's capacity.
- It helps to build team spirit.
- It has a greater impact with the uses of multimedia.
- It helps to improve problem solving skills of learner.

Limitations

- It is not economic in terms of money, time and effort.
- It may lack group control, if size is large.
- It demands special facilities or materials.
- Generally follow up is difficult in workshop technique.

COMPUTER ASSISTED LEARNING

CBI, computer based information, CAI, computer assisted information/instruction, CBT, computer based training etc. are all the forms that are used to provide educational information through computer.

Computer assisted learning (CAL) emphasizes on student-centered learning using content through a digital medium, where content is presented and one can progress on completing a task and performance is evaluated/accepted as correct or stated as in correct response.

Types of Computer Assisted Learning

- Distance Learning/Education:
  - Web-based education (internet and WWW)
  - Computer and video technologies
- Computer-mediated courseware (interactive CD-ROM)
- **On-line Classes:** may use a combination of any or all of the above
- Telemedicine.

Types of Computer Assisted Learning Software

There are number of CAL softwares that include Drill and practice, Games, Simulations, Tutorials, Tools, Hypermedia, CMI software (tests), etc.

- **Drill and practice:** This is supplementary to the normal teaching process. It is good for mastery of a subject like mathematics, where computer generates problems that are solved by students. The computer indicates right or wrong answers and sometimes may indicate the reason of wrong response. It can be thought as flash card system of stimulus response, where computer immediately indicates success on completion of a task and keeps giving problems to solve. Speed is important. It provides the feedback and keeps students' performance record.

- **Game format:** It includes point scoring and can be individual or team format. This pattern is apt for a motivating environment.
- **Simulations:** It provides all details of patient situation and asks student to assess the patient and arrive at a diagnosis, plan intervention and evaluate the care. Simulations can also demand decisions in emergency situation and indicate if the results are a good or a poor decision. Simulations are safe, inexpensive, fast, slow, clean, and possible.
- **Tutorials:** It presents students with information on a selected body of knowledge and asks questions, giving hints if student gets stuck. It may also provide remedy only when concept is clear and correct. It again tests this process until content is learned. They are good for teaching material at concept level. It involves application programs used by students for learning.
- **Tools:** Spreadsheet programs, statistics packages, hypermedia software, desktop publishing software, presentation software, CAD software, etc.
- **Hypermedia:** It can be thought of as "chunks" of information (nodes), stored in a structure, and accessed by links (buttons). They may use hypertext i.e. use textual information structured by use of links and nodes. Hypermedia would use textual information but also use sound, video and/or animation, whereas multimedia would use more than one media with text, graphics, sound, video and or animation etc. Multimedia provides sensory rich environment for learning. Interactive multimedia provides human interaction via the computer.

Settings in Which CAL can be used

- **Home:** Educational CD's, Distant education, WWW educational sites
- **Colleges/Universities:** Videos, educational CD's, distance education, simulation activities
- **Computer labs:** Webinar, interactive software CD's
- **Organizations/Corporations:** Webinars, teleconferencing, annual mandatories, HR/training modules
- **Hospitals:** Patient simulation models, Skill CD's, Tele-health
- **Testing Centers:** Computer testing modules (Common registered nurse practitioners)
- **Senior Centers:** Health CDs, videos, WWW educational sites
- **Libraries:** Reading activity CDs, videos, interactive educational program

Advantages of CAL

- It provides multiple modes of communicating data and opportunity to learn variety of skill and knowledge
- Students can learn at their own pace, work and acquire next academic level
- Simple and can be managed by a student in his/her own time
- Provides a two-way flow of information
- Supplement traditional classroom or lecture materials
- Gives prompt feedback
- More accurate monitoring of learner progress.

Limitations of CAL

- Lack of computers or resources
- Must be internally or self-motivated

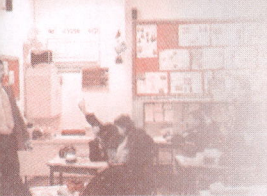

- Hardware or software problems/internet connectivity
- Must be familiar computer hardware and software
- Time commitment is required to prepare and complete simulations
- Resistance of learners and teachers to utilize CAL resources
- Individual differences in learning styles.

Evaluating the Effectiveness of CAL

To evaluate the effectiveness of CAL the following questions can be asked.
- Does the content matches the learning objectives?
- Have the different mediums/techniques been used appropriately?
- Is it easy to navigate through the program or CD?
- Do learners' perceive the program or CD helpful for gaining knowledge?
- Does it enriches or adds to the existing learning resources?
- How beneficial is it from the teachers' and students' point of view?
- How the CD or programs will enhance skills? Is it a better method of learning as compared to what is available?

PROBLEM-BASED LEARNING

Problem-based learning (PBL) is a method where students learn through solving problems and implementing strategies for better results. It involves analytical and critical thinking skill to reach a solution. In today's progressive academic world, where learning is self-directed, problem-based learning plays a very important role.

Concept

The concept is based on proactive participation of the students into the learning activity. It involves use of innovative methods to draw conclusion for improving standards of practice or living. Here, students apply findings in their real life situations to constantly explore, question and generate newer ideas which provides a sense of achievement.

PBL provides opportunity to uses newer techniques where the student sets his/her own direction to gain knowledge and skills. It is essential to mould the thinking process of students to think critically and make choice to learn through a proactive process. It contributes to proactive educational system where students try to find solutions to problems that they face and increase their body of knowledge.

Importance in Nursing

It prepares nurses to deal with issues and problems independently. It helps in developing analytical skills, which are useful in providing evidence-based care. It helps in developing a questioning attitude to explore and come up with innovative strategies and team spirit if working in group.

Principles

Teacher should function as facilitators and allow students to find solutions independently. Each member in the group works around an identified problem, and contributes solutions; every alternative

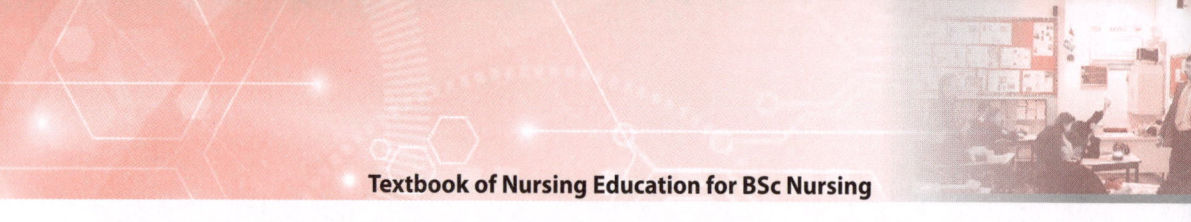

is listed until a solution is shortlisted. It is aimed at inculcating an inquiring temperament. An issue may be identified from theory or clinical area. Issues may be interdisciplinary requiring an interdisciplinary approach to understand and reach as answers. Teacher and students interact at regular intervals until problem is resolved.

Requirements of Problem-based Learning

There are certain essential steps that should be followed by students while using problem-based learning.

- **Understanding the Problem:** At the beginning, the learner should clarify their concepts regarding the problem at hand. They state the problem meaningfully in an objective manner and identify their strengths or lacunae to solve it.
- **Learning about the Problem:** Learner must judge the difficulty and hindrance that may be encountered. They also assess the adequacy of knowledge and skills required to deal with it and evaluate the availability and accessibility of resources. All group members should share gathered information and knowledge and ensure all are at same wave length.
- **Solving the Problem:** After recognizing the actual problem, the learner should: enumerate identified solutions; prioritize the possible solutions; and lastly select best alternatives. The whole process is documented: newly identified solution; situations where applicable and method of disseminating for use.
- **Reflecting on the Process:** In this stage, learner has to do SWOT (S-strength, W-weakness, O-opportunity, T-threat) analysis to build ones confidence in the process and overcome hurdles next time. They must evaluate its utility value for practical application.

Role of Teacher in Problem-based Learning

- Since its student-centered activity, teacher gives her feedback wherever required.
- Teacher has to create opportunity to develop problem solving skills so that students can fine tune their skills.
- Teacher identifies variety of situations/cases requiring problem-solving strategies.
- Teacher performs the role of mentor, guide, and a protagonist when required and makes funds and data accessible. Teacher has to motivate student to take the risk.
- Teacher consciously links the process with situations/cases to give an authenticity to the problem. Learning activities is connected designed problem situations. Teacher acts as a facilitator, guide, preceptor, etc.

Role of Student in Problem-based Learning

- Participate actively to complete the task.
- Students need to regularly evaluate their performance.
- Keep gathering information to solve the problem.
- Perform peer evaluation.
- Listen and develop positive attitude to receive feedback.
- Develop skill to reach a resolution and grow.

Comparison of Problem Based Learning

Problem based learning	Problem solving
Method of gaining newer data when need is felt	Reaching/drawing conclusions based on earlier learning

Problem based learning	Project based learning
Learning to solve a problem existing in the real world by undertaking exercise of identifying a solution with help of different disciplines	Student learns to complete an assigned task through syntheses of theory with practical activity, which is planned so as to implement what is learned

This method can be implemented at various academic levels as students need to master learning through problem solving. It can be used at different points in the curriculum special technical learning should be problem-based learning, writing nursing care plan should be problem-based; thereby students learn and generate a new body of knowledge. Learning, which occurs due to research activity, is to a large extent problem-based learning gain deeper insight for the learner.

Steps in Problem-based Learning Tutorial Process

- **Step 1:** Look for unclear concepts, which need to be simplified and discussed.
- **Step 2:** Enumerate issues to be tackled, take into consideration difference of opinion, and make notes and points of agreement.
- **Step 3:** "Brainstorming" to clarify the existing knowledge, reasoning, and judgments of the situation, solutions, lacunae and the discussion will be documented.
- **Step 4:** Review previous steps and organize the points in priority and it may be rearranged.
- **Step 5:** Obtain consensus on the objectives laid for the learning experience, while the mentor ensures they are feasible, holistically framed and age/group appropriate.
- **Step 6:** Each member of the study group independently gathers data to achieve the goal
- **Step 7:** Each member comes back to pool in what they have gathered, thereby increasing their resource. The teacher monitors the activity to see if it is going as per plan and if learning is taking place.

Stages of Problem-based Learning

- **Stage 1— Definition (10 mins):** Choose a team leader who will record the discussion generated by the lead question.
- **Stage 2 — Analysis (30 mins):** Encourage spontaneous and ingenious ideas to the problems under study, identify possible answers and reasons that students can provide with applicability.
- **Stage 3 — Research Aims (15 mins):** Recognize need to seek more data to clarify/support the generated solutions or to reach a new one. Chalk out a schedule of activity and assign task to be completed and reported.
- **Stage 4 — Research:** Scheduling time frame for works to be done individually and in group, for example, preparation of list of resources or equipment and place of availability.
- **Stage 5 — Synthesis (1-2 hours):** In this session, need to reflect on the freshly acquired data with the team under the guidance of the mentor, reach a common understanding and consensus on

the subject matter understudy and summary of the learning experience are shared. PBL provides a powerful means of opportunity to learn and apply solutions to real world events and problems and deal with changes in the clinical area.

Advantages

- Gives freedom for students to plan and organize their learning experience.
- Improves interpersonal interaction.
- Motivates students to explore and use their potential.
- Helps students to get focused and build positively on their errors.
- Prevents mechanical learning through an interactive process.

Limitations

- This method can be used in small groups.
- Structured/objective evaluation becomes difficult.
- Inexperienced teacher or student may not want to deviate from traditional method.
- Both faculty and students may find it exhaustive.
- Weak students may find difficulty to match up to the group and assignment.

SIMULATION

Simulation is defined as "the process of designing a model of a real system and conducting experiments with this model for the purpose of either understanding the behavior of the system and/or for evaluating various strategies used for the operation of the system."

Simulation is one of the most popular methods adopted to teach humanities and social science. Simulation involves imitation of process of the real world. It is the most widely used tool for decision making.

Uses of Simulation

Simulation is widely accepted method of teaching. In manufacturing industry, simulation can be used to understand and learn assembly line, production process, inventory control process, etc. In nursing, simulation can be used to understand the delivery process at birth, administration of intravenous drugs, cardiopulmonary resuscitation, etc.

Value of Simulation in Nursing

The true value of simulation lies in its ability to offer experience throughout the educational process that provides students with opportunity for repetition, pattern recognition and faster decision making. Simulation - based education should be part of normal training process. The student needs to participate in simulations in addition to their patient care experience to learn and deal with clinical problems. Simulations are essential to minimize harm and practice safely because only 10% of employers thinks that students joining them are safe to practice in clinical area.

Types of Simulation

There are five different types of simulation methods.

- **Task trainer simulation:** Task trainer simulation allows the students to practice basic skills, which are required for their professional practice area. It improves student's visual, tactile and coordination skills. Example-Drawing blood, insertion of I/V channel.
- **Manikin-based simulation:** Manikin-based simulation refers to simulation where manikin is used. It may include low, mid and high fidelity simulation manikins and the level of fidelity refers to the technological abilities of the equipment. Manikin may be static or dynamic. Dynamic manikin may show the vitals, blinks, cries etc.
- **Standardized patient simulation:** Standardized patient simulations facilitate interactive teaching through the innovative combination of technology and patient actors. The patient actors are called Standardized Patients.
- **Virtual reality simulation:** In virtual reality simulation, unique state-of-the-art virtual devices are used. It enables learner with high fidelity training procedural simulation enhancing with true-to-life tactile sensations.
- **Tissue-based simulation:** It provides opportunity to practice procedural skills outside of the clinical environment.
  Example: wound dressing, episiotomy stitching, endotracheal intubation. This not only benefits the learners but also ensures patient safety and quality clinical care.

Advantages

- The biggest strength of simulation is to obtain answers to the unknown situation.
- Simulations help in creating the real scenario in class without interrupting ongoing process.
- Feasibility can be tested before procuring any device or making changes in the system.
- Allows controlling time and avoiding bottle neck.
- Allows gaining insight of situation that may not be anticipated.
- Relatively straightforward and flexible.

Limitations

- Building simulators requires skill to replicate and have them in working condition.
- Findings from simulation are difficult to interpret as they are merely close to reality.
- It is not economical in terms of cost.
- Invalid model would result in providing wrong results.
- Results may differ with repeated use.
- Each simulator has different features and operation instructions, therefore training on one does not assure mastery on all models.

SELF INSTRUCTIONAL MODULES

Self-Instructional Modules are those which contain organized learning content to help a student to learn unassisted or with little assistance from teacher. A self-instructional module is a method of teaching where students can learn at their own pace.

Characteristics of Self Instructional Module (Fig. 2)

- Self-explanatory
- Self-contained
- Self-directional
- Self-evaluation
- Self-learning

Phases of Self Instructional Module

- **Preparatory phase:** This phase is concerned with data collection, data analysis and interpretation in the area of curriculum, educational program, priorities. Secondary information required for the background of target group, their learning needs and interests. Learning resources are also identified in the preparatory phase.

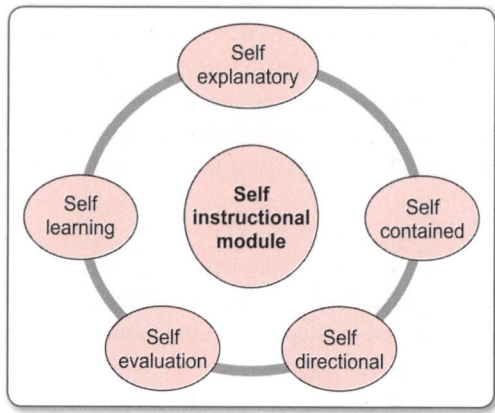

Fig. 2: Characteristics of self instructional module

- **Implementation phase:** After the preparatory phase implementation phase is started and it includes the following sub phases.
    - **Preparation:** The self-instructional module is prepared by organizing the content under suitable number of unit. At the beginning, it is introduced to the learner describing its purpose, use and learning objectives. Every unit contains the structure, objectives, introduction, elaboration of learning materials, checklist of self-evaluation and answer key.
    - **Production:** After preparation the self-instructional module is reviewed, formatted, printed and developed.
    - **Dissemination:** It is distributed to the target groups timely.
    - **Utilization:** The self-instructional module is utilized by the learners.
- **Evaluation phase:** In this phase the self-instructional module is evaluated in the format of input, process and outcome or product. Input evaluation mainly refers to the learner's previous knowledge on the subject or topic that is included in self-instructional module. Process evaluation mainly refers to the way of preparation, production, dissemination and utilization. Outcome or product evaluation is concerned to what extent learner has attained the educational objectives in terms of knowledge gain.

Advantages

- Students can learn at their own pace.
- Useful in choice-based learning system.
- Student can test their learning output from a given exercise.
- It is a very structured method of teaching.

Limitations

- Suitable only for highly motivated learner.
- It has no scope with learner teacher interaction.

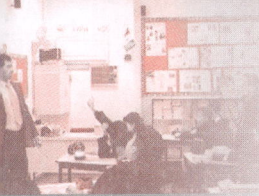

- Communication/language problem may arise.
- Takes a lot of time to design the module.

EXHIBITION

Exhibition is a widely accepted method of teaching throughout the world, starting from secondary level, graduation and post-graduation level. It is used by the learner to fulfill the requirement of curriculum.

Definition

An exhibition is a systematic display of models, specimens, charts, posters etc. to convey some significant information based on single theme to the target audience, thereby achieving learning objectives.

Purposes

- To disseminate health information using multimedia
- To create interest among large number of people
- To motivate people for adopting better health practices
- To minimize health problems
- To stimulate self-learning among students.

Characteristics of Exhibition

- Exhibition is a type of presentation in which a concept is displayed using varieties of appropriate audio visual aids.
- An exhibition should have a central theme that includes some subtheme.
- The entire interrelated subtheme is presented in such a way that integrity is maintained.
- All the displayed learning material should be self-explanatory.
- Appropriate number of demonstrations is also used to achieve desired results.
- Multi-channels are used to impart educational information for a greater impact.
- It is aimed to catch the attention of large group of people.
- The selected venue, date and time should match with the interest of target audience.
- Attention should be paid to color,, flow and style of presentation.

Types of Exhibition

Based on learning needs, it is decided whether exhibitions will be conducted at group level or individual level.

Teacher's Role

According to the curricular requirement and learning needs of students, a topic is selected for exhibition. Basic guidelines are given to students for developing a framework of exhibition and the deadline for preparation phase. On completion of preparation phase, students have to rehearse under supervision of teacher. Lastly, the exhibition is conducted by students when teacher are physically present.

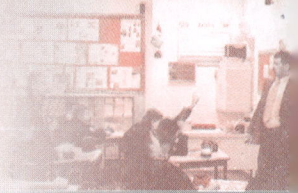

Advantages

- It facilitates self-learning.
- It stimulates creativity of the students to prepare and present the topic.
- It facilitates group dynamics.
- Exhibition is one of the methods of teaching, by which information is delivered to a large audience.
- Exhibition has publicity value where a new project or activity is being communicated.
- Exhibitions caters to the needs of a mixed group.
- Exhibitions fit into festive occasions and can serve recreational requirements.
- Exhibitions can stimulate healthy competitive spirit when assigned as group activity.

Limitations

- It is not economic in terms of time, cost and human effort.
- A lot of investment of resources is involved.
- Exhibitions cannot be used repeatedly at the same place without making substantial changes.

MICROTEACHING

Microteaching as a teachers training method is used worldwide. It advances teaching skills of teachers by promoting real-time teaching experiences. Most of the pre-service teacher education programs widely use microteaching. Other than general education it is also accepted by many disciplines including Medical science, Health science, Social science and Nursing. It helps a student to develop presentation skill that is the core skill of microteaching. This method involves the steps of Planning, Teaching, Observing, Re-planning, Re-teaching and Re-observing.

Microteaching is prepared on a single concept and practiced to a less number of students. It minimizes the complexities of real teaching, as immediate feedback can be sought after each practice session.

Definition

It can be defined as a method of teaching which is focused on a single theme or small scale content for a smaller group of learners involving the steps of preparation, presentation and immediate feedback in a non-threatening environment.

Uses of Microteaching

Micro teaching exercise provides opportunity to the teachers to evaluate and critically look at their own performance, without criticism. It boosts the morale of the teacher. Given a chance to practice different aspects of teaching skills, budding teacher not only gets feedback of their own teaching skills but also learn to evaluate others in the group, which makes them comfortable and open to critical review of their skills.

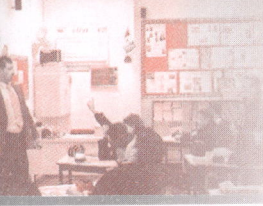

Equipment for Microteaching Session

To record, a hand cam and to visualize the recording, TV or computer with LCD projector are needed. To write the points of discussion, chalk board may be used.

One-day Plan for Microteaching

A schedule can be prepared for every student to present his/her skills for evaluation by the mentor and peers. A list of topic can be assigned using either different skill for every student or all skill to be performed by all students breaking a large content and evaluate one skill at a time. Each skill may be assigned 10–15 minutes and maximum 20 minutes (in case of demonstration). This depends on the available time allocated in teacher course for microteaching and number of student teachers in a group.

Steps in Microteaching

- **Preparation:** Every student teacher prepares the content to be taught before her peers and mentor. The session begins with the objectives of the presentation of a specific skill. This would help the audience to focus and ensure all dimensions of that skill are performed well like pace of presentation, clarity of explanation, use of AV aids, voice and body language.
- **Presentation and observation:** Every student teacher is allotted specific time duration to present one teaching skill, using the appropriate A.V aid. The peers function as students as well as use a guideline to evaluate the presentation so as to provide feedback. The checklist/guideline helps to objectively observe the teaching, note down points, so as to contribute in the analysis and to provide constructive feedback.
- **Videotape viewing:** The student group uses the recording to go back and review the presentation as well as helps the presenter to observe her/his own performance and make required improvement and incorporate the strong points in the next session. As a team, they draw conclusions of the entire teaching episode.
- **Discussion and analysis:** The student teacher views her recorded teaching either with the group or independently. With the help of the mentor, her peers summarize their observations, and prepared anecdote to give the feedback to the student teacher of her teaching style and weaknesses. Skills requiring modifications or deletion are suggested to enhance teaching. Objective of lesson as well as of microteaching if achieved are assessed.
- **Giving and receiving feedback:** The student teacher first in front of the peer group and mentor does self-evaluation after completing the presentation of the skill and viewing the recording. Then one of the peer group members gives positive criticism/feedback and appreciation, inclusive of the points generated during discussion and analysis so as to motivate the student teacher. It also provides opportunity for the presenter to clarify doubt.
- **Giving feedback:** Points one should keep in mind when providing feedback:
  - Instead of being vague, be specific: i.e. point the exact aspects done well and not up to the mark, by quoting instances.
  - Don't be judgmental but stick to the point: Judgmental words may create a feeling of inferiority that decreases self-confidence.
  - Highlight those aspects, which are possible to improve: Giving realistic suggestions such as to maintain eye contact for individuals, who are introvert.

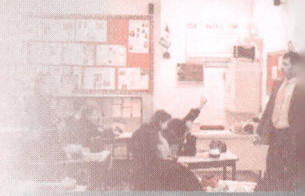

- Suggest few selected areas on which the person can work on: Instead of drawing conclusion, giving constructive suggestion. i.e. "You were not trying to catch the attention of audience.", it's better to state that tone modulation can catch the attention of the group.
- Give positive feedback before telling shortcomings: As it may get the person feel dejected and block the mind so that appreciation may not get registered.
- **Receiving feedback:** When student teacher receiving feedback, he/she must-
  - Listen to the feedback rather than reacting to every comment.
  - Keep an open mind so that the feedback can be used to enhance teaching skills rather than taking it as fault finding and block one's growth.
  - Write down points briefly so that the list of comments can be referred before the next presentation.
  - The most critical feedback is the most beneficial for improving.
  - Obtain feedback to the point so that exact aspect can be focused supported with anecdote.
  - Do not take all feedback as face value but try to understand each person's genuine remarks.
- **Appendices:** An assessment sheet is prepared, which includes the aspects to be evaluated by the peer member, comprehension by students, type of visuals used to support the teaching, appropriateness of introduction, duration of time taken to introduce, punctuality in starting and completing session, depth of the content, organization of content, any specific observation made can be noted in the remarks column. It should also elicit the standard/quality of teaching reflecting the style and overall impact of the session.

Advantages

- It increases the confidence level of the student teacher.
- It provides comfortable environment for practicing teaching than real classroom situations.
- It helps to refine and fine tune to groom effective teachers.
- Micro teaching program is budget-oriented or economic in terms of money.
- It lessens the chances of mistakes.
- Helps to develop positive attitude towards any criticism.
- Micro teaching enables the teachers to gain instant feedbacks from the supervisors and peers.

Limitations

- It does not promote creativity due to restricted time period of teaching.
- It requires competent mentors for conducting microteaching.
- Teacher may lose interest due to less number of students.
- It is a teacher-oriented activity therefore, student learning is ignored.
- Artificial situations do not help in preparing teachers for real time situations.
- It does not facilitate to develop all teaching skills in a single session of microteaching.

VIRTUAL LEARNING

Virtual learning is also known as digital learning or e-learning. It is moving away from the classroom or traditional method of teaching, where the presence of a teacher is not mandatory. Virtual learning brings the real world in to the classroom via the computer or web or using software designed in a

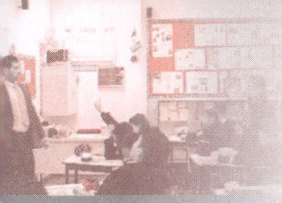

manner to permit interaction or get an opportunity to interact with a facilitator in a different setting. Virtual learning method provides students to take up additional courses or choice based course. Many university programs are integrating virtual learning into the system to enhance learning experience.

Definition

It is a method of learning which uses computer software, internet or both to deliver instruction to students without requiring a teacher or classroom.

Forms of Virtual Learning

- **Computer-based:** Instruction is provided by a computer where a software is installed that can frequently be customized with suitable learning material and it also meets the learning needs of students.
- **Internet-based:** It is similar to computer-based instruction, but here the software is delivered by Web and stored on a remote server.
- **Remote teacher online:** In this method of virtual learning, instruction is provided by a teacher, and he/she interacts with the student either via Internet or online video, online forums, e-mail and instant messaging. The teacher is not present physically.
- **Blended learning:** It is a combination of virtual and traditional method where the teacher is physically present and provides face to face instruction with the help of at least one virtual learning methods.
- **Facilitated virtual learning:** This is a computer-based, internet-based or remote teacher online instruction that is supplemented by a human facilitator. The human facilitator does not involve in giving instruction but facilitate through supervising learning process.

Advantages

- Learner gets the chance to study in their own pace.
- It gives the freedom to choose the time for study.
- Learner gets the opportunity to receive up to date information.
- It allow to access additional learning material.
- It allow to control their own learning experience.
- It does not have restricted physical boundaries.

Limitation

- It requires responsible learner.
- Learner should have the higher level of self discipline.
- It does not offer human interaction.

MASTERY LEARNING

According to Bloom (1985) the students have to be helped to grasp the content before proceeding to the next. Traditionally, a teacher continues to teach in the classroom based on course outline and

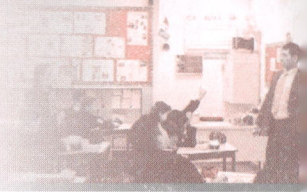

periodically evaluate the students. Irrespective of their performance, the teacher continues teaching the remaining portion of the syllabus. In mastery learning, total learning content is divided into parts with specified objectives. Learners have to proceed from each block of content in a series of sequential steps. Each student should demonstrate a high level of success on tests before progressing to new content.

Definition

Mastery learning refers to a category of instructional methods, which establishes a level of performance that all students must master before moving on to the next unit (Slavin, 1987).

Principles of Mastery Learning

Mastery learning is based on the principle of collaborative learning, peer tutoring and standard learning. It becomes effective when students learn in groups or teams by supporting each other's progress. Mastery learning may also be more effective when used as an occasional or additional teaching strategy. For mastery learning, challenging topics are selected rather than regular lessons. Low scoring pupils may gain more from this strategy than high scoring students.

Focus of Mastery Learning

- **Behavioral objectives:** Specific or behavioral objectives are stated clearly to the students before teaching a portion, therefore student become aware about their own role as well as teachers expectation.
- **Small learning segments:** The subject matter of a unit is broken into small segments and each segment contains self-assessment questions which allow learner self-evaluation.
- **Self-spacing:** Considering the teaching principle of individual difference each learner is allowed to learn the study units according to their own speed but the degree of mastery remain same.
- **Individual attention:** In the process of teaching learning, if any portion of study material is not clear to any student, then individual instruction is provided.
- **Criterion referenced testing:** According to the philosophy of mastery learning, each student must have a standard level of performance. Each learner is expected to perform a certain level, which is specified therefore criteria reference test is used in student evaluation.

Advantages

- It facilitates learning collaboratively.
- It emphasizes on achieving higher score.
- It motivates student to assume their responsibility.

Limitations

- All types of lesson are not suitable for mastery learning, challenging topic is more suitable.
- It is not suitable for all group of learner; it is more effective for lower scoring students.
- It is not very practical to use for a large and mixed group of students with varieties of learning skill.

CLINICAL TEACHING METHODS

Nursing is a professional course and it has a strong service orientation. In nursing, psychomotor skill attainment is vital along with theoretical knowledge. After completion of any nursing program learner is expected to take care of a person towards achieving optimum level of health. Health and illness have multiple dimensions and health care is provided in a team approach. Therefore, a nurse's role is not simple. To perform multirole in clinical and to provide safe care to client in number of settings, a student nurse must develop psychomotor skills. To develop desired level of skills, students are exposed to actual patient setting and supervised by competent instructor. Clinical instructor plays an active role in skill development of students. A variety of clinical methods need to be employed to build and sustain clinical skills which is vital for professional development.

Definition

Clinical teaching is a method of teaching adopted by nurse educators or clinical instructors to mentor a single student or small groups of students to ensure safe delivery of nursing care.

Focus of Clinical Teaching

Clinical teaching helps to understand the relationship between health, illness and the health care system. It enable student to recognize how to respond in different clinical situations. Students also understand the role and function as a health care team member and develop competency in critical thinking, reasoning, and implementing evidence-based nursing care. They become committed to patient care and grow professionally.

Steps in Clinical Teaching

- Formulating objectives and plan of clinical experience.
- Conducting clinical teaching based on the objective of the clinical posting.
- Allocating patient in clinical setting.
- Assessing the student performance by conducting ward test.

Purposes of Clinical Teaching

To attain learning objectives, student's nurses are taught various nursing activities using different clinical teaching methods in actual clinical setting. The purposes of clinical teaching methods include:
- To practice different techniques, procedures and approaches necessary in patient care.
- To teach in maintaining harmonious relationship with health team member.
- To maximize sensitivity among nursing students.
- To teach managerial skills necessary in effective organization of nursing service.
- To develop technical skill that necessary for monitoring of client health.
- To develop professional skill among nursing students.
- To meet clients health needs.
- To improve standard of nursing practice.

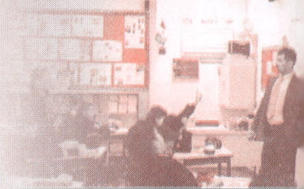

Types of Clinical Teaching

There are a number of methods used to teach nursing students in clinical setting and all these methods have some specific purpose, advantages and limitations. Commonly used clinical teaching methods are Nursing care plan, Case study, Nursing care conference, Bedside clinics, Nursing rounds, Demonstration, Process recording, Care analysis etc.

NURSING CARE PLAN

Nursing care plan refers to a projected plan for delivering patient care on regular basis. It includes a systematic process of assessing client's health, identifying health problems, planning and implementing nursing care, evaluating effects of nursing intervention and modifying the process based on changes of health status.

Purposes of Nursing Care Plan

- To provide a means of communication among nurses and other health care provider.
- To provide nursing care in an organized manner.
- To provide patient care consistently.
- To meet client health needs.
- To monitor client's health status on regular basis.
- To maintain quality of patient care.

Types of Nursing Care Plan

- Standardized care plans: It specifies the nursing care for groups of clients with common needs.
- Individualized care plans: It is used to meet the unique needs of a specific client.

Steps in Nursing Care Plan

- **Patient identification:** In this step, a student nurse is allocated to a patient for preparing nursing care plan and providing care on a daily basis. The student nurse collects information about patient that includes: client's name, age, gender, date of admission, occupied bed number, unit name, name of treating doctors, provisional diagnosis etc.
- **Chief complaints:** It is the patient's description about his illness for which he is seeking treatment or health advice. The hospitalized patient may inform about the reason of hospitalization.
- **Health history:** Health history includes details about health related information in terms of present health history, past health history, health habits (food habit, sleep habit, bowel and bladder habit, other habits i.e. smoking/alcohol consumption/drug addiction) dietary history, psychosocial history, family history etc. If the client is a child, then birth history, growth and developmental history are also important. In case of pregnant and nursing mother, antenatal, intranatal and postnatal history needs to be included.
- **Physical examination:** The client is assessed thoroughly and findings may be recorded system wise or in head to foot direction.

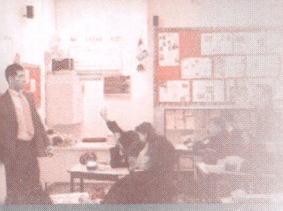

- **Reviewing laboratory records:** All laboratory investigation reports are assessed and relevant information is recorded in nursing care plan.
- **Medical/Surgical management:** The student nurse has to summarize the medical or surgical management of client because many nursing activities are dependent on medical and surgical management.
- **Forming nursing process:** After analyzing the health information obtained from health history, physical examination, and laboratory reports data are clustered in terms of subjective and objective data. These subjective and objective data are used to form nursing diagnosis and objectives. To attain each objective, number of nursing activities are planned and the plan is executed by student nurse under supervision of clinical instructor or nursing tutor. After carrying out nursing action, the client is evaluated for changes of health status. Every day care provided by student nurse uses same format of nursing process. If any new health problem arises that is added and similarly any nursing diagnosis may be eliminated, if previous health problem subsides.

Format of Nursing Process

Assessment	Nursing diagnosis	Objectives	Planning	Intervention	Evaluation
Subjective data-					
Objective data-					

- **Health education:** Every day during interacting with client relevant health information is provided to client and family member. While giving health advice, student nurse has to remember that information should be relevant and appropriate.
- **Conclusion:** This is the last step of nursing care plan and it is used to summarize nurses interaction with client, significant events that promotes or decorates health status, ultimate attainment of health objectives etc.
- **References:** To develop a nursing care plan, student nurse has to refer or review literature for enriching theoretical knowledge that is essential in providing nursing care. The list of references is included here.

Advantages

- It guides in providing patient care.
- Using nursing care plan, individualized patient care is possible.
- It allows a student nurse to provide complete, unified and need-based care.

Limitations

- It increases dependency on theoretical concept.
- If nursing care plan is not modified at regular basis, it become less effective.
- It is time consuming and interrupts patient care.

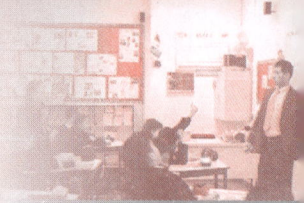

CASE METHOD

It refers to in-depth analysis of patient health status and response to treatment in relation to personal characteristics, socio-economic characteristics, health habits and provided care. It also allows the comparison with actual patient status with theoretical information.

Types of Case Method

Nursing Case Study

Nursing student is assigned a patient by the mentor or preceptor based on the learning objective in that area. Student provides care for at least a week or two that allows understanding and helps in gaining confidence in caring of the patient with a specific condition. She assesses and plans need based care to resolve felt and perceived needs/problems. She also attempts to apply innovative nursing care strategies to improve quality of care and early recovery. At regular intervals, she consults with the teacher regarding the plan, intervention and outcome of care. On completion of care in the stipulated time period, she submits the case study for evaluation.

Patient Care Analysis

It is similar to nursing case study but additionally it involves complex patient condition when patient is studied from time of coming to the unit until discharged/transferred/dies. Duration could be a month. Two or more patient with same disease are assigned for analysis.

Incidental Case Study

A patient with unusual condition or rare case is assigned to student for a short duration of time with the intention to understand. The student provides care to patient for one to two days until complete information is obtained and discussion is initiated during a nursing round.

Teacher's Role

Teacher guides a student in patient selection, providing format in advance, and supervise regularly. Teacher should guide the student as and when needed to enrich the learning experience. Under supervision of teacher it is ensured that the care is provided as planned. She initiates discussion at the end of the stipulated period of care so that other students learn and can contribute towards improvement of care.

Advantages

- It helps to grow interest among student in patient care.
- It provides opportunity for an in-depth understanding of disease process.
- It helps to understand the impact of nursing care on patient and family.
- Student learns to correlate theoretical information with actual patient status.
- It builds skill in using problem solving approach.

Limitations

- Learning is limited only in one area or disease process.
- It is time consuming.
- Benefits are more for the individual learner.

CASE PRESENTATION

It is a widely accepted method of clinical teaching that allows student nurse to take care of a patient on regular basis and study thoroughly. After an in-depth study, formal presentation further increases confidence and clarify their doubts.

Case presentation refers to a formal presentation of an assigned case, starting from patient identification, assessment, medical & nursing diagnosis, details of disease process, medical & nursing management, and advance level of management, response, complication and prognosis.

Process of Case Presentation

At the beginning, a student is assigned to a patient and instructed to provide care regularly. Before providing care details, health information is collected through interviewing, examining and reviewing investigation report. The gathered information is utilized to diagnose health problems, to determine objectives and to plan nursing course of action. Based on planned course of action nursing care is provided, changes of health status is noticed, monitored for complication and prognosis is noticed. The case details are also compared with existing literature. The details of this activity are recorded in a given format. Lastly, student is allowed to present the case before peer groups and also invites them to clarify doubts. Under the supervision of teacher, a constructive discussion takes place.

Advantages

- It allows in-depth study of a case.
- Student gets the opportunity to interact with health team member.
- It helps to gain confidence in patient care.
- It facilitates in improving communication.
- It promotes decision making and problem solving skill of student.

Limitations

- It restricts learning in one disease process only.
- Individual student is more benefited than the group.
- Inadequate communication skill of student lengthens the duration.

BEDSIDE CLINIC

Bedside clinic refers to a discussion of client's health involving a mixed group of health team members in the presence of patient.

It is conducted at the bedside centering the patient and usually lasts for 30 minutes. Prior to the discussion patient is informed and all the students in the group are introduced to the patient. It helps student to understand better through facilitating direct interaction and clinical demonstration.

The patient selected for bedside clinics is mostly typical rather than unusual condition. The student who cares for the patient would present the patient picture and course of medical treatment and plan for home care and problems encountered while caring. The other participants in group may clarify, provide suggestions for improvement of care or share their own experience if they too have cared for patients with similar conditions.

Steps in Conducting Bedside Clinic

Unit Preparation

The unit or place where bed side clinic would be conducted is prepared in terms of space, ventilation, light, comfort and privacy, so that it can accommodate the desired number of people for defined period of time. Generally bedside clinic is conducted in teaching corner or demonstration room.

Preparation of Patient

Patient is informed before conducting the clinic at bedside. To prevent harm and maximize patient cooperation, all kinds of support is provided to patient. The purpose of conducting bedside clinic is explained to the patient and introduced with audience. Patient should not be kept in the discussion room throughout the clinic, especially when sensitive issue is discussed.

Preparation of the Group

Groups are well informed about their roles and responsibilities. Active listening and participation is expected from each group member.

Phases of Bedside Clinic

- **Introductory phase:** where students get acquainted with the patients background, nursing care received and type of questions that are needed to be asked.
- **Working phase:** In the second phase, discussion is initiated either by clinical instructor/Nurse Educator or Head nurse. The function of this phase is information gathering and sharing to understand the case. It is ensured that patient should not be embarrassed/fearful or sick. Once required information is collected, patient is allowed to go back to his allotted bed.
- **Evaluation phase:** The discussion moves in to the last phase, which is post clinic evaluation. It provides the opportunity to evaluate the problem, care and various aspects of patient care. The students may be evaluated on their ability to contribute in discussion. After that an interaction occurs between the groups, the key points are highlighted before concluding.

Advantages

- There is better retention of knowledge as students participate actively.
- It also improves their ability to care for another patient.
- Encourages students for closer contact with reality.
- The discussion allows comparison with theoretical concepts.
- It helps to gain confidence.

Limitations

- Puts the patient in a difficult position as he/she has to express his problem in front of many individuals.
- There is poor standardization in bedside clinic.
- It is restricted to a small group.

NURSING CARE CONFERENCE

It is similar to bedside clinic except the act of consultation is conducted in the absences of the patients. In the process of nursing care conference, a group of nursing students and their supervisor meet together for an informal discussion of patient's health problem.

Types of Nursing Care Conference

Nursing care conference is categorized as individual conference and group conference.

- **Individual conference:** The individual conference can be planned or incidental. The unplanned conference is often initiated by student/instructor or ward sister. The teacher guides an individual student to understand disease process, planning and implementing care for the purpose of improving nursing skills and thereby improving patient care. It provides opportunity to mentor the student and develop positive attitude to patient care. It is focused on development of clinical skills and over all change.
- **Group conferences:** They involve a group of students who discuss on a common area of interest under the guidance of the teacher. It stimulates innovative ways to deal with issues of concern in the clinical area.

DEMONSTRATION

It is a practical exhibition and explanation of how something works or is performed.

The most effective way to teach an occupational skill is demonstration. It requires two most essential teaching skills, one is the ability to demonstrate; and the other is the ability to explain. Both are vital to the success of either an operation lesson or an information lesson. In nursing, class demonstration is of vital importance as the teacher performs procedures step by step, which the students are expected to master.

Definition

Demonstration is display of the sequential flow of technical skill, an activity, mastering manual dexterity or skill in maintaining the principle while involved in a scientific activity.

Purpose of Demonstration

- To teach the students regarding organization of required resources at right time and right place.
- To use the resources appropriately without misuse.
- To teach the appropriate level of communication with client and family members.

- To teach patient safety by adopting various safety measures.
- To teach about environmental control.
- To teach to follow the steps systematically maintaining scientific principle.
  - Return demonstration may be used at end of a session taken by teacher to review the steps of the procedure and achieve mastery of skill in doing the procedure.

Preparation before Demonstration

- Practice before demonstrating procedure in front of the class.
- Be aware of possible hindrances.
- Collect all articles required to demonstrate and ensure they are in working condition.
- Arrange all articles in order of use and keep near at hand.
- Do planning about time management to avoid unnecessary time waste.
- Organize students to sit/stand around in a manner that permits visibility to see the demonstration as well as articles used.
- Go as per the plan and wherever possible get students to participate in steps they are aware of, for example, informing patient about the procedure.
- Explain preparation of the environment, i.e. the demonstration room, so that students get clear idea of the preparation they will need to do in clinical area while performing a procedure.
- Explain preparation of patient even if procedure is done on a manikin.

Presentation of Procedure

- Ensure the activity is visible to the all students in the group and teacher is loud enough.
- Perform the procedure with interest, efficiency and yet professionally.
- Avoid getting hyper and anxious, use anecdotes to make it look easy and enjoyable learning.
- Maintain caution while performing the procedures.
- Maintain eye-contact with the students; and interact with them.
- Look at the patient directly and communicate with patient during demonstration, if procedure is being demonstrated on an individual or manikin.
- Enact each step supported with a commentary so that they know the rationale.
- Have a brief recapitulate of the procedure demonstrated.

Precautions

- Ensure that each student gets the chance to observe the procedure.
- Avoid demonstrating the procedure when student is doing return demo.
- Plan time for students to do return demonstration within the frame work of class time.
- Don't demonstrate too many skills at one time.

When Carrying Out a Demonstration

- Confidently perform the steps as students will role model the teacher.
- Give a running commentary of the step as you perform the procedure.

- Ensure students can get a good view.
- Highlight key aspects, have questions that will tie up the key aspects as you move forward in the procedure.
- Emphasize safety rules while demonstrating time to time.
- Use variety of visual aids to illustrate.
- Involve students during the demonstration to make it a participating activity.
- Ensure mistakes are avoided as students may retain them instead of the correct step.
- Summarize and emphasize the main points.

After Demonstration

- Ensure if students have understood the steps of the demonstrated procedure.
- Clean and replace articles used in their allocated place.
- Plan for return demonstration so they can practice the newly learned skill.
- Observe the performance of students and give feedback.
- Encourage them to repeat the procedure until they achieve dexterity.
- Mentor weak students so that they become skillful.
- Assess students' performance for acquisition of skill.
- Allow sufficient time interval before re-demonstrating.

NURSING ROUNDS

It involves moving around in the patient area from bed-to-bed discussing the patient's history, present health status, line of management and the effect of care. It is usually conducted by clinical instructor/ ward sister with staff and student nurses for clear understanding of disease and the effect of nursing care for each patient. Clarifications are provided by the student nurse attending on the patient and suggestions/feedback received from the peer group and mentor.

Rounds may extend only up to one hour. For the success of nursing rounds, student and teacher should know each patient as the rounds are to be completes in an hour's time. The student nurse caring for the patient with the staff nurse will discuss shortly about patient's condition, care offered and response of patient.

Purposes of Nursing Rounds

- To inspect each patient's health status
- To get verbal report about patient care and response to treatment
- To evaluate the effect of nursing care
- To ensure patient safety by noticing unusual response or changes of health status
- To teach staff or student nurses regarding specific part of patient care
- To modify any plan of nursing care for maximizing patient benefit.

Types of Nursing Rounds

Based on purpose, nursing round is of three types: Informational rounds, Instructional rounds, and Problem solving rounds.

Advantages

- It facilitates understanding of disease process and appropriate nursing care.
- Improves and motivates group interaction.
- It emphasizes on individualized patient care.
- It gives the opportunity of correction.
- Ensures patient safety.

Limitations

- This method is not useful to teach a large group.
- It not equally beneficial for all, especially those who are unaware about patient.
- It may create anxiety to some patient.

PROCESS RECORDING

Process recording is a clinical teaching learning method required largely by students in the psychiatry unit. Process recording is the written report of the exact conversation between the student nurse and the patient during the time of interaction with patient, including details of observation regarding the verbal and nonverbal behavior of client, mood, effect, insight etc. Student nurses interact with patient to understand the disease process, patient's perception towards illness and treatment and also to recognize the response to treatment.

Definition

Process recording is defined as a method of recording of nurse-patient conversation including verbal and nonverbal that helps to understand and analyze patient's perceptions, thoughts, feelings and moods.

Purpose of Process Recording

- To establish rapport with the patient
- To understand psychodynamic of illness
- To identify patients' needs and problems
- To develop an awareness about the pattern of communication and its effect to client
- To develop skills in making conversation with student.

Uses of Process Recording (Fig 3)

Steps in Process Recording

Introductory

In the first step of process recording, student prepares self and identifies the purpose of the interaction before approaching patient.

Interaction Step

In this step, the patient stimulates interaction with the patient and records the conversation. Here, the teacher may guide the student to observe for cues and assess her own feelings during the interaction.

Recording Step

Students writes out the exact conversation that has taken place, her impressions of patient's feelings and her own feelings. Student also records her experience and learning. On completion of the exercise, student and teacher evaluate the recording for deeper understanding of the behavior of the patient.

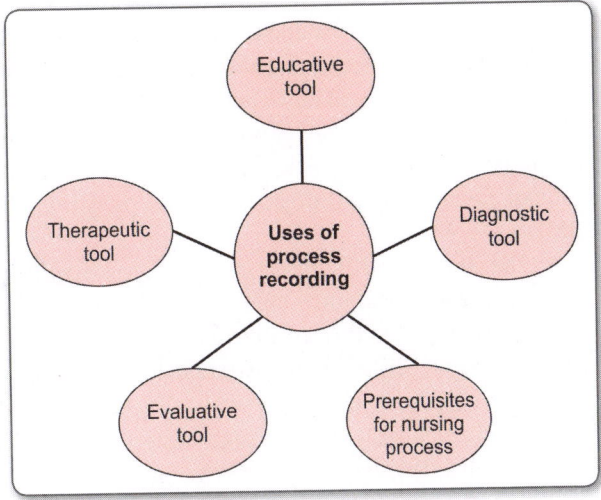

Fig. 3: Uses of process recording

Advantages

- In process recording, available information is used for review and analysis.
- It improves documentation skill.
- It promotes analytical thinking.
- It offers a useful means of relating communication theory to practice
- It encourages the user to analyze his or her practice, behavior and decisions.
- It provides opportunity to engage in reflection on their practice in a structured way.

Limitations

- Poor recording may fail to serve the purpose.
- Poor language or written skill may affect the transcriptions of the data in process recording.
- It requires a great deal of time to prepare.

SUMMARY

Teaching is not providing knowledge required by students neither advising regarding a specific learning content, but it could be referred as an interaction between student, subject and the mentor to bring out a new learning experience. It is a process by which the mentor molds her prodigies' character in any one through intellectually, socially, emotionally and physically. Teaching may take place formally or informally, it may be one way method or two-way method and today teaching uses multi-way i.e. students are not exclusively dependent on teacher; they have access to not just text books but the multimedia. Hence, learning constantly places challenges to the teacher to make teaching effective and interesting in the classroom.

Given this scenario, teaching should follow some principles and a teacher should organize teaching experience from: simple to complex, definite to indefinite; concrete to abstract; particular to general; using both deductive and inductive thinking process, and the psychology of the learner.

There are a **number of teaching methods** that a teacher can select based on learning objectives. Teaching methods are mainly categorized into classroom method and clinical method of teaching. Classroom methods of teaching include: lecture method, discussion, seminars, role play, project, assignments, symposium, field trips, exhibition, computed based/assisted learning, micro teaching, problem based learning (PBL), simulations, programmed instruction, and self-instructional modules (SIM).

In the clinical area, different group of teaching methods is selected for the purpose of attaining higher level of technical and professional skills that are essential to serve the community and profession. Clinical teaching methods mainly include: nursing care plan, case method, nursing round, bedside clinics, process recording, demonstration and nursing conference.

It does not matter which method would be adopted by teacher but teaching should be integrated with all influencing factors and highest level of learning is expected through minimizing the gap between high performers and low performers; thereby certain standard is maintained.

ASSESS YOURSELF

ESSAY ANSWER QUESTIONS

1. What is teaching? What are the principles involved in teaching? Describe each with suitable example.
2. Describe the characteristics of good teaching. Discuss the style and steps of lecture method.
3. What are the different methods of teaching a teacher can employ to ensure learning? Discuss briefly discussion as a method of teaching.
4. Discuss the role of a teacher that can be incorporated to make lecture interesting. Compare lecture and discussion methods. Describe different types of discussion method.
5. What is the meaning of discussion? Write down the types & use of discussion? How to conduct discussion? List down the advantages & limitations of discussion method.
6. Discuss project as a method of teaching? When project is appropriate to select as a method of teaching? Write down the student's role in project method.
7. Enumerate the features of workshop. Discuss steps involved in workshop. Describe the teachers role in workshop method.
8. What is computer assisted learning? Describe the types, advantage and disadvantage of Computer assisted learning.
9. State the meaning of bedside clinic. How to conduct bedside clinic? Discuss the advantage & limitation of bedside clinic.
10. What is case method? What are the different types of case method? Briefly discuss any one case method.

Contd...

SHORT ANSWER QUESTIONS

1. Write down the uses of role play in nursing.
2. What are benefits of tutorial method?
3. How field trips facilitate teaching?
4. Why virtual learning is important?
5. What are the merits of demonstration method?
6. What are the uses of micro teaching?
7. Why problem based learning is selected?
8. What are the roles of teacher in symposium?
9. How care plan helps a student?
10. What are the differences between case presentation and case study?

SHORT NOTES

1. Seminar
2. Exhibition
3. Field trips
4. Assignment
5. Nursing conference
6. Process recording
7. Programmed instruction
8. Self instructional module
9. Mastery learning
10. Simulation

MULTIPLE CHOICE QUESTIONS

1. **Lecturing is an oldest method of teaching and highly:**
   A. Individualized
   B. Student centered
   C. Effective
   D. Motivating
2. **Steps of lecture method is sequenced as:**
   A. Set Induction, Explaining, Stimulus variation and Closure
   B. Set induction, Closure, Stimulus variation and Explaining
   C. Stimulus Variation, Set Induction, Explaining, and Closure
   D. Explaining, Closure, Stimulus variation and Explaining
3. **In brain storming number of new concepts and ideas are possible to generate within –**
   A. Fraction of time
   B. Wide range of time
   C. Short period of time
   D. Long time gap
4. **Problem Based Learning (PBL) provides opportunity to uses:**
   A. Newer technique and innovative ideas
   B. Newer technique and older problem
   C. Older problem and traditional method
   D. Newer problem and conservative ideas
5. **In a classroom level of seminar, group generally consists of:**
   A. 5 to 10 participants
   B. 10 to 15 participants
   C. 15 to 20 participants
   D. 20 to 25b participants

Contd...

6. Process recording is used mainly to understand:
   A. Psychology of an patient
   B. Psychology of student
   C. Psychodynamic of illness
   D. Nature of psychosocial environment

7. A teaching method that involves displaying the sequential flow of technical skill following scientific principle is known as:
   A. Seminar
   B. Symposium
   C. Demonstration
   D. Field trips

8. The teaching method involves a series of speeches on single aspect of a topic is known as:
   A. Seminar
   B. Symposium
   C. Panel discussion
   D. Workshop

9. In bedside clinic groups are well informed about their roles and responsibilities and participation with active listening is expected from:
   A. Each group member
   B. Each group leader
   C. Each patient
   D. Each staff nurses

10. In micro teaching focus is on a single theme or small scale content for a smaller group of learner involving the steps of preparation presentation and immediate feedback in:
    A. A calm and quiet environment
    B. A non threatening environment
    C. An unknown environment
    D. Distracted environment

ANSWERS TO MCQs

1. (A)	2. (B)	3. (C)	4. (A)	5. (B)	6. (C)	7. (C)
8. (B)	9. (A)	10. (B)				

BIBLIOGRAPHY

1. Candela, Lori and Edmunds, Johnna, "An online Doctoral Education Course Using Problem Based Learning", Journal of Nursing Education, February, 2009. 48(2). Page No. 116 to 119.

2. WilkieK. "The nature of problem-based learning", in Glen S and Wilkie K (editors), Problem-based learning in nursing: a model for a new context, 2000, London: Macmillian.

3. Cannon R, Newble D. (2000) A handbook for teachers in universities and colleges. A guide to improving teaching methods (4th edition), London: Kogan Page.

4. Bastable, S. (2008). Nurse as Educator: Principles of Teaching and Learning for Nursing Practice. Sudbury, MA: Jones and Bartlett Publishers.

5. "Clinical Teaching Strategies in Nursing", Kathleen B. Gaberson, Marilyn H.Oermann, 3rd edition, Springer Publishing Company.

6. "Fast factors for the clinical nursing instructors", Eden ZabatKan, Susan Stabler-Hass, Springer Publishing Company, New York.

7. "Virtual Learning Environments", Pierre. Dillenbourg, University of Geneva, EUN Conference 2000. Education for Health, Vol.17, No.2, July 2004, 236-39

8. DeYoung.S; Teaching Strategies for Nurse Educators, 8th edition; Pearson education, prentice Hall, 2003, New Jersey.

9. Neeraja K.P; Text book of Nursing Education, 1st edition, Jaypee Brothers Medical Publishers; New Delhi, 2009.

10. Sankaranarayanan B, Sindhu B, Learning and Teaching Nursing 2nd edition, Brainfill, 2008;Kerala.

11. Kumar. N. Educational Technology Theory and Practice; 1st edition; AITBS Publisher; 2009, Delhi.

12. Devi Sanatombi Elsa, Manipal Manual of Nursing Education, 1st edition, CBS Publishers and distributors, Pvt. Ltd, New Delhi, 2008.

13. Maude B.A Principles of progressive Education applied to Nursing Education, 1st ed, The Macmillian company.

14. S Priya, Nursing Education, Vora Medical Publication, Mumbai.

15. Heidgerken.E. Loretta, Teaching and Learning in Schools of Nursing, Konark Publications, 3rd Edition, 2005 New Delhi.

Unit 7

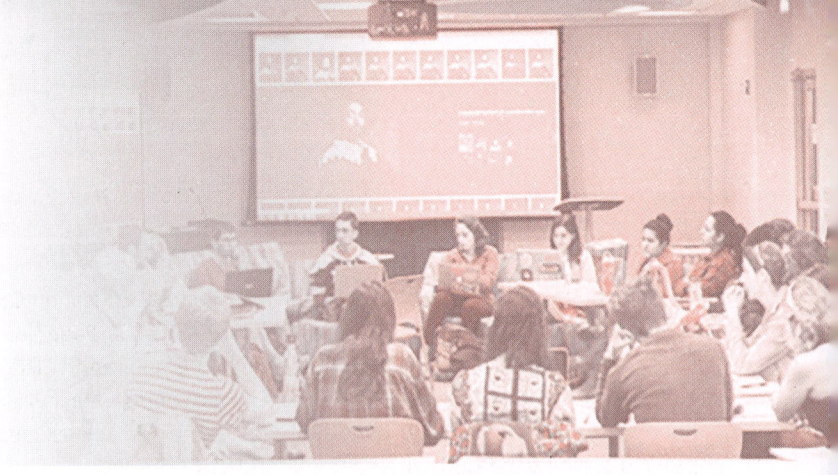

Review of Educational Media

— Piti Kaul, Jagadheeswaran P

CHAPTER OUTLINE

- **Understanding of Educational Media**
- **Classification of Educational Media:**
  - Display Materials: Black Boards, Chalk Boards
  - Printed Materials: Textbooks, Dictionaries, Newspapers, Magazines
  - Graphic Materials: Graphs, Charts, Diagrams, Posters, Maps
  - Audio Visual Aids: Radios, Telephones, Television And Tape Recording
  - Projected Aids: Film Strips, Projectors, Micro-Projector, Opaque Projector, Overhead Projector.
- **Introduction of AV Aids**
- **Objective AV Aids**
- **Purpose of AV Aids**
- **Selection and Source of AV Aids**
- **Advantages of AV Aids**
- **Principles of AV Aids**
- **Guidelines for Effective use of Educational Media**
- **Types of AV Aids**
  - Audio Aids
  - Visual Aids
  - Audio-Visual Aids

LEARNING OBJECTIVE

The learner will be able to

- Classify educational media:
  - Display materials; such as black boards, chalk boards
  - Printed materials; such as text books, dictionaries, newspapers, magazines
  - Graphic materials; such as graphs, charts, diagrams, posters, maps
  - Audio visual aids; such as radios, telephones, television and tape recording
  - Projected aids; film strips, projectors, micro-projector, opaque projector, overhead projector.
- Define the AV aids
- Describe the objective AV aids
- List out the purpose of AV aids
- Make out the selection and source of AV aids
- State the advantages of AV aids
- Explain the principles of AV aids
- Understand the guidelines for effective use of educational medias
- Explain the various types of AV aids
  - Audio aids
  - Visual aids
  - Audio-visual aids
- Answer the questions as an exercise for self-assessment in learning the unit

INTRODUCTION

Educational media is the media that is used to educate someone on a topic. It can be used at home or in the classroom to supplement lessons in formal education. Some examples include primary documents, documentaries and music. The media are usually used in combination. The six key building blocks of media are face-to-face teaching, text, graphics, audio (including speech), video and computing (including animation, simulations and virtual reality).

Educational media and multimedia technology are the channels of transmitting information to learners. There are various types of educational media and multimedia technology that are currently utilized in teaching and learning processes, which are: computer system, microphone, mobile device, interactive whiteboard, digital-video, online media stream, digital game, podcast and so on. The use of computer system in the classroom allows teachers to demonstrate a new lesson, animate, present new materials, illustrate how to use new programs and show new websites. In a noisy classroom or large classes, learners will be able to hear their teachers' instruction clearly and in the process learn better with the use of microphones.

Mobile devices such as clickers or smartphones can be utilized in enhancing feedback activities during and after instruction delivery by the teacher. An interactive whiteboard provides touch control of computer applications, which enhances the experience in the classroom by displaying visuals that can be viewed on a wider screen by learners'. This assists in visual learning, and interaction for learners to draw, write or manipulate images on the interactive whiteboard. The digital video eliminates the need for in-classroom hardware players and allows teachers and learners to access video clips immediately without the internet access. Online media streams can enhance streamed video websites for classroom teaching and learning processes. The digital game motivates the learners in learning a particular concept at hand and its use is increasing every day. Podcast is relatively new invention that allows teachers to publish files to the internet where learners' can subscribe and receive new files from people by a subscription.

EDUCATIONAL MEDIA

Educational media refers to channels of communication that carry messages with an instructional purpose. They are usually utilized for the sole purpose of learning and teaching.

Classification of Educational Media (Fig. 1)

There are different ways to classify media: print media, non-print media, and electronic media.
- *Print media*: They include, books, journals, magazines, newspapers, workbooks and textbooks
- *Non-print media*: They include, projected and non-projected media.
- *Electronic media*: They include audio media, visual media and audio-visual, projected media and non-projected media
  - **Projected media**: They require light source for projection, for example, film projector slides.
  - **Non-projected media**: They do not require light source and include 3-dimensional objects, 2-dimensional objects, prints, charts, models.
- *Audio media, Visual media and Audio-visual media*:
  - **Visual media**: These are the ones that can be seen. For example, television, computer and white board.

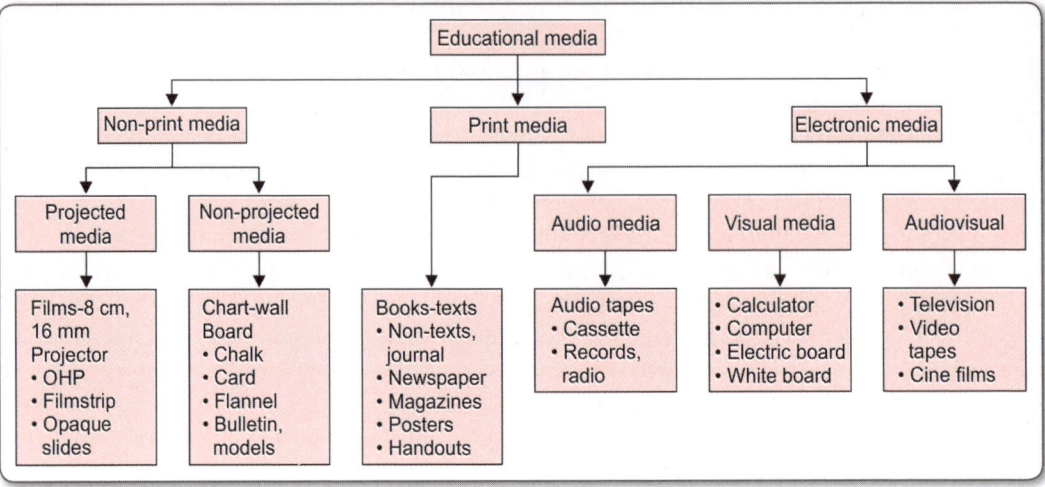

Fig. 1: Classification of education media

- **Audiovisual media**: This term refers to those instructional materials, which provide learners with audio and visual experiences by appearing to the hearing and seeing senses at the same time, for example television, video tapes, and closed circuit television (CCTV).

AUDIOVISUAL AIDS

Audiovisual materials must be seen in their relationship to teaching and learning process as a whole. Audiovisual education is an instructional method where particular attention is paid to the audio and visual presentation of the materials with the goal of improving comprehension and retention of learnt subjects. These educational materials are designed in such a way that they appeal to the students' senses, facilitate quick learning and clear understanding of the subject.

Audiovisual aids are multisensory materials, which motivate and stimulate the individual's interest. They make dynamic learning experiences more concrete, realistic and specific. Also they contribute significantly in developing creative thinking. It is commonly known that maximum retention of any learnt subject is by a combination of hearing, seeing and doing. Hence, audiovisual aids are also termed as teaching aids. They supplement the unidirectional didactic lecture method which is more interactive and interesting.

This reminds us of a famous proverb: "**I see and I forget, I hear and I remember, I do and I understand.**" The percentage of learning has been listed in the Figs 2A and B.

Definition of Audiovisual Aids

- Visual aids are those sensory objects or images which initiate or stimulate and reinforce learning.

—**Burton**

- Audiovisual aids are anything by means of which learning process may be encouraged or carried on through the sense of hearing or sense of sight. —**Good's dictionary of education**
- Audiovisual aids are any device, which can be used to make the learning experience more concrete realistic and more dynamic. —**Kinders James**

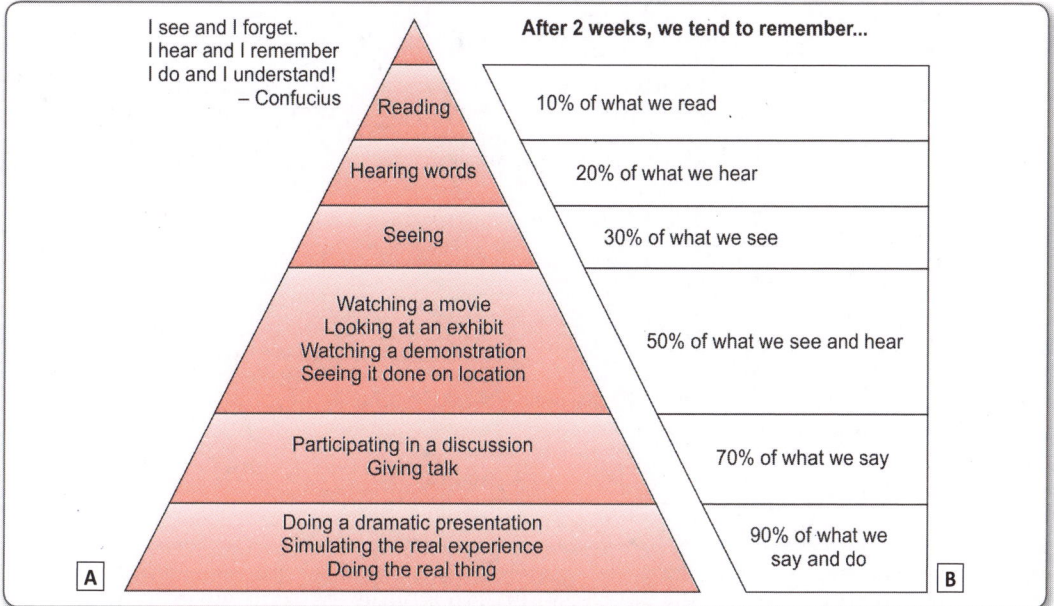

I see and I forget.
I hear and I remember
I do and I understand!
– Confucius

Reading	10% of what we read
Hearing words	20% of what we hear
Seeing	30% of what we see
Watching a movie / Looking at an exhibit / Watching a demonstration / Seeing it done on location	50% of what we see and hear
Participating in a discussion / Giving talk	70% of what we say
Doing a dramatic presentation / Simulating the real experience / Doing the real thing	90% of what we say and do

After 2 weeks, we tend to remember...

Figs 2A and B: (A) Various components of audio-visual aids; (B) Percentage of learning

Objective of AV Aids (Fig. 3)

- Improves the teacher's skills in making teaching-learning process more effective
- Grasp and reverts the learners' attention
- Facilitates the interest in all levels of students
- Provides strong foundation to facilitate the lesson plan contents on teaching
- Creates more interest in class room teaching
- Breaks the teacher - centered approach and facilitates the activate participation of the learners
- To be an antibody to the disease of verbal instructions
- To provide effective motivation to the learners

Purpose of Audiovisual Aids

- To make clear changes on concepts of teaching learning process
- To offer the stunning experience in teaching learning process
- To give variety of stimulations to the learners in learning activity
- To attract and retain the learners attention
- To provide opportunity to handle and manipulate the various teaching aids
- To create interest to the teachers and learners
- Provides positive rewards to the learners

Selection of Audiovisual Aids

Selection of audiovisual aids is dependent on:

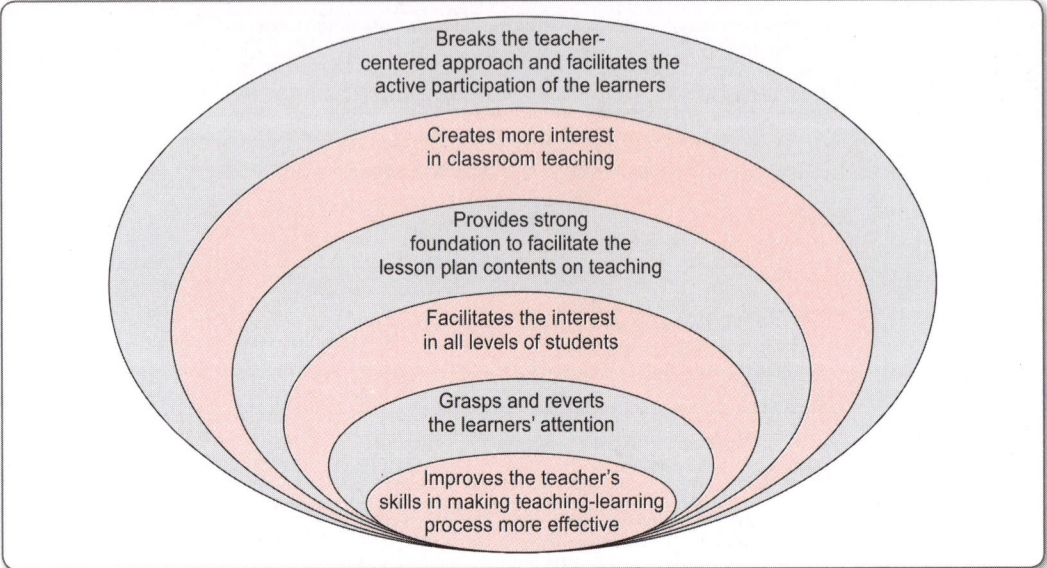

Fig. 3: Objectives of audiovisual aids

- Teaching objective
- Nature of subject matter
- Nature of audience
- Size of audience
- Availability of equipments, materials and funds
- Skills and experience of extension agents in preparation and use of audio visual aids

Advantages of Audiovisual Aids (Fig. 4)

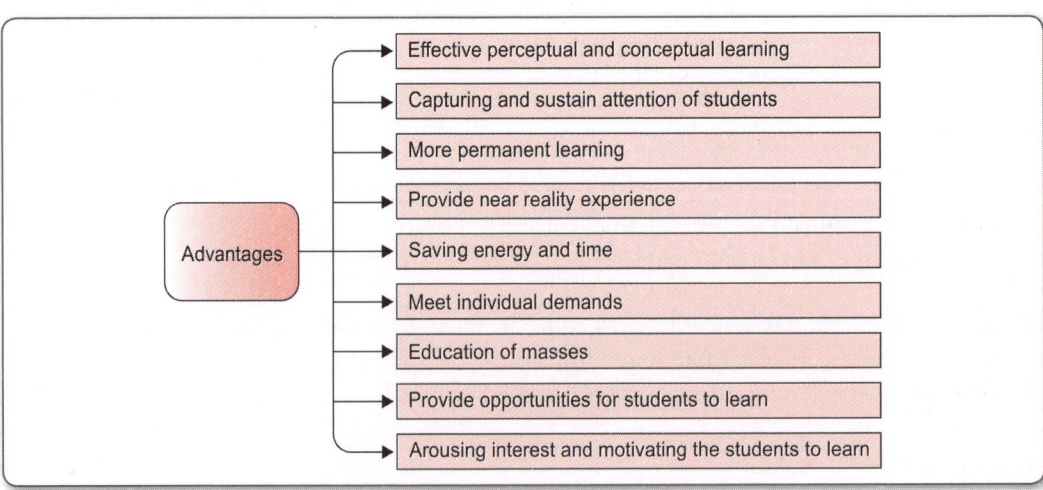

Fig. 4: Advantages of audiovisual aids

Principles of Audiovisual Aids

Audiovisual aids are dependent on following principles:

- *Principle of selection*: They should suit the age level, grade level, and other characteristics of the learners. They should be interesting and motivating and should be the true representative of the real things. They must focus on the realization of desired learning objectives.
- *Principle of preparation*: As far as possible, locally available materials should be used. The teachers should receive some training in the preparation of aid and should prepare some of the aids themselves. Students may be associated in the preparation of aids.
- *Principle of handling*: Arrangement of keeping aids safely and to facilitate their lending to the teachers for use.
- *Principle of presentation*: Teachers should carefully visualize the use of teaching aids before their actual presentation and should be fully familiar with the use and manipulation of the aids. Adequate care should be taken to handle an aid in such a way so that no damage is done. It should be displayed properly so that all the students are able to see it, observe it and derive maximum benefit out of it.
- *Principle of response*: Teachers guide the students to respond actively to the audiovisual stimuli and master it.
- *Principle of evaluation*: Continuous and ongoing evaluation is necessary.

Guidelines to use Proper Audio Visual Aids

- Make them to summarize or show the sequence of content first.
- Make them to visually interpret statistics by preparing charts and graphs that illustrate what you will deliver.
- Make them to illustrate and reinforce your support statements.
- Make them to add visual clarity to your concepts and ideas.
- Make them to focus the attention of the target group on key points.
- Donot make use of the project copies of printed or written text. Instead, summarize the information and show only the key points on the visual aids. If the group must read every word, use handouts for reading, either before or after your presentation.
- Never put yourself in the role of aiding your visuals. A presentation is primarily an oral form of communication. If your only function is to read the information on your overheads or slides, the target group will become easily bored.
- Never use copies of your transparencies as handouts. They reinforce what you are saying; they don't say it for you. If you want your target group to remember what you meant, you'll need to provide written text in addition to any key point summaries or charts that you need for your transparencies.
- Never use charts, graphs, or tables that contain more information than what you want to provide. The group will have difficulty focusing on the point that you're trying to make.

Types of Audio Visual Aids

Audiovisual aids can be classified as follows:

- **Audio aids**: The instructional device through which message can be only heard are known as audio aids like tape recorder, radio and telephone

- **Visual aids**: The instructional device which helps to visualize the message are known as visual aids.
  - Projected visual aids like slides, overhead projector and power point slides
  - Non-projected visual aids like posters, charts, graphs, models, specimens, chalkboards, picture and photographs, graphic aids, cartoons, chalkboard, flashcards, bulletin boards
  - Display type: Visuals which are spread before the audience for viewing to get the message by looking at them like poster, models, exhibits and specimens
  - Presentation type: Visuals presented or projected before the audience for viewing but at the same time, one explains or presents the message of the visuals, so that the message gets a meaningful understanding like slides, overhead projectors, charts and power point slides.
- **Audiovisual aids**: The instructional devices through which the message can be heard and seen simultaneously are known as audiovisual aids.
  - Projected Audiovisual aids like video and cinema
  - Non-projected Audiovisual aids like drama, puppet show and street play.

Non Projected Visual Aids

Graphic Aids: Cartoons (Fig. 5)

The cartoon is a visual graphic aid which illustrates in the form of symbols of an object, organization, an opinion and a situation. It make use of humor, fantasy, saltire and exaggeration, which helps to summarize the major content and convey the message. If the cartoon is made in a simple and clear way, they save time in reading and explanation. Cartoons are primarily designed to influence public.

Quality of drawing is also a important while making a cartoon, the student make sure about the correct interpretation of any theme in cartoon such as what it tells. Many a times they present the realities and ultimately change the behavior of people and opinion builder, Students can also apply graphic aid in their study such as to portray the right and wrong ways to do a procedure, in hospital setting to portray the right and wrong body mechanics.

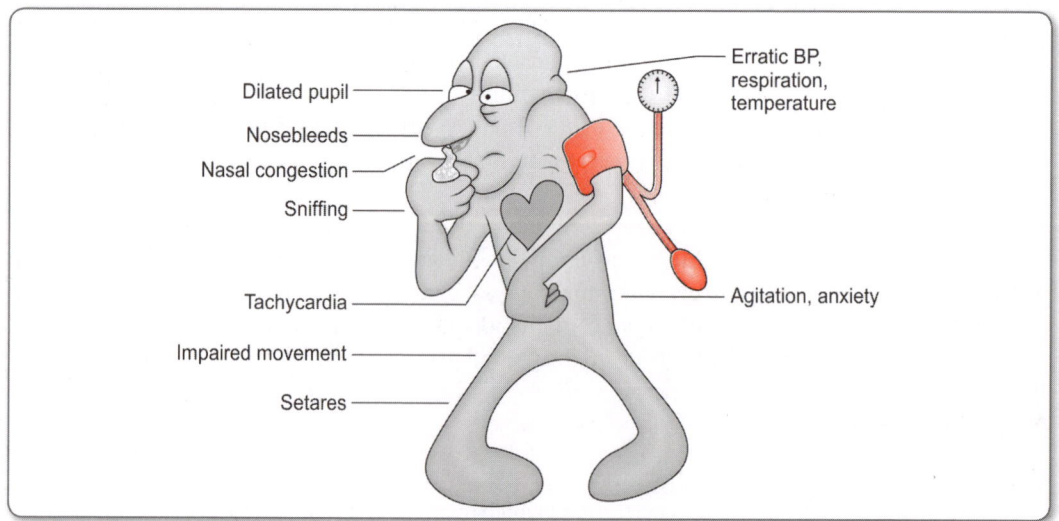

Fig. 5: Example of cartoons

Characteristics

- It must be in proper size so that everybody can see them.
- Presentation of the cartoons depends upon the learner age and educational level.
- Wording should be minimal and meaningful.
- It should always self-explanatory.
- It should be humorous and funny.

Advantages

- Motivates students to engage with the lesson's teaching point
- Make activate to students in a particular idea or topic
- Capture and maintain attention
- Promote innovative thinking on different aspects
- Encourage students to use their ideas and concepts
- Relieve boredom and help to interpret the meaning in easy way
- Make students laugh and, smile which minimized stress
- Help to maintain teacher relationship with students

Chalk Board/Black Board/ White Board (Fig. 6)

It is one of the common types of audio-visual aids. Chalk board or black board is a simple and effective visual aid used for presenting varieties of material.

Definition

A chalk board/black board/white board is any dark coloured or white, flat, smooth surface on which one can write or draw with chalk or any material such as marker pen. It is one of the oldest and simplest visual aids.

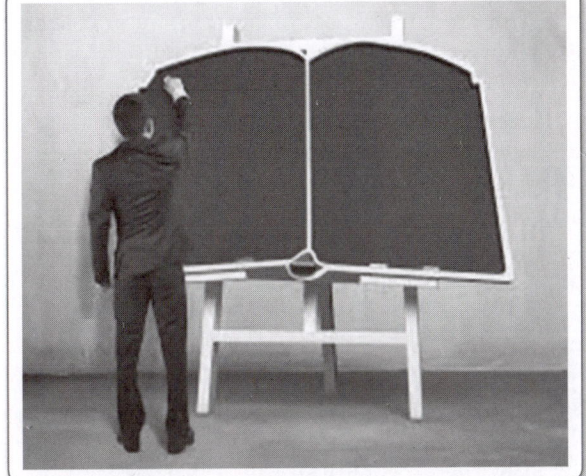

Fig. 6: Chalk board

Chalk Boards can be fixed or portable and can be made of materials such as wood, slate, glass, magnetic materials, sun mica.

The purpose of the white board is to record in semi-permanent form the key points and explanations during teaching session. This enables the students to see as well as hear and to copy the points for future reference. Most white boards use dry pens that can be wiped off with a dry cloth. Others can be wiped with some spirit also.

Advantages of Using a Chalk Board

- It is simple to use and needs little practice.

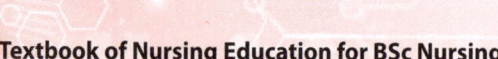

- It is easily available, economic and reusable and can be used any time.
- It can be used in a wide variety of ways, for example, simple outlines, drawing, summary of main points, etc.
- It encourages active doing and seeing on part of the audience.
- Mistakes can be quickly erased and is a natural supplement to all other aids.

Disadvantages of Chalk Board

- Written materials cannot be saved or preserved
- Cannot be used for a large audience
- Requires imagination, initiation, practice, and preparation
- Cannot illustrate moving parts.

Technique For effective use of Chalk Board

- Stand on the left side and not in front when writing.
- Do not turn your back to the audience for a long time.
- Use the board cleanly so that it is readable to all.
- Write or draw in advance, if you have to write many things or do complicated drawings.
- Write in an organized way and avoid crowding the board with words or figures.
- Writing should be legible and straight.
- Write down new words you want to stress on, in capital letters with even pressure.
- Write at an eye level of audience and begin writing from the top down.
- Use a proper eraser in up and down motion. Erase the matter you have written first. Don't clean the black board with hands.
- Before erasing the board, ask the students in the class whether they have noted down the important points.
- When writing on the board you should avoid talking and verbal discussion, as the words are lost to the class.
- Face the students always when addressing them.

Flash Cards

Flash cards are a set of pictured paper cards of varying sizes that are flashed one by one in a logical sequence. Flash cards can be self made or commercially prepared and are made up of chart or drawing paper: plain paper using colors or ink on them for drawings.

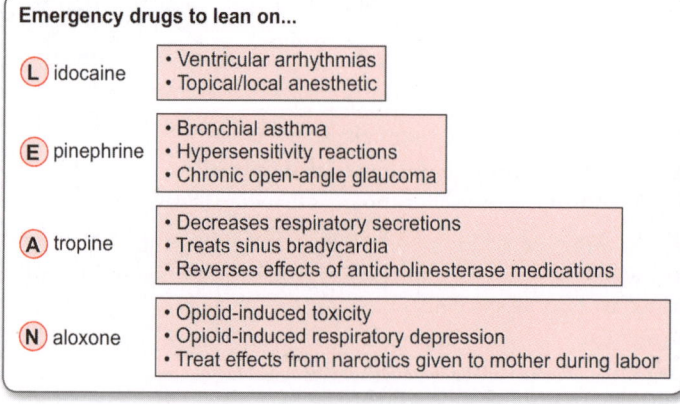

Fig. 7: Example of a flash card

Purposes of Flash Cards

- To teach the students in class room

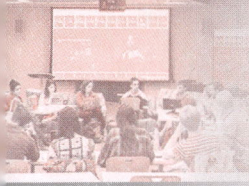
- To give health education to small group of people
- To organize group discussions.

Principles

- The messages should be brief, simple, clear and visible to audience. It can be in the form of a line drawing or photographs or cartoons. The content is written in few lines at the back of each card.
- The size of card is usually 10" × 12" or 22" × 28".
- For one talk, 10–12 cards can be used. It should not be less than 3 and more than 20.
- Picture for each idea should be prepared, which will give visual impact to the idea.
- The height of writing on the flash card should be approximately 5 cm for better visualization.

How to Use the Flashcards

The following steps should be used while displaying flash cards.
- Give brief introduction about the lesson to students.
- Give instructions to students about their actions while you flash the cards.
- Flash the card in front of the class by holding it high with both your hands against chest or use folding or frame or box, so that all the students can see it.
- It can also be displayed in a bulletin board or on a wall.
- Allow the students to respond as per instructions given already.
- Review the lesson by selectively using flash cards.

Advantages

Flash cards can be used to
- Introduce and present topics
- Apply information already gained by students to new situations
- Review a topic
- Drill and practice in elementary classes
- Develop the cognitive abilities of recognition and recall of students
- Work as a useful supplementary aid and can be effectively used with other material.

Disadvantages

- Cannot be used for a large group
- Prone to get spoiled soon
- Preparation is time consuming.

Posters

Posters are the graphic aids with short quick and typical messages with paintings that capture attention. The message can be conveyed to many people at many locations.

Purposes

- To communicate a more general idea to a large populations
- To thrust the message for leading to action for the class room and community

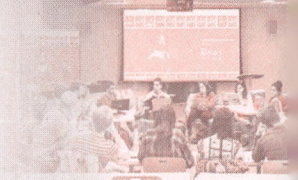

- To provide general motivation
- To create an aesthetic or atmospheric effect.

Preparation and Rules

- To convey a specific idea or content
- To focus on one point
- To support local demonstration
- Planned for specified people
- Convey the message at single glance
- Use bold letters
- Use attractive colors
- Place in locations, where people pass or gather.

Features of a Good Poster

- It should be brief.
- It should be simple so that message can be easily understandable.
- It should be relevant and based on single idea.
- It should have suitable colors and color combinations should be used to make the poster attractive and eye catching.
- While displaying the poster, one should be sure to find a place where there is adequate light and where the larger population can see it.

Advantages

- It conveys the message very quickly to large number of people.
- It attracts attention of people.
- It can stand alone and is self-explanatory.
- Good poster leads to action with good motivation.
- It does not require a detailed study or preparations.

Disadvantages

- Poster does not always gives enough information.
- When a poster is seen for longer time, it may not be attractive. So it should be dynamic.

Flannel Graphs/Khadi Graph/Felt Board

Flannel Graphs are rough felt boards covered with skin tight flannel/wool or khadi on to which cutouts, writings, symbols, figures made out of light card board are pasted. (Figs. 8 and 9)

Advantages

- Flexible, dynamic, portable, convenient and reusable

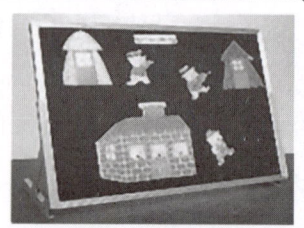

Articles required:
- Wooden or plywood boad
- Khaddar cloth or velvette cloth
- Flannel pictures
- Gum

Fig. 8: Articles required for flannel graphs

- Locally produced, in-expensive, and attract attention easily when properly displayed
- Promote step by step logical and orderly presentation, which can be referred again for classifying
- Simple to make; its use saves time in teaching
- Helps in communicating ideas to students. Students can use them effectively too
- Adds variety to visual aids and can be used where other methods cannot be employed.

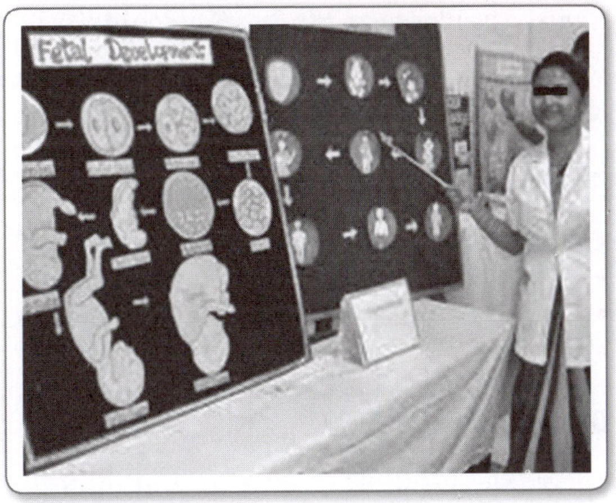

Disadvantages

- Mostly useful for small groups and not for large groups.
- Not useful for abstract learning.

How to use it Effectively?

- Be thorough with the script, try it out and rehearse it.
- Keep the pieces in sequence.
- Tilt the board at 45° angles to stick better.
- Place the piece with little downward pressure.
- Commentary must be used for each piece.
- Do not overcrowd the board.

Bulletin Board

Bulletin Board is a device for displaying study material or current news in a visualized form. It is the work of the student by the students and for the students. This device is often the most effective and exciting display element in a classroom (Fig. 10).

Purposes

- Motivates the learner
- Broadens the sensory experience and provides experience outside the students' environment
- Gives the correct initial information
- Supplement and correlates the instructions and saves time.

Fig. 9: Flannel graph

Fig. 10: Bulletin board

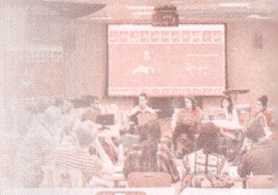

Items to be Placed on the Bulletin Boards

Various items that can be placed on bulletin boards are photographs, newspaper cuttings, all kinds of creative work of the students, group activities, announcements, etc.

Advantages

- Serves as an introduction to a particular topic
- Explains important events, announcements
- Reports special activities in the school, shares knowledge, and stimulates curiosity
- Summarizes and highlights events.

Disadvantages

- Not effective for illiterate group.

How to use a Bulletin Board Effectively?

- The theme message conveyed should be clear, simple, interesting and balanced.
- Arrange the information in neat and orderly way using appropriate material.
- Do no crowd the bulletin board.
- Give suitable title, large enough to be seen from a distance.
- Use neutral color for the background.
- Layout should be attractive, simple, and easy to understand.
- The information conveyed should remain for a limited period.

You cannot compel a person to look at a bulletin board; the display itself must have the power to hold attention of the looker.

Charts

Chart is a visual aid which depicts pictorial and written key information in a systematic way. It is a combination of pictorial, graphic, numerical or vertical material, which presents a clear summary of the content. They are symbols which are used for summarizing, comparing, contrasting and explaining subject matter (Fig. 11).

Purposes of Charts

The main purposes of charts are to:
- Visualize an idea/content, which cannot be effectively explained in words
- Highlight important points and to provide outline for materials covered in presentation
- Show continuity in teaching process.

Advantages

Advantages of charts are as follows:
- It is an effective tool for teaching – learning.
- It arouses interest.
- It involves low cost.

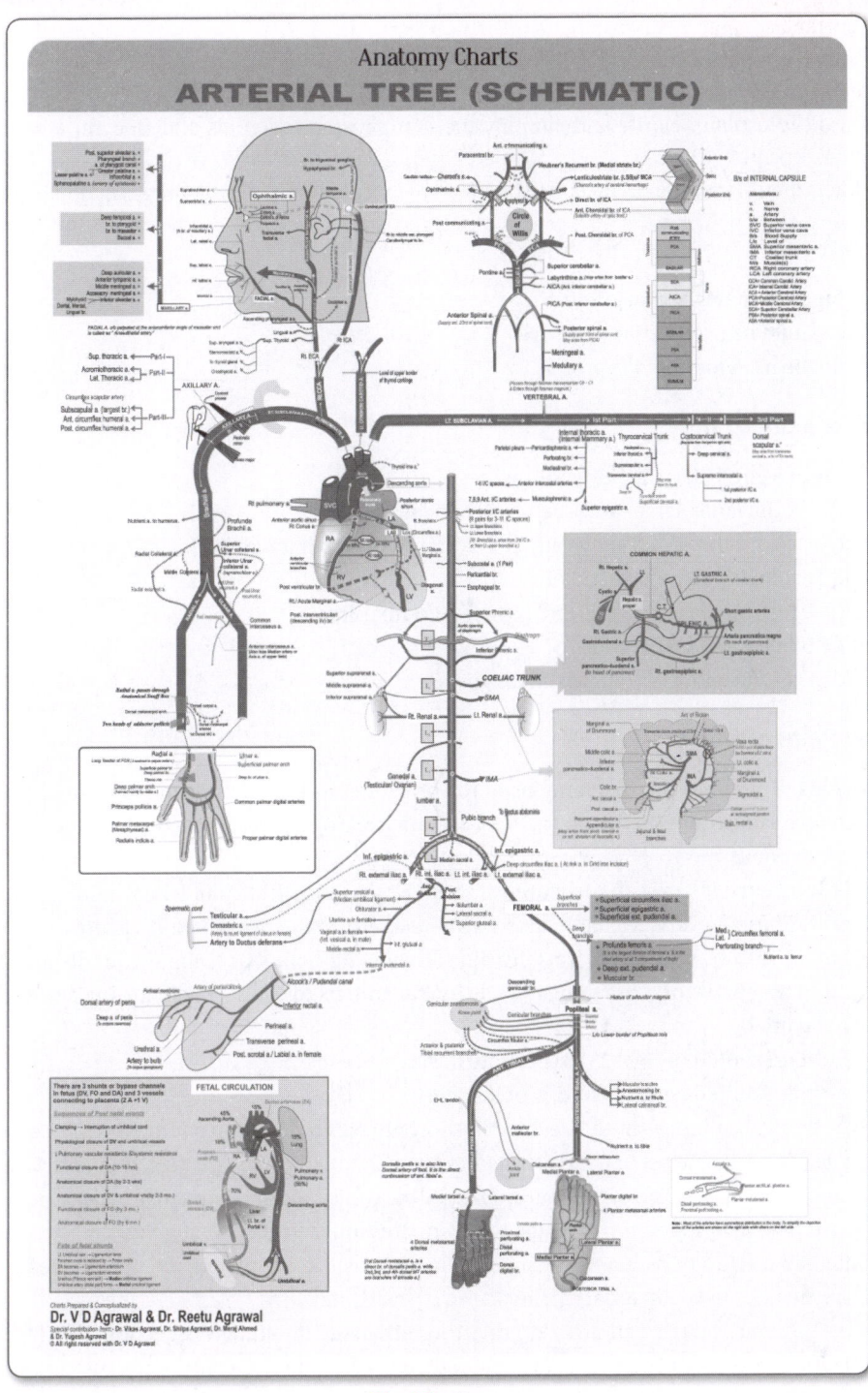

Fig. 11: Charts

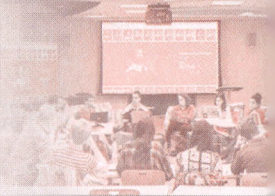

- It is portable.
- It is easy to prepare a chart.
- It can be used and reused.
- It is used to explain, clarify and simplify the complicated materials and to compare and show relationships.
- It attracts attention, reduces the amount of verbal explanation and encourages action.

Disadvantages

Disadvantages of charts are as follows:
- Charts cannot be used for large groups.
- It cannot be used for illiterate groups.

Features of a Good Chart

The features of a good chart include following:
- Should be sufficiently large to be seen easily by the audience
- Should be clear, simple, attractive and not overcrowded with too many facts
- Should tell about the theme in detail
- Should be in symbols and words and have few comparisons
- Should highlight the main points
- Should be strong enough to stand the rough use.

Common Types of Charts

- **Flowchart**: These are the diagrams used to show organizational elements or administrative or functional relationships. In this chart, lines, rectangles, circles, are connected by lines showing the directional flow.
- **Tabulation chart**: It shows the schedule of an activity or of an individual. For example, time-table of a class. These are very valuable aids in the teaching situation, where breakdown of a fact or a statement is to be listed. It is a useful aid for showing points of comparison, distinction, and contrast between two or more things. While making the table charts, the following points must be kept in the mind.
    - The chart should be 50 × 75 cm or more in size.
    - The chart should be captioned in bold letters.
    - The vertical columns should be filled in short phrases rather than complete sentences.
- **Flip chart**: These are a set of charts related to specific topic, which are tagged together and hung on a supporting stand. The individual charts will carry a series of related materials or messages in sequence. The salient points of specific topic are presented. These are large note pads that can be mounted on a stand or over a white board. When a sheet is completed, it can be folded over and next sheet can be used. Material can be prepared in advance.
- **Pie chart**: In this, a circle is drawn and divisions are made into different sections. Each section is coded differently and code keys are given at right corner of the chart as legend. The circumference is divided into suitable sections. It is relevant for showing the component part.

Pamphlet (Fig. 12)

The pamphlet form of literature has been used for centuries as an economical vehicle for the broad distribution of information.

A pamphlet is an unbound booklet (that is, without a hard cover or binding). It may consist of a single sheet of paper that is printed on one or both sides depending upon the objectives of message. It can be folded in half, in thirds, or in fourths, called a **leaflet**, or it may consist of a few pages that are folded in half and saddle stapled at the crease to make a **simple book**.

Pamphlets can contain information, which may be general and specific to subject area. Pamphlets are very important in marketing because they are cheap to produce and can be distributed easily to consumers.

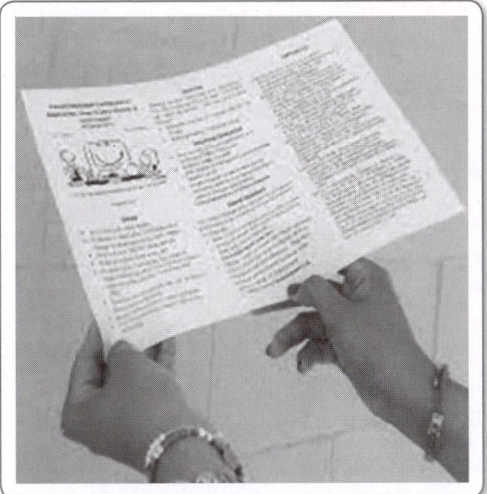

Fig. 12: Example of a pamphlet

A pamphleteer is a historical term for someone, who produces or distributes pamphlets, especially for a political cause.

Due to their low cost and ease of production, pamphlets have often been used to popularize political or religious ideas.

Pamphlets have also long been an important tool of political protest and political campaigning for similar reasons.

Commercial Use

The pamphlet has been widely adopted in commerce, particularly as a format for marketing communications. They can be used for the purpose of:

- Product descriptions or instructions, relevant information, event guides and are used in the same way as leaflets, brochures.
- Of recent, pamphlets are used most by corporations looking to extend offers or promotions such as Direct TV. They are found in shopping bags in popular retailers such as bed, bath and beyond.

Projected Visual Aids

Camera

It is a device to take photographs (Fig. 13).

Types of Camera

- Fixed fox simple box camera with single speed shutter
- Box camera with two speed shutters
- **All metal reflex:**

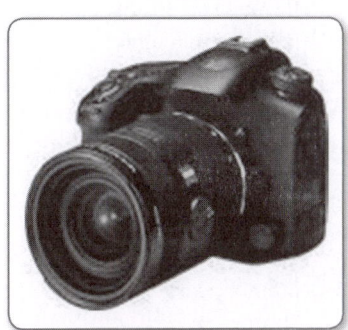

Fig. 13: Camera

- ▪ Single Lens Reflex
- ▪ Double Lens Reflex
- Miniature cameras with couple plates
- Old model field cameras using plates

Advantages

- It create high quality images.
- It easily conveys message.
- It draws attention of a large group of people.
- It provides direct experience to the events, objects.
- Students get motivation while organizing photography events.

LCD Projector (Fig. 14)

LCD projector has more advanced features than the conventional method projectors. Educational institute are equipped with LCD projectors. Every Class rooms are equipped with projectors, which give the outcome and meet the objective. It helps to view the educational film and present the topic through slides.

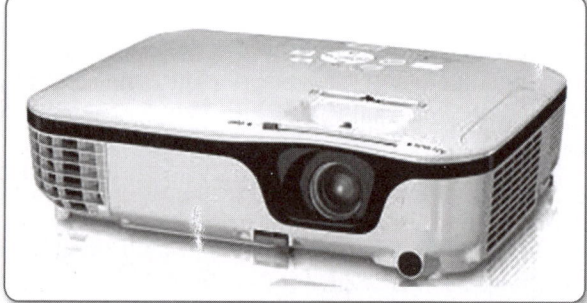

Fig. 14: LCD projector

Liquid crystal display (LCD) is a device, which sends light from metal halide lamp through a prism that separates light to 3 polysilicone panels – one each for the red, green, and blue components of the video signal

Advantages

- It has high contrast and brightness.
- It is permanently mounted in class room without specific arrangement.
- It is less expensive and affordable.
- Students can be attentive in class room while the presenting topic.
- It can be accessible by large group of people.
- It is easy to handle.
- It is easy to prepare the teaching material and shows the educational film to the students.
- Lecture becomes more effective and interesting.
- Teacher can face the students while teaching in the class.

Parts

- Lens
- Memory card
- Shutter
- A set of rechargeable batteries and a battery charger.

- Press button
- Zoom
- AC Adapter.

Microscope

The term microscope is **derived from** Ancient Greek: *mikrós*, "small" and skopeîn, "to look" or "see". Microscopy is the science of investigating small objects and structures using the microscope. Microscopic means invisible to the eyes unless aided by a microscope. It is an important instrument for diagnosis of disease.

Parts of Microscope (Fig. 15)

- **Eyepiece lens or ocular**: The lens at the top of the microscope that a person can look through. They are usually had magnifying power of 10X or 15X.
- **Eye piece tube**: Connects the eyepiece to the objective lenses.
- **Arm**: Supports the tube and connects it to the base.
- **Objective lenses**: There are three to four objective lens on a microscope, they consist of 4X, 10X, 40X and100X Powers. Objectives can be forward or rear-facing.
- **Base**: The bottom of the microscope, used for support.
- **Illuminator**: It is a light source for microscope located at the base. Most light microscopes use low voltage.
- **Stage**: It is used for mounting the specimen. The flat platform where slides are kept on stage. Stage clips hold the slides in place. It is beneath the revolving nosepiece.

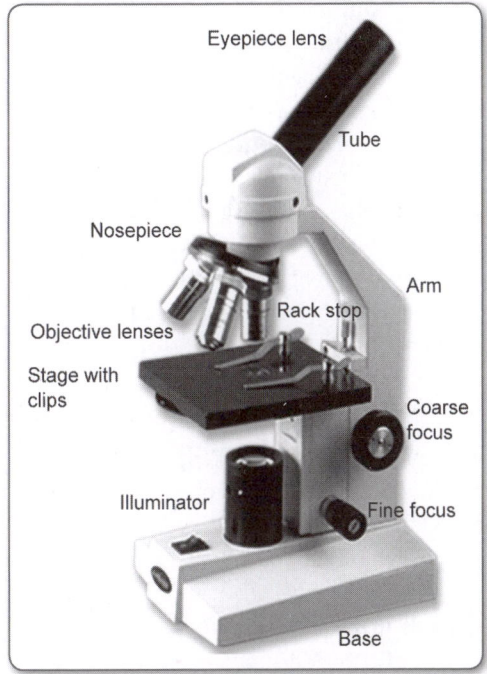

Fig. 15: Parts of a microscope

- **Condenser**: The purpose of the condenser lens is to focus the light onto the specimen. Condenser can be raised and lowered. It is located under the stage often in conjunction with an iris diaphragm.
- **Diaphragm**: It is used to adjust the amount of light coming through the condenser. The wider the diagram the greater the numerical space and the smaller the detail seen.

Types

- **Simple Microscope**: Microscope contains only one magnifying lens. Images become larger than the actual objects size while using magnifying glass.
- **Compound Microscope**: It contains more than one magnifying lens. Microscope magnifies the size of the object about 1000 times.

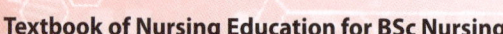

- **Electron Microscope**: Electron microscope uses an electron beam as source of illumination and magnet to focus to beam. It has greater resolution power than compound microscope. There are two types of electron microscopes:
  - Transmission electron microscope
  - Scanning electron microscope.

Over Head Projector (OHP)

The overhead projector is the commonly used audiovisual aids. It is a machine that projects large images of clear acetate sheets called overhead transparencies onto a screen. It is designed for use in daylight. The teacher can write or draw diagrams on the transparency sheet while he/she teaches and these are projected simultaneously on the screen by the over head projector. Transparencies can be prepared from various sources such as hand written/hand drawn by teacher or computer generated. They can also be produced by teachers using a photocopier or commercially produced (Fig. 16).

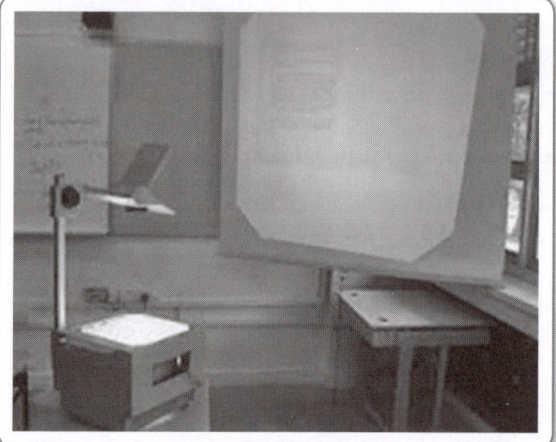

Fig. 16: Over head projector

How to Use the Transparencies during Presentation

- Ensure that screen is kept above the head and is in full view of the audience.
- Make sure that the teacher does not block the view of audience while presenting.
- Darken the room appropriately by blocking out sunshine and dimming nearby lights.
- Switch off the projector, if you are going to discuss the important points or during the change of transparency.
- Talk to the audience, not to the screen.

Purposes of Transparencies

- To enable the audience to develop concepts and sequences in a subject matter area
- To help the teacher to prepare marginal notes on the transparencies for their use without exposing them to the class
- To assess the performance of learners, while other classmates observe
- To use contrast color of the content while showing relationship of various content areas.

Advantages

- Enables the teacher to point out features appearing on the screen by pointing to the materials at the projector itself.
- Helps to observe the students' reactions to the discussion of teacher.
- Encourages attention of the student and creates interest.

Opaque Projector

Opaque projector is the only projector on which you can project **non-transparent materials** such as book pages, objects, coins, postcards, or any other similar flat material that is non-transparent. The projector helps to project and simultaneously enlarge the image directly from the original material, printed matter, all kinds of written or pictorial matter in any sequence desired by the teacher. It requires a dark room, as projector is large and not movable (Fig. 17).

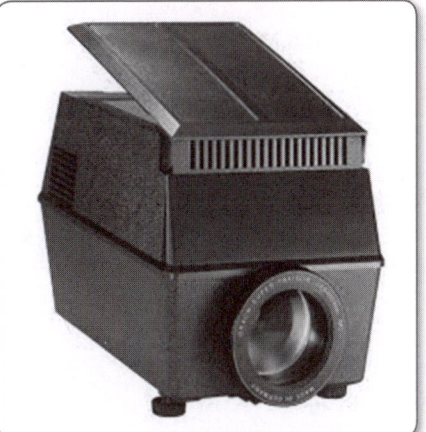

Fig. 17: Opaque projector

Advantages

- Stimulates attention and arouses interest can project a wide range of materials like books, stamps, coins, specimen etc. when only one copy is available.
- Helps in enlarging drawings, pictures and maps etc.
- Helps in projection of hand-written materials, if typing material is not possible.
- Helps students to retain knowledge for longer period.
- Can be operated easily.

Disadvantages

- The equipment is costly.
- It needs to be handled and used with care.
- It needs a dark room for projection.

Slide Projector

A slide is a small piece of transparent material on which a single pictorial image or scene or graphic is reproduced or photographed slides of still pictures on positive film which you can process and mount individually yourself or send to a film laboratory. The standard size of the slides is 2" × 2". You can prepare good slides with any 35 mm camera.

Slides can be prepared by both teachers and pupils from photographs and pictures taken by them during field trips undertaken for various purposes such as historical, geographical, literacy or scientific excursions. The slides need to be arranged in sequence, while using them for teaching.

Slide projection is used for showing still pictures to an audience using 35 mm slides. It is necessary to operate slide projector in darkness in order to obtain a clear image. Slides can be obtained commercially or teachers can make their own slides using modern 35 mm camera with a close up facility.

Types of Slides (Fig. 18)

The slides can be of two types
- **Photographic slides:**
  - These can be 2" × 2" or 3" × 4" size

- They can be black and white and
- Colored

- **Handmade slides**: These can be made with following material
  - Acetate sheet
  - Cellophane
  - Etched glass
  - Plain glass
  - Logarithm

Advantages

- It only requires filming, processing and mounting by self or laboratory
- Results in colorful, realistic, reproduction of original subject
- It can be prepared with any 35 mm camera for most of the uses
- It can easily be revised and updated
- It can be easily be handled, stored and rearranged for various uses
- It is easy to combine with tape narration and can control time for discussion
- It can be used for individual purpose or can be adopted for group use.

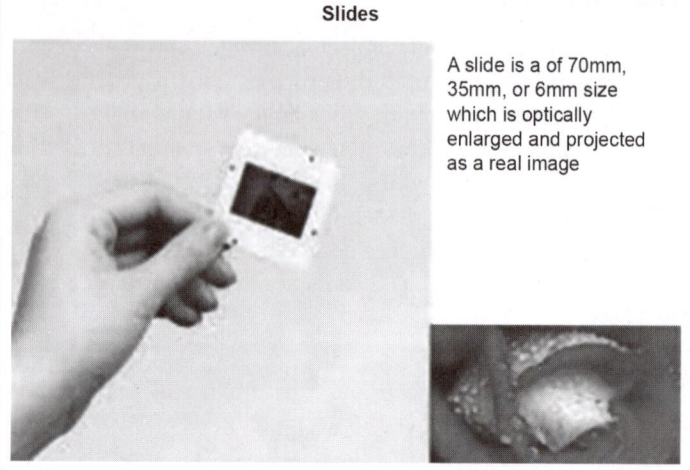

Slides

A slide is a of 70mm, 35mm, or 6mm size which is optically enlarged and projected as a real image

Fig. 18: Slide

Filmstrips

Film strips are sequence of transparent still pictures with individual frames on 35 mm film. It is a fixed sequence of related stills on a roll of 35 mm film or 8 mm film. Each strip contains from 12 to 18 or more pictures (Fig. 19).

Principles

- A tape recorded narration can be synchronized with film strip before using them and selected carefully to meet the needs of the topic to be taught to learners.
- They should be carefully selected for teaching purpose.
- If more specific study is required, it should be shown again.
- Filmstrip should be used to stimulate emotions, build attitudes and to point out problems.
- It should be introduced appropriately and its relationship to the topic of the study should be focused.
- Always use a pointer to show specific details on the screen in order to direct attention of learners.

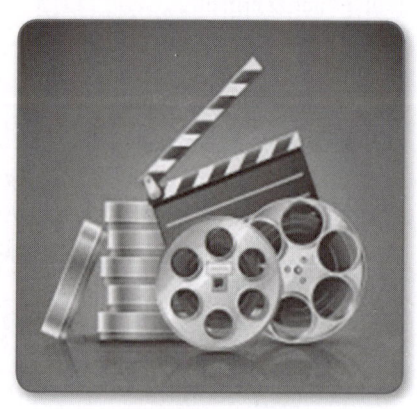

Fig. 19: Film strips

Types of Filmstrip

They can be of two types.

- **Discussion filmstrip**: It is a continuous strip of film, which consists of individual frames that are arranged in sequence usually with explanatory titles.
- **Sound slide film**: It is similar to filmstrip. In this, recorded explanation is audible, which is synchronized with the pictures rather than explanatory titles or spoken discussion.

Advantages

- They are compact, easily handled and always in proper sequence.
- These can be supplemented with recordings.
- They are inexpensive when quantity reproduction is required.
- They are useful for group or individual study because projection rate is controlled by instructor or user.
- They can be projected with simple light weight equipment

Motion Pictures

What are Motion Pictures?

Motion pictures are recognized as one of the most powerful media for education. Films can be of two types, Motion Films and Sound Films. In Sound Films, the action is stimulated by projecting a series of still pictures at a rapid succession. In sound films, 24 frames are projected per second.

The films are available in standard sizes of 8, 16, 35 and 70 mm. Sixteen millimeter films are best accepted for educational purposes in schools and colleges and eight millimeter for individual instructions. They can be projected in the classrooms and do not require special booths to project. However, 35 mm and 70 mm films are best used for entertainment purposes in theaters and require special booths to operate them.

When using the motion pictures following head to be kept in mind:

- The teacher must have the 'Know-how' of the best utilization of these materials and help students to acquire skill in its effective use.
- Legal aspects should be considered in production of educational communication media such as television program. Permission must be obtained from authorities to avoid possible legal involvement.

Advantages

- Promotion of the viewers through motions, movements and activities.
- Enlarge or reduce the actual size of object by combining a camera and microscope to photograph objects and actions too small to be seen by naked eyes, for example, Amoebae.
- Condense time and space by omitting unnecessary material and concentrating on important aspects are focused.

- Provide an easily reproducible record of an event or an operation, for example, how a counselor handles a behavioral problem, events of deaths due to a particular disease such as plague, etc.
- Creates reality and allows revealing the invisible through animated drawings, for example, functioning of an eye or ear, working of a machine, etc.
- Influence and change attitudes of the learners which are not yet firmly established.
- Overcome barriers of literacy, even the slowest learning person can react to the message presented.
- Promote an understanding of abstract relationships by clarifying ideas, events through visual and auditory devices for example, photographs combined with animated drawings, charts and diagrams.
- Provide supplementary or enrichment experiences for individual student.
- Provide a review of summary of the information learned in other ways by the class.
- Provide an occasional break for entertainment.

Limitation

- Projecting equipment is heavy.
- Darkening and electricity facilities are required.
- Both hardware and software are very costly.
- Has a fixed sequence, difficult to update.
- Often seen as recreational device.
- Audience variability in relation to age, educational background and sociocultural factors may affect its effectiveness.
- Film literacy is required.

Categories of Educational Films

The educational films can be classified into:
- **Entertainment Films:** The entertainment film aims at emotional rather than intellectual appeal. This may or may not have educational contribution because it is designed particularly for entertainment. However, there are entertainment films that do make contribution towards the educational objectives of the curriculum for example, "Eye of the Blind", Woman in White" films.
- **Advertising Films:** The primary purpose of these films is selling of the goods of the advertiser sponsoring the films. Recently, many industrial films are also prepared in a way that they have utility and the course of studies also.
- **Documentary Films:** The documentary film is one which deals with a social situation. It attempts in a realistic, undisguised and authentic manner, to interpret the events, the cultures or the problems of the day for the purpose of assisting man to understand his place in society and to stimulate thinking and planning for the future. Many documentary films may be used for instructional purposes and are excellent teaching aids in the field of social problems for example, preventing AIDS etc. and case studies.
- **Text Films:** These films are specifically prepared for integrating in a course. These may provide information, show a process and demonstrate a skill or any other activity. These are also called "How to do films". Training can be provided through these films by their proper selection and utilization.

Videotape Recording and Videodisc (Fig. 20)

It is a medium in which images are recorded electronically on magnetic tape along with sound. Video can be prerecorded as off-air recording of television program or commercially produced videos. The teachers must brief the students in advance so that students understand and note down the points. It is important to brief the learners after video.

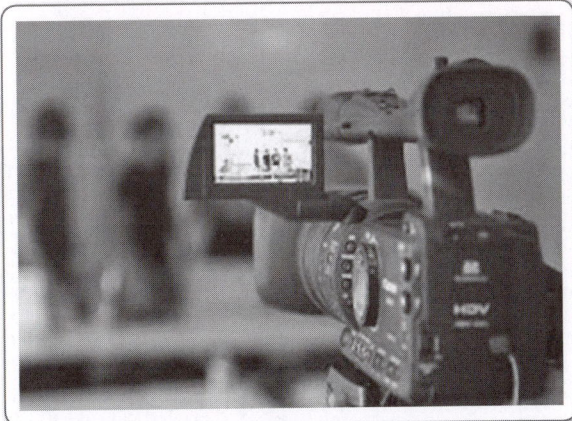

Fig. 20: Videotape recording

Recording the Video

Teachers and students can make their own video recording with video camera. This enables the reality of the learning material or the workplace to be brought into the class room and provides acultientric interest for discussion. For making a video, permission needs to be taken from authorities.

Advantages

- Are useful in describing motion, showing relationships and giving impact to topic.
- Allow immediate replay of video recording.
- Can be reused and is cheaper than films.
- Easy to record sound and pictures together.
- May include special recording techniques.
- Can combine still and motion on video disc.
- Is convenient to make duplicate copes of video tape recording.

Limitations

- High cost for studio production equipment.
- Has reduced the value of films in teaching.
- Master disc is expensive to produce.

Educational Television (Fig. 21)

Television is the presentation of an image on an electronic screen. The message on the screen may be 'Live', when the event is occurring while the viewers see it or the message may not be live, when it is presented by a film or videotape prepared directly for television viewing or films, filmstrips, drawings, slides and photographs are examples of prepared messages to be later used on Television.

Advantages

- It is an important media in communication of information, ideas, skills and attitudes.
- Media for achieving educational and family goals.

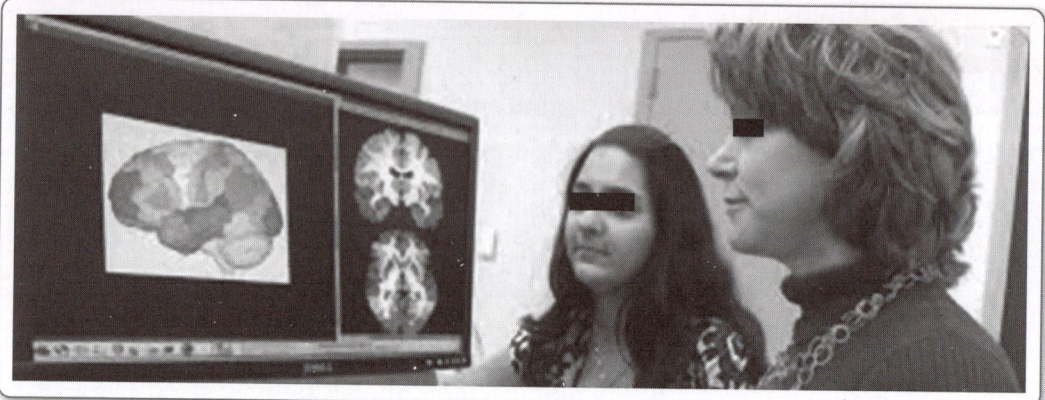

Fig. 21: Educational television

- Provides real life experiences and gives a feeling of presence at the scene.
- Enriches students knowledge by transmitting wide range of experiences through still pictures, films, objects, specimen and dramas.
- Brings models of excellence to the classroom. Viewers can hear and see the great scientists and creative teachers.
- Make programs understandable and appealing to persons different in age, education or maturity.
- Disseminate ideas and information to people of similar interests and maturity for example, nurses, doctors, lawyers and teachers.
- Saves time by eliminating the repetitions by editing and enable the students to learn more in less time.
- Provides both instructive and enjoyable experiences by making it interesting and providing variety of experiences.
- Can reach thousands of students and viewers at the same time and also enables the teachers to improve his communication skills.
- The teaching can be incorporated with class room's techniques.

Limitations

- It is a one way communication device and moves at a constant speed.
- Television Program cannot be scanned. Viewer/learner has to match the tempo of learning to the tempo of TV presentation.
- Small screen size in comparison to motion pictures enables to classify detailed information.
- Lack of personal contact with the teachers which deprives the students from guidance and motivation.
- Learner remains a passive spectator and not an active participant.
- Fixed timing of presentation may not match with schedule of learners.
- More abstract than the exhibits.
- One can observe the compressed experiences but cannot touch, handle or see a material at one's own pace.

How the Television can be Effectively used in Teaching?

It can be made effective by:

- Making it instructor guided – giving proper experiences.
- Systematic broadcasts related to course of study or syllabus with objectives and planned learning experiences.
- Ordered and sequential broadcasts presented at regular intervals in sequence, one building upon another.
- Integrated broadcasts related to other learning experiences such as practice reading, discussion, and labs.

Televisions can be used in three basic ways as given below:

- **Total Television Teaching**: There is no teacher in the classroom to complement and supplement the TV teachings and sight assistance is given by a 'Live' teacher through teleconferencing. This is used to carry on independent study by providing rich contents.
- **Television as a Complementary Basic Resource**: This functions as a part of regular curriculum, just as textbooks and workbooks.
- **Television as Supplementary Enrichment**: This has special value in bringing very latest information to a topic of class room for discussion, for example, events recorded by films or videotapes. It is built on the concept or enriching the knowledge and experiences.

AUDIO CASSETTES

These are useful resources in teaching; however, they should be used appropriately.

The purpose of making an Audio Cassette recording is to capture specific content and make it available to audience. However, it should not be used for long periods in lecture sessions as it can be boring.

Advantages

- They can be prepared by teachers themselves by making their own recording in a audio or video studio.
- They can serve as a good medium for adding interest to sessions on nursing care if they are prepared by capturing the feelings and experiences of patients.
- They can stimulate discussion when played in classroom.

Computer Assisted Learning (CAL) (Fig. 22)

Computer assisted learning (CAL) refers to a wide variety of teaching application. It includes posting learning material on World Wide Web to allow students to prepare for tutorial and access online materials.

The teacher instead of writing on black board or chalk board takes notes on computer and projects on to the screen and displays to whole class.

It enables the student to read easily than hand writing. It can be saved and sent by email to all students or posted on web. Students can work in small group and use laptop to take notes on their group discussion. They can further transfer or copy the content on computer.

Course ware or teaching material can use a single computer or computer can be used in combination with wide range of media i.e. multimedia.

The teacher prepares course ware or it can be obtained from other sources also. The learners select the material and load in the computer and it forms a learning experience for student. Computers do have the potential to produce high quality graphics, displays, data storage and retrieval and other effects, which is not possible for teacher to use in normal classroom teaching.

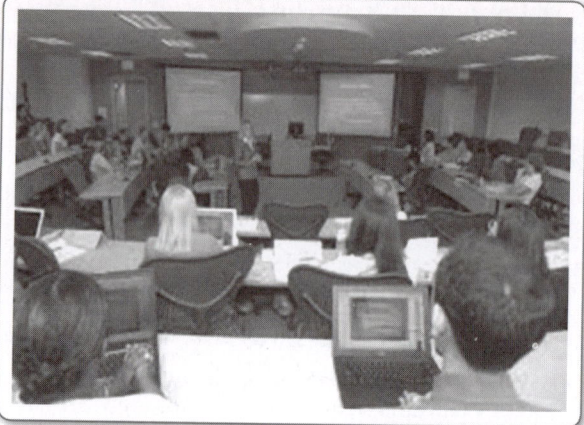

Fig. 22: Computer-assisted learning

The student using computer can take the material at own pace and refer back to previous section as per his requirement. They can answer questions. It posts problem solving. Students can use it to make own presentation in class and for presenting assignments. It creates own presentation for class and upload this to course webpage.

Advantages

- Learning is individualized and self-paced
- There is instant feedback on student response.
- Program are written by experts and undergo vigorous editing before publication.
- It is most effective.

VIDEO CONFERENCING

Video conferencing has become an important media of education. It utilizes live video– links between geographically separated campuses. This facility allows groups of students and teachers to interact who would otherwise have to travel long distances to meet and interact with faculty and teachers. For example, students who live at a distance from a campus are able to register for a program which is taught in a very distant location from students. Learners participate in teaching learning process and experiences by means of video conferencing.

Video conferencing is useful for conducting tutorials or teaching sessions for the learners who live in geographically distant locations. This can be used for all types or meetings and are viable for programs that recruit small numbers of students from distant locations.

Power Point Presentation

This is a form of visual presentation which replaces the overhead projector as the medium of choice for teaching and presentation to a large as well as small group. Microsoft Power point is a graphics package (a part of Microsoft office computer software). It enables a teacher to produce highly sophisticated slides or overhead transparencies for making presentation. It creates teacher notes and handouts for students. If a teacher has basic computer skills, it can be easily used.

NONPROJECTED THREE DIMENSIONAL VISUAL AIDS

After black boards, three dimensional Aids are most widely used teaching aids. Let us, therefore, discuss each of these separately.

Objects

Objects are samples of real things. These are visible, tangible aid which are complete in itself, for example, a book, a syringe with needles, a thermometer, a blood pressure apparatus, a stethoscope etc. (Fig. 23).

Replica is a full sized copy of an object. It looks, feels and act like the object itself. It is useful when the original happens to be fragile or inaccessible. Examples are chase dolls, dummy, pelvis, and fetus etc.

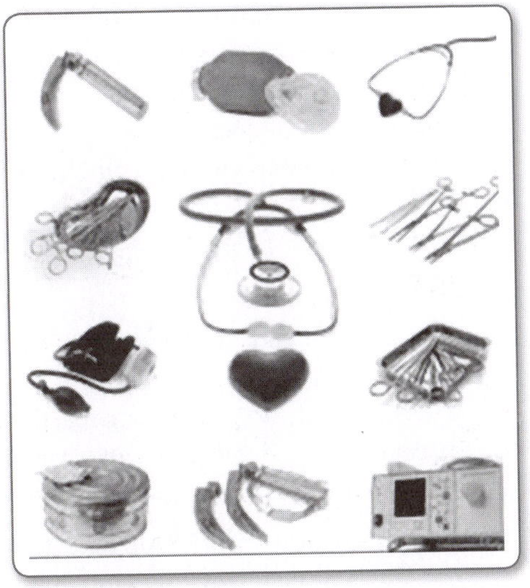

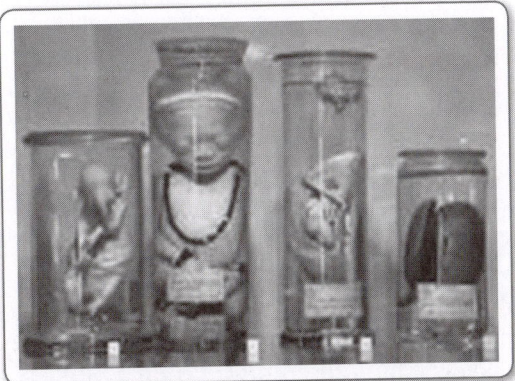

Fig. 23: Examples of objects

Advantages

- It gives an accurate picture of finer points and details
- It presents multisensory approach in learning.

Disadvantages

- Can be used for small groups only.
- May get damaged easily.
- There is a problem for their storage.

Specimens

A specimen is a part taken as an example of a whole for example, specimen of organs of the body such as heart, lungs, kidneys, uterus etc., can be used to teach anatomy. Loose bones and particular muscles can also be shown as specimens. In teaching about varieties of pulses and cereals in nutrition class, a handful of each of these can be shown as specimens. The students get firsthand information by looking at them or handling them (Fig. 24).

Fig. 24: Examples of specimens

Models

A model is three dimensional recognizable imitation of a real object (Fig. 25). It can be handled, operated and seen from a number of angles. This quality makes the use of models in teaching more interesting, effective and instructive than a chart or picture which has only two dimensional representations.

Models are a replica of a real object. It may be of same size, smaller or larger than the things they represent. Model is used when the use of real object as a visual aid is not applicable and when sight or sometimes touch in understanding of the subject is needed.

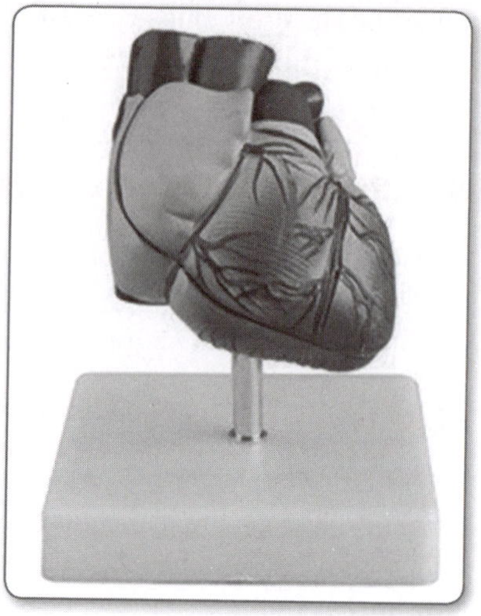

Fig. 25: A model of heart

Purposes

- To give first-hand information about an idea to the participant.
- To inspire people to work on the real thing.
- To help in easy understanding and explaining a subject this is very difficult or sometimes impossible to bring to the classroom such as a paddy field or a human heart.

Models for teaching can be used for various purposes such as in relation to:

- **Size**: when something is too large to be used, for example, a large hospital project, a plan for a building for school of nursing.
- **Time**: If we want to teach something of the past or future.
- **Physical inaccessibility**: Places we cannot visit or see, for example, models of pyramids
- **Unusable reality**: Real materials that cannot be studied, for example, it is easier to study models of human heart, human eyes, kidneys etc.
- Models are used to simulate resuscitation procedures that are invaluable and enable the nurse to practice the skills of external cardiac massage and expired air ventilation.
- **Process**: Use of three bottles suction method or the working of the Wangestine apparatus for continuous gastric suction can be taught easily by use of models.

Types of Models

- **Scale models**: Represents external form and shape of original object and are prepared either smaller or larger than the original for example, Tajmahal, insect etc.
- **Crosssectional models**: Reveals internal structure of real object for example, heart mechanism, oil engine etc.
- **Working models**: Show operational or essential parts of real objects for example, working telephone, oil engine etc.
- **Simplified models**: Shows simple features of the external form of the real objects without reproducing the original in precise proportion. For example, Animals, birds, fruits etc.
- **Mock-ups**: A mock-up refers to a specialized model or working replica of the object, which is being depicted. In a mock-up, a certain element of the original reality is emphasized or highlighted to

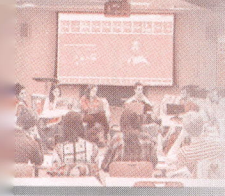

make it more meaningful for the purpose of instruction. Mock-ups are often used in technical institutions for training purposes.

Principles of using Models

- Arrange display of models to stimulate interest and arouse curiosity.
- Secure models when real objects cannot be brought in to the classroom.
- Use mock-ups or synthetic devices to show functioning of complete units.
- Explain that any model or mock-up is incomplete or out of its natural setting.
- Encourage making of models and mock-ups in certain subjects.
- Avoid too large, unorganized or over-elaborate displays of models.
- Avoid using models or mock-ups too complicated for maturity of the group.

Advantages

- Allows learners to see the equipment or operation in real life.
- Other senses are also brought into play.
- Helps to stimulate reality. The three dimensional form affords a back for concrete experience.
- Reduction/enlarging of objects to a convenient size is possible.
- Provides interior views of objects, which are normally invisible.
- It's easier to use models of human heart, eyes and kidney. They afford dissection and assimilation of parts.
- A working model explains the various processes of objects and machines.

Disadvantages

- Many items obviously cannot be brought into the classroom.
- Models are not available for many items.
- It is useful only for teaching in small group.
- Good models are expensive or very time consuming to make or have made.
- Sometime wrong concepts are conveyed to learners.
- Need more storage space.
- Time and money usually limit the number of learners who can work with items individually.

RESEARCH ON AUDIOVISUAL AIDS

Relevance of Educational Media and Multimedia Technology for Effective Service in Teaching and Learning Processes

Omodara O.D. (M.Ed.); Adu E.I. (M.Ed)

Department Of Curriculum Studies Center For Educational Technology College Of Education Ikere Ekiti, Ekiti State Nigeria Department Of Curriculum Studies Center For Educational Technology College Of Education Ikere Ekiti, Ekiti State Nigeria

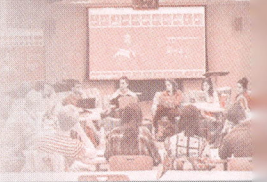

Abstract

This study was focused at examining the relevance of educational media and multimedia technology for effective service delivery in teaching and learning processes. It also highlighted the various classifications of educational media and multimedia technology with diagram and tabular illustration. Using relevant content analysis method, pertinent empirical evidences that revealed positive effects on learning from computer and television technology programs were re-visited. Relevant conclusion and recommendation were made that educational media and technology is inestimable in teaching and learning activities and the Federal and State Governments, Non-GovernmentalOrganizations and School Administrators should embrace it.

Keywords

- *Media, Multimedia, Service, Teaching and Learning.*

WHY EDUCATIONAL MEDIAS ARE IMPORTANT FOR NURSING STUDENTS

- Educational Media increases the student's motivation by sensory stimulation through using attractive materials in class room teaching.
- To provide basis for more effective perception and conceptional learning in every aspects of nursing theory and practical.
- It increase and sustains the attention and concentration of students.
- Provides realism in the teaching learning situations.
- Explicate the meaning fullness in every nursing concept.
- It rectifies the language barriers of students in teaching learning process.
- Provides accurate and usual images for easy learning.
- Helps to symbolizing the each factors which is in the part nursing curriculum to the nursing students.
- Educational media gives ready-made handouts in all class Room teaching.
- Helps to introduce the opportunity for situational or field types of learning in class room.

SUMMARY

This chapter has been explain in enthusiastic manner for the nursing students to acquire the various aspects of educational Medias which will be used in class room setting including the objectives, classification, purpose ,advantages, principles and importance, guidelines to use for the nursing students in an attractive and illustrative manner as per the CET syllabus of Indian nursing council.

ASSESS YOURSELF

LONG ANSWER QUESTIONS

1. Describe the non-projected AV aids with suitable examples.
2. Explain the projected AV aids with suitable examples.
3. Explain the importance of importance of AV aids in nursing education and nursing research, with suitable examples.
4. Describe LCD briefly.
5. Explain the principles and purpose of AV aids.
6. Write short essay on graphic aids.

SHORT ANSWER QUESTIONS

1. Define AV aids
2. Define model
3. Mention the various type of charts
4. What are the motion pictures?
5. What is opaque projector?

SHORT NOTES

1. Flash cards
2. Computer assisted nursing education
3. Posters
4. Pamphlets
5. OHP

MULTIPLE CHOICE QUESTIONS

1. **An educational aid in which there is a flannel covered board and illustration:**
   A. Flannel graph   B. Flash card
   C. None of these   D. puppet show
2. **Film is an example of what approach in education:**
   A. Group   B. Individual
   C. Mass   D None of these
3. **Consists of series cards which are flashed one after another while teaching:**
   A. Flannel graph   B. Flash card
   D. None of theses   C. Puppet show
4. **Radio talks should not exceed how many minutes:**
   A. 15   B. 20
   C. 25   D. 30

Contd...

MULTIPLE CHOICE QUESTIONS

5. **Form of play acting using puppets:**
   A. Drama
   B. Puppet show
   C. Role play
   D. Street play

6. **Combined audio visual aid is:**
   A. All
   B. Computer
   C. Film
   D. TV

7. **Mike publicity is what type of media:**
   A. Audiovisual communication
   B. Audio aid
   C. None of these
   D. Visual communication

8. **We can communicate large number of people through:**
   A. All
   B. Mass media
   C. Print Media
   D. TV

9. **Health education cannot be effective without:**
   A. A. Vaids
   B. Concept
   C. Group
   D. Learners

10. **A teaching aid in which each card is "flashed" as the talk is in progress:**
    A. Computer
    B. Flannel graph
    C. Flash card
    D. Chart

11. **Three groups of audiovisual aids:**
    A. All the above
    B. Auditory
    C. Combined AV
    D. Visual

12. **A group teaching method in which group members enact the roles as they have observed:**
    A. Drama
    B. Film
    C. Puppet show
    D. Role play

13. **Give three examples of mass media:**
    A. All the above
    B. Film
    C. Poster
    D. Radio

14. **A mass media in which message should be short, direct, noticeable at a glance and easy to understand:**
    A. Computer
    B. Radio
    C. Poster
    D. TV

15. **A teaching method in which students are given the opportunity to experience at firsthand what they learn in the class room:**
    A. Chart
    B. Field trip
    C. Flannel graph
    D. Poster

ANSWERS TO MCQS

1. (A)	2. (C)	3. (B)	4. (A)	5. (D)	6. (D)	7. (B)
8. (A)	9. (D)	10. (C)	11. (A)	12. (D)	13. (A)	14. (C)
15. (B)						

BIBLIOGRAPHY

1. Jaspreetkaur R Sodhi.Comprehensive text bookof nursing education. 1st edtion.New Delhi: jaypeePublishersPvt. Ltd.; 2017.

2. Dr.S.L Goel, Health education in theory and practice 1st edition.Newdelhi: DD publisher's pvt Ltd; 2013.

3. Dinesh Kumar Sharma, Communication and education technology for nurses. 1st edition. Jalandhar: lotus publishers; 2007.

4. Loretta Heidgerken, Teaching and learning in school of nursing principles and methods. 3rd edition. Newdelhi: konark publisher's pvt ltd; 2002

5. ASHA MAHESWARI, communication and education technology for nurses1 st edition.Indore: N.R.Brothers; 2005.

6. K.P Neeraja text book of nursing education 1st edition. Newdelhi: jaypee publisher's pvt Ltd; 2003.

7. B.T.Bavantappas,nursing education, first edition. New Delhi: Jaypee brothers' publication; 2003.

8. Francis M. Quinn's, the principles and practice in nursing education, third edition. United Kingdom:Stanley thrones publications ltd;1997.

9. Stephen M. Coney, "Using Instructional Materials," N.E.A. Journal, No. 2, February, 1948.

10. Volume 37:

11. Bell, Walter S."Audio-Visual Anniversary", Educational Screen, (November, 1947)6 Oct 1992. Journal volume 3:

12. Ode, Elijah Ojowu). "Impact of audio-visual (AVs) Resource on teaching and Learning some selected private secondary schools in Makurdi." International journal of Research in humanities, arts and literature; 2014

13. DeBernardes, A Olsen, EG (1948). Audio-visual and community materials – some recent publications." Education Leadership: 256–266.

14. Mathew, NG;Alidmat, AOH. "A study of the usefulness of Audio-visual aids in EFL classroom: implications for effective instruction". InternationalJournal of Higher Education. : 86–92.

15. M.Marwalows. Different types of A.V aids are available from: http://www.studylecturenotes.com/curriculum-instructions/audio-visual-aids-in-education-definition-types-objectives

16. Deepathi S, some details about teaching aids available from: https://www.slideshare.net/deepati1/teaching-aids-39749045

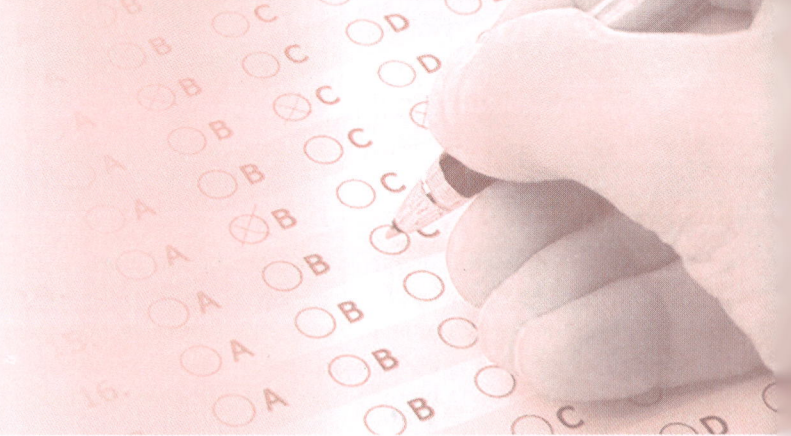

Unit 8

Educational Assessment

— Assuma Beevi TM

CHAPTER OUTLINE

- Common Terminologies Related to Educational Assessment
- Purposes of Evaluation/Assessment
- Scope of Evaluation
- Principles of Student Assessment
- Types of Assessment/Evaluation
- Factors Influencing on students assessment
- Evaluation Process
- Measuring Instrument

- Essay Questions
- Short Answer Questions (SAQs)
- Multiple Choice Questions (MCQs)
- Viva Voce or Oral Examination
- Clinical Evaluation
- Written Assignments
- Attitude Assessment
- Questionnaires
- Tool Used for Observation Methods

LEARNING OBJECTIVE

At the completion of the chapter, the be able to:

- Implement the concepts and principles of assessment appropriately in evaluating the performance of the students
- Differentiate the uses of formative, summative and confirmative evaluations
- Use appropriately the criterion and norm referenced evaluation.
- Differentiate between measurements, tests and assessments.
- Identify the importance of course objectives in student assessment.
- Identify the uses and purposes of assessment.
- Select appropriate evaluation methodology to determine student achievement.
- Describe various instruments used in student assessment in theory and clinical practice.

INTRODUCTION

Evaluation is an important process to measure learning and health-related outcomes, monitor performance, determine competence to practice and arrive at other decisions about individuals, and organizations. Evaluation also makes us accountable for the quality of education and service provided to our students, patients, governing boards, and society. Student evaluation is the systematic process of collecting and interpreting information as a basis for decisions about learners. Through evaluation, the teacher determines the progress of students toward meeting the educational objectives and developing competencies. Evaluation is a continuing, open-ended process closely interwoven with learning and teaching.

KEY TERMS IN EDUCATIONAL ASSESSMENT

Evaluation

Evaluation is a process that includes measurement and value judgement. It may be related to any material, process or product. In teaching learning situation, involved teachers, teaching content, audiovisual aids, organizational infrastructure are evaluated as input; teaching methods are evaluated as process and student's performance is evaluated as outcome. If a teacher conducts class test and computes the score based on correct responses, it is called measurement but when the obtained score is interpreted after adding values like first class, second class, pass and unsatisfactory is known as evaluation.

Evaluation is an act of judging the learner's behavior based not only on attainment of learning objectives but also their personality changes such as social attitudes, interest's, ways of thinking, work habits and personal and social adaptability.

In the process of evaluation, value of an object, event, or person is determined either by comparison to similar things or to a standard.

- 'Evaluation is defined as 'a systematic process of determining the extent to which educational objectives are achieved by pupils'
  —Gronlund NE
- *'Evaluation is the process of determining to what extent the educational objectives are being realised.'-*
  —Ralph Tyler
- *'Evaluation in education is systematic process which enables the extent to which the students has attained the educational objectives to be measured. Evaluation always includes measurements plus a value judgment.'*
  —J.J. Gulbert

Measurement

Measurement is concerned to the quantitative description of learner's behaviors. Evaluation is the process of assigning numbers to an event, individual or object-based, on their characteristics according to specified rules. In the process of measurement, value judgement is not required. A group of first year BSc nursing students are asked to show the return demonstration of simple bed making and allotted time was same for all the students. It was observed that out of 50 score, they obtained 18, 20, 25, 28, 30, 35, 38,....49, etc. It indicates the measurement of student's performance on bed making.

Two types of referencing standards are used in measurements that include criterion-referenced and norm-referenced standards.

- **Criterion referenced standards** are absolute, not related to peer performance and must have standard set of criteria prior to examination with defined level of performance.
- **Norm referenced standards** are relative, based on peer performance, varies with each group and cut-off point is not related to competence.

Assessment

Assessment is a systematic process, by which information is obtained relative to some known objective or goal. It is the process of defining, selecting, designing, collecting, analyzing, interpreting, and using information for the purpose of recognizing and improving students' learning and development. Students knowledge, attitudes, skills, values and behavior can be assessed at the beginning, mid or end of session in any educational program.

Purpose of assessment is to determine the student's or the program's quality of work over a period of time. Examples of assessment are development of portfolios, achievements, projects, observations, etc.

Tests

Tests are indirect measures of achievements. Tests consist of a set of questions that require a correct response or answers from the student either in writing or orally.

PURPOSES OF EVALUATION

Assessment is an important part of the curriculum. It is an integral part of the learning process, in which students are informed of their quality of performances. Student assessment follows instruction and impetus for reflection, evaluation and curricular improvement. In an educational setting, one of the key elements of survival for a student is passing a test. The student assessment has various purposes. It may be for the benefit of the students, teachers, institution and society.

For the Students

- **To recognize student's learning:** Students are evaluated after completion of a lesion or unit basically to recognize how students have learned. Teacher can analyze the results to know whether majority of students scored well or not?
- **To assess the student's progress throughout the session**: How consistently students are following teaching session and performing is assessed through the use of repeated evaluation .
- **To identify student's strength's and weaknesses:** Evaluation can be done to identify student's strengths and weaknesses. Evaluation is usually conducted at the beginning of educational program or at the beginning of unit as pretest.
- **To meet student's needs**: Formative evaluation is not only done to recognize student's weaknesses but it also helps to meet student's needs through changing the approach of teaching, modifying teaching methods, repeating the teaching content etc.

- **To encourage student learning:** Frequent evaluation gives the feedback to students about their progress or deterioration that act as reinforcement.
- **To help students in acquiring appropriate level of knowledge, attitude and skill:** In case of formative evaluation, students gets repeated feedback regarding their acquisition of knowledge, attitude and skill. It gives the opportunity for corrective measure so that desired level of knowledge, attitude and skill is acquired.
- **To determine recipients of awards and recognition:** Students are evaluated at the end of educational program for determining the recipients of awards and recognition. Course completion certificate is provided to those students, whose performance is up to the mark or more than desired criteria.
- **To compare the level of competency among students:** Student's performance score is compared with reference group.

For the Institution

- **To take decision about promoting student for higher level of learning:** Both the short and long-term educational program, students are evaluated in number of occasion either semester, half-yearly or yearly basis. Specially the result of summative evaluation helps to take decision whether all will be promoted or not.
- **To appraise teacher performance:** Evaluation can be conducted to evaluate teaching skill of teacher and the test result is used to appraise teacher performance.
- **To change/modify teaching, learning method based on evidence:** Test score of student evaluation is used for research purpose that indicates the more or least effective method of teaching; compare two or more teaching method thereby appropriate method of teaching is adopted, eliminated, accepted or changed.
- **To report student's progress to parents:** It is the responsibility of a teaching institution to communicate with parents regarding student's motivation, progress or deterioration.
- **To fulfill the requirement of university:** Every university have some set of guidelines in relation to student evaluation which is followed by each teaching institution.
- **To change/modify curriculum based on evidence:** The impact of curriculum is reflected in students evaluation as it is not only based on value judgment but also includes the numerical value of measurement.
- **To evaluate the teaching program:** The teaching program is evaluated for its beneficial effect, draw back etc.
- **To gain college credit:** The result of summative evaluation indicates college credit. Being a teaching institution a school or college takes the responsibility to run it with smooth functioning. The number of pass out students and their percentage of marks bring credit to college.
- **To develop and revise curriculum**: Using various techniques and tool of evaluation the strengths and weaknesses of an existing curriculum is identified and realized the need for revision.

For the Teacher

- To identify areas for improving instruction
- To document instructional outcomes for faculty promotions
- To evaluate the extent that educational objectives are realized
- To estimate the effectiveness of teaching method
- To estimate the effectiveness of audiovisual aids
- To predict the outcome of teaching.

For the Society

- Demonstrating quality standards for the public institution or profession
- Articulating the values and priorities of the educational institution
- Informing the allocation of educational resources
- Selecting the right candidate for right discipline
- Preventing the society from incompetent professional
- To improve the standard of education
- To enrich the wealth of society.

SCOPE OF EVALUATION

Nursing Education

- **Selection of students:** To find suitable candidates each educational program of nursing has some set of criteria for the learner that is assessed before admission in terms of entrance test. Entrance test may include written test, viva or other comprehensive test and all these are different kind of evaluation.
- **Feedbacks to students:** Throughout the session students are evaluated with varieties of test. The level of engagement in learning, learning difficulty and progress in learning is assessed at different occasion and feedback is given so that corrective is taken by the students.
- **Feedback to parents:** Parents is the person who develops their child with basic education through formal and informal way. Parent expects the progress in learning from institution. Based on comprehensive evaluation periodically parents are informed about progress in learning as well as specific difficulty.
- **Feedback to teachers:** Teacher plays important role in teaching learning process. They need to plan how to teach a group of learner with more or less similar level of knowledge, different types of attitudes, social behavior and motivation. They not only plan and organize the teaching learning experience but also conduct it and for all these activity evaluation is important to run the system.
- **Motivation of learning:** Evaluation plays important role in student's motivation as it helps to realize the result of positive effort. When student achieves the target it motivates further for setting higher level of target.
- **Certifications on course completion:** Based on summative evaluation, students are awarded that certify specific level of competency attainment. Course completion certificate also indicates the students rank and relative position in the group.

Nursing Management

Various methods of evaluation is used to select and recruit staff nurse, to place in appropriate unit, to assess their learning needs, to appraise their performance, to promote in higher position and for disciplinary action.

Nursing Practice

At every aspect of nursing practice evaluation is used: to identify client's health problem; to recognize client's health perception; to analyze client's health behavior; to find the effect of nursing care and to estimate the changes of client's health status.

Nursing Research

Different tools of evaluation are widely used in nursing research. Nurses are interested: to describe health behavior, health practices, symptom variation among people; analyze the causes of illness; recognize the relationship among socio-demographic variable, environmental variable and clinical variable; find the effect of nursing care. All these are possible with the appropriate use of evaluation techniques and tools.

PRINCIPLES OF STUDENT ASSESSMENT

- *Principle 1, Assessment should be valid:* Assessment tasks and associated criteria should measure the intended learning outcomes of the student at the appropriate level.
- *Principle 2, Assessment should be reliable and consistent*: Assessment instrument and task should be reliable, clear and have consistent processes for the setting, marking, grading and moderation of assignments and examinations.
- *Principle 3, Information about assessment should be explicit, accessible and transparent:* Clear, accurate, consistent and timely information on assessment tasks and procedures should be made available to students, staff and others concerned with assessment.
- *Principle 4, Assessment should be inclusive and equitable:* Assessment should ensure that tasks and procedures used for assessment should do not be disadvantageous to any group or individual. It should not dilute or compromise academic standards.
- *Principle 5, Assessment should be an integral part of all educational endeavors and should relate directly to the program aims and learning outcomes:* Assessment process and procedures should primarily reflect the nature of the discipline or subject and help to develop a range of generic skills and capabilities for the students in that particular discipline.
- *Principle 6, The amount of assessed work should be manageable:* There should not be overloading of assignment schedules and should be based on what is required for profile achievement.
- *Principle 7, Formative and summative assessment should be there in each program:* It serves different kind of purposes.
- *Principle 8, Timely feedback to promote learning:* Students are entitled to receive feedback as early as possible after each type of assessment. Student should be informed about the nature, extent and timing of feedback for each assessment task in advance.

- *Principle 9, Student assessment policy and protocol should be a part of staff development policy:* All those involved in the assessment of students must be competent to undertake their roles and responsibilities. It should be ascertain before employing teachers or academicians. Regular training on modalities of assessment should be part of continuing education for academic staffs.
- *Principle 10, Assessment or evaluation should be a continuous process:* To plan, organize, conduct, and continue educational program evaluation is continued throughout the course.

TYPES OF EVALUATIONS

Formative Evaluation (Fig. 1)

Formative evaluation refers to evaluation methods that are intended to measure student's progress towards a specific goal and allow the teacher to adjust instruction on a frequent basis. There are many type of formative evaluation that are used in classroom such as direct questioning, class test, response logs etc

Benefit of Formative Evaluation

- It helps to recognize student's engagement in learning.
- Formative evaluations are easy to conduct.
- Formative assessments are easy to score.
- The test results of formative assessments are easy to use.
- It require a limited amount of time to complete.
- It helps in setting individualized goals for students.
- It helps to monitor progress on regular basis.
- There is no single type of formative evaluation.
- Identifies areas in which additional instruction or assistance is needed.

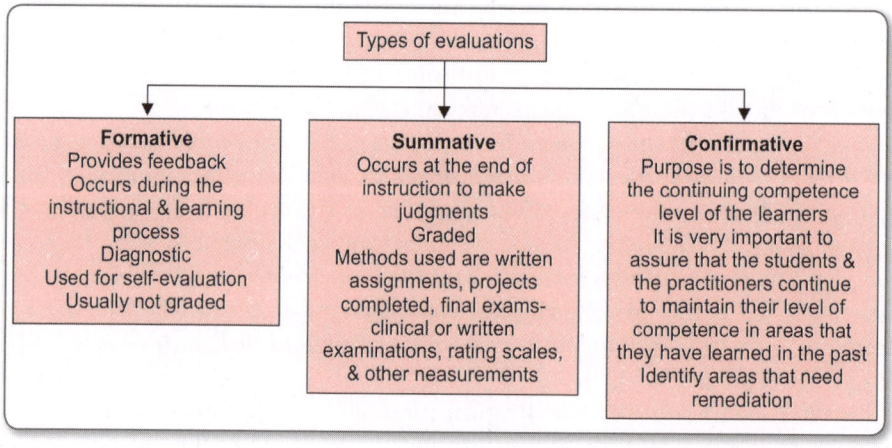

Fig. 1: Types of evaluations

Summative Evaluation

Summative evaluation refers to the assessment strategies used at the end of instructional unit by comparing it against some standard or benchmark, Example, end of semester examination or a final project. Difference between formative and summative's evaluation are given in Table 1.

Benefits

- It helps to guide teacher's effort for next session.
- It gives credit to student's hard work.
- It has much broader content scope.
- It gives credit to the organization.

TABLE 1: **Difference between formative and summative evaluation**

Characteristics	Formative	Summative
Purpose	Detect strengths and weaknesses	Find overall achievements
Frequency	Frequency is more than summative evaluation. • During or end of unit	Frequency is less than formative evaluation. • At the end of educational program
Area covered	One unit or some portion of teaching content	Cover whole course
Administrative utility	Advisory requirement	Decisive requirement
Feedback to students	Done immediately	Within the time frame of course completion
Feedback to faculty	Facilitate to take corrective action	Does not facilitate for corrective action

Confirmative Evaluation

Confirmative evaluation refers to the type of assessment that enables evaluator to verify the competence level of the learners. It is more comprehensive in nature and the test score is used for keeping permanent record.

Benefits

- More comprehensive than other methods of evaluation
- Varieties of skill are evaluated
- It guides to make concrete decision.

FACTORS INFLUENCING ON STUDENT'S ASSESSMENT

Course Objectives

It is the criteria or standard or yardstick against which performance is evaluated. Evaluation criteria are developed based on course objectives. Mager (1984) suggested the importance of educational objectives as the performance to be exhibited by a learner before being considered competent. So an educational objective is the intended result of instruction rather than the process itself. A useful objective will relate to: The task the student has to perform; conditions under which the performance should be exhibited; level of performance that will be considered acceptable.

Course objectives should follow the principle of SMART and it is important in planning of authentic assessment. The specific objectives that are smart will indicate the behaviors expected of the students and will act as spring board for developing a suitable assessment program. The teacher should think about the assessment process in advance. But most of the teachers thinks about content at first and then secondly develops the assessment instruments. Output measures are not thought naturally by most of the teachers. It is important to consider output measures that contain a knowledge component, a skill component and essentially an attitude component.

- Input (lesson content)
- Process (e.g. Teaching)
- Output (e.g. Student Performance in terms of knowledge, attitude and skill) (Fig. 2)

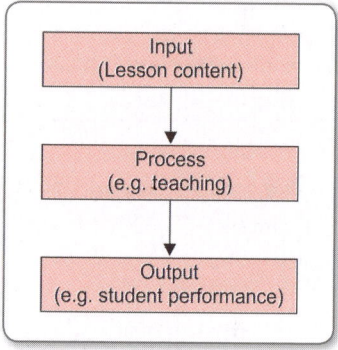

Fig. 2: Assessment process

The knowledge component relates to the learner's ability to remember and understand. The skill component encompasses the psychomotor tasks that are essential for professional competence. The attitudinal components are the key personal qualities for a professional. In essence, before choosing an instrument the faculty should define what exactly need to be assessed. Some instruments appropriate for testing knowledge may not be suitable for measuring skills and vice versa. It is appropriate for the faculty to look into various categories of objectives put forward by Bloom (1956) Harrow (1972) Krathwahl, Bloom and Masia (1964).

Availability of Resources

- Student assessment or evaluation is influenced by the availability of resources. Resources may be in terms of setting where assessment will be conducted, people who will assess the students, equipments and tools that are used for measuring performance, Time within which assessment is completed. Beside these resources, some cost is associated with each evaluation process.

Teacher's Competency

- If the evaluator or assessor is not aware about the purpose, learning outcome, student's background, method of administration, analysis and interpretation of test results then assessment is not successes due to various type of error.

Organizational Support

- Teachers intention or competency is not sufficient for a successful assessment, organization support also important. Organizational support in terms of culture of fairness, promptness, quality concern is essential for effective evaluation.

Learner Motivation

- Lack of student's motivation may leads to failure of evaluation or assessment. Demotivated students do not assume their responsibility thereby inappropriate preparation causes substandard results.

The Evaluation Process

Evaluation is a process and it requires that the evaluator should follow the steps of the process properly. The following are the steps for any evaluation process.

- *Step-I, Specify the purpose:* At the beginning of any evaluation, purposes need to be identified that guide us to select the appropriate methods and tools for evaluation. Example- To assess student skill on oral medication administration.
- *Step-II, Determine what is to be measured:* The answer is obtained from learning objectives. The learning objectives or specific objectives are derived from general objective which indicates the learning outcome. Example-Measurable behavior is *skill* on oral medication administration to an infant.
- *Step-III, Define each element in operational terms:* When specific objective is stated with measurable term then it is easy to identify the learning outcome. Learning outcome is expressed with list of behavior that is observed or demonstrated by learner. Skill is the psychomotor activity that includes:
  - *Preparation* (patient preparation, unit preparation, medication preparation)
  - *Administration* (assuring all rights of drug)
  - *Termination* (observing clients response, recording, reporting, replacing used article for reuse, discarding other non reusable items)
- *Step-IV, Select appropriate data collection method and instruments:* To assess skill on oral medication administration the most appropriate methods of data collection is observation in natural setting and the tool will be observation checklist.
- *Step-V, Administer the tools:* In this step the selected method and tool is used. Before using the tool the examiner or evaluator should be familiar with the tool and students are informed about the test.
- *Step-VI, Record the results:* As the method is observation, immediate recording is important with a separate record sheet for each student.

- *Step-VII, Analyze the test results:* Score on each area is summated and total score is obtained. The total score of individual students either converted to percentage or gradation according to organization practice.
- *Step-VIII, Summarize and report results:* In this step the test result is summarized and communicated to concerned faculty member and students.
- *Step-IX, Make a judgment:* It is the last step of evaluation which concern with judgment. Based on test results it is decided whether any one or group of students need to repeat the test or not. In case of summative evaluation, either student is promoted for next level or remains in same level.

CHOICE OF ASSESSMENT METHOD

There are a number of questions to be asked before making a choice of assessment method. The first and foremost question is what should be assessed? And why to assess?

When selecting assessment instrument, the faculty must ascertain that the instrument is valid, reliable and feasible. Faculty concerned must make decision on what students should learn and the reasons for making those decisions must be established first. Then the type of assessment should be determined. For example, if a teacher wants his or her student to read a chapter and find the answer of a series of multiple choice questions at the end. Here Method of assessment can be self-assessment and the instrument could be multiple choice questions. Faculty should be able to make a distinction between assessment method and assessment instrument.

MEASURING INSTRUMENT

Measuring instrument or tool is the device which measure learning behavior of students. Every tool has some strengths and weaknesses. It is the evaluator's responsibility to select the right tool for measuring learning behavior with minimum bias and error.

Appropriateness of Measuring Instruments

For assessing or evaluating a student, one needs to select appropriate measuring instruments according to the objectives that need to be achieved. A tool that measures the cognitive domain may not be suitable to measure the skill of a student. These require a different set of instrument. One must be cognizant what need to be measured of and how it should be measured. The following guideline can be used to select or develop appropriate instruments.

- For information, seeking use of MCQ, Essay and Oral examinations
- For eliciting Understanding, one can use Essay and Oral examinations
- For performance appraisal, the assessor can use Observation check list, Rating scales, Check lists and Anecdotal reports
- For measuring Attitudes, examiner or evaluator can use, Observation, Special Scales and Interviews.

Qualities of Measurement Devices

Whatever may be the instruments used, one should ascertain that the instruments or measurement device should satisfy certain criteria. These are:

- **Validity:** Does it measure what it is supposed to measure?
- **Reliability:** How consistently measuring?
- **Objectivity:** Do independent scorers agree?
- **Practicality:** Is it easy to construct, administer, score and interpret?

Important Points on Test Construction

- Examination content should match theory and practical objectives
- Important topics should be weighted more heavily than less important topics
- The testing time devoted to each topic should reflect the relative importance of the topic
- The sample of items should be representative of the instructional goals
  Miller's pyramid describes how an examiner should prepare tests for professional competence. **(Fig. 3)**

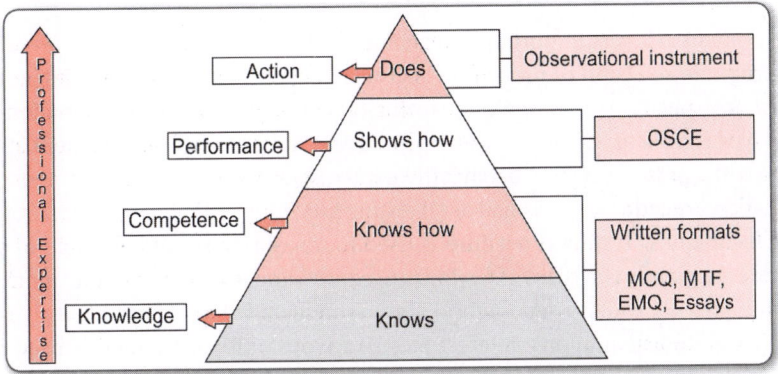

Fig. 3: Measuring behavior and uses of Tool (Miller's Pyramid)

Bloom's Taxonomy of Educational Objectives

Bloom's taxonomy of educational objectives has described six cognitive levels: Knowledge, Comprehension, Application of knowledge, Analysis, Synthesis and Evaluation.

Levels of Cognitive Domain

The cognitive domains have two levels of thinking. Level 1 can be tested with recall and factual questions using multiple choice questions, short answer questions and Level 11 can be tested with essay questions and modified essay questions.

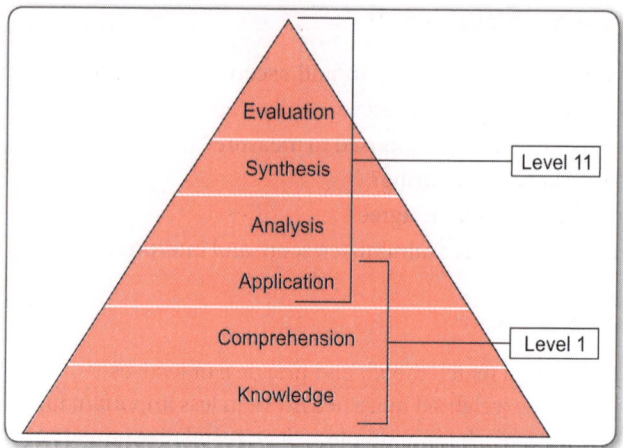

Fig. 4 : Levels of cognitive domain (Bloom's Taxonomy)

EVALUATION PROCEDURE (FIG. 5)

The process of evaluation is very important in teaching and learning. To evaluate the learning outcomes of student appropriate selection of procedure is crucial. Learning outcome may include knowledge, attitude, skill or any specific skill. Based on learning outcome to be assessed evaluation procedure is two types: first type is used to test person's abilities such as Aptitude and achievement and the second types is used to test a person's typical behavior like interest, attitude, social adjustment etc. Based on methods evaluation procedure is classified as (i) testing procedure, (ii) Self report techniques, and (iii) Observational techniques. Testing procedure is used to measure a set of behaviors of a person at a given time. There are mainly two types of testing procedures, one is written test and another is oral test. Self report techniques is a widely used method of measurement where the evaluate gives information regarding his/her attitudes, opinions, interest etc. Two types of tools are mainly used in self report technique that includes questionnaire and interview. Observational technique is mainly used to obtain information about one's usual and specific behavior through using checklist, rating scale, anecdotal records etc.

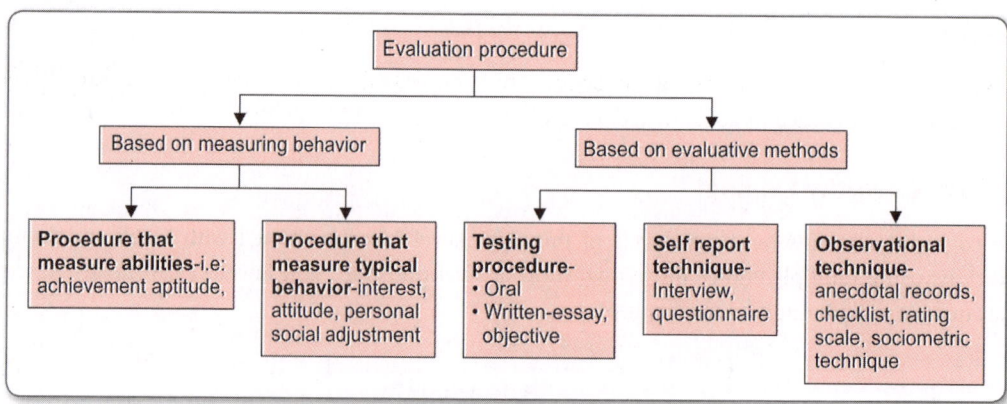

Fig. 5: Types of evaluation procedure

Testing procedure

Essay Questions

"A test item which requires a response composed by the examine, usually in the form of one or more sentences, of a nature that no single response or pattern of responses can be listed as correct, and the accuracy and quality of which can be judged subjectively only by one skilled or informed in the subject."*(John M. Stalnaker (1951, p.495).*

Criteria

- Requires examinees to compose rather than select their response
- Elicits student responses that must consist of more than one sentence
- Allows different or original responses or pattern of responses
- Requires subjective judgment by a competent specialist to judge the accuracy and quality of responses
- It allows students with an indication of the types of thinking and content to use in responding to the essay question

When should Essay Questions be used?

It is appropriate to use essay questions for the following purposes:
- To assess students' understanding subject-matter content.
- To assess students' reasoning skill
- To assess students complex thinking and constructed responses.
- If teacher's skill in writing objective items is poor but adequate resource is available (Time, personel e.g., small classes, grading assistants).

How Should Essay Questions Be Constructed?

- Clearly define the intended learning outcome to be assessed by the item
- Avoid using essay questions for intended learning outcomes that are better assessed with other kinds of assessment
- Clearly define the task and situate the task in a problem situation
- Scope of the task must be delimited
- Construct the problem or problem situation precisely and specifically
- Present a realistic and acceptable task to students
- The task can be either in the form of a question or a statement
- Specify the marks or grade and approximate time for each item precisely
- Specify the criteria for valuing the questions
- It is better to use several short essay questions instead of one long essay
- It is better to avoid options while giving essay questions for assessment or evaluation.
- It is advisable to preview and review essay questions before using to improve the framing of questions

- Preview (before)
  - Foretell student responses
  - Make a model answer
  - Get a knowledgeable staff to evaluate the question and model answer with learning outcome
  - Review after critically analyzing the answers written by the students to the particular essay question.

Checklist for Writing Essay Questions

- Look whether there is a better option to ask question on the topic?
- Is the essay question is appropriate for the intended learning outcome?
- Is the essay of appropriate length and do it need to be split into several short essays?
- Is the question specific and limited to specific tasks?
- Is the questions framed well and possess clarity?
- Is the problem realistic?
- Is the problem presented in an innovative manner?
- Do the students know the allotted time for each question?
- Is the student aware about grade or points allotted for each question?
- Have you avoided optional questions?
- Do you prepare the model answers and whether it is aligned to the intended learning outcomes?
- Have you had somebody knowledgeable to review the items for suitability?

Scoring Answers of Essay Questions

Holistic Method

In this method, an ideal essay for the question may be prepared as a standard. The scorer will read each essay in full first and form a general impression of it. Then the essay as a whole will be compared with the model answer. The essays will be categorized according to different degrees of quality before assigning grades. Then each essay is read for a second time carefully to ascertain its quality. All essays within each category are assigned same points in a three point scale as good, very good and not as good or mediocre, better than acceptable and not acceptable or poor, not as poor and very poor.

The Analytical Method

A model answer for each essay is prepared totally or its key points. The key points should include major ideas such as accurate factual information, suitable examples, relevant rationales, compact organization etc. the scorer reads each essay and search for key points or major ideas. Each key point should be rated separately. This method is more reliable than holistic method. This method also gives room for to the teacher to give proper feedback as the teacher can pin point what was left by the student in organizing the essay.

Guidelines for Scoring Essays

The scorer should decide which method he or she is going to use in scoring the essay. It can be holistic method or analytical method. Whatever may be the method it should be consistent. Check the scoring key or model answer beforehand to ascertain that the scorer is using the correct method. If needed, revise the key or model answer. One needs to decide before hand how to handle irrelevant and inaccurate answers. One should be careful not to identify the student during the assessment and also should be vigilant to be consistent in following the scoring method and should not change in between the method. All students should be graded with same method. Rate all answers to same question before starting to rate the next question. Score the answer for a particular question without interruption. If the scorer is rating question number 3 for a student, he or she should score question number 3 of all students without any interruption. Shuffle the answer sheets in between so that the order will be changed so that certain amount of bias can be avoided. It is better to have two evaluators for essay questions and an average of the two evaluation will give a better and unbiased results.

Advantages

- Relatively simple to construct
- Assess complex learning outcome and thought processes
- Tests writing skills
- Encourage the organization of knowledge, integration of theories and expression of opinions
- Students can submit an organized coherent essay of relevant material
- Stimulates increased studying
- Stimulate realize tasks
- Assess higher-order or critical thinking skills
- Evaluate student thinking and reasoning
- Provide authentic experience.

Limitations

- Reliability is a major concern. There is a need to assure consistency of scoring over time and when multiple individuals are involved
- Scoring of written response is more likely to be affected by general subjective biases of the scorer
- Halo effects occur when given the benefit of doubt more often than other students
- More time is required for scoring
- Like essay questions, it also requires at least minimal written communication skill
- Lack of written communication skill limit student's ability to score
- Grading may be influenced by content effects, expectations or grading fatigue
- Time consuming to answer
- Grading may be influenced by factors extraneous to the content
- Promote original thinking
- Scoring is more subjective and time consuming
- Assess a limited sample of the range of content
- Provide practice in poor or unpolished writing.

Misconceptions

- Assess higher-order or critical thinking skills regardless of how they are written
- Essay questions are easy to construct
- The use of essay questions eliminates the problem of guessing
- Essay questions benefit all students by placing emphasis on the importance of written communication skills
- Essay questions encourage students to prepare more thoroughly.

Modified Essay Questions (MEQ)

Modified essay questions in effect are an account of a series of events in evolution of a case study, narrated as they occurred. Points are selected at suitable junctures in the narrative to invite responses which can then be compared with a summary of the reactions of experienced practitioners. It provides a brisk learning experience and careful preparation can give a measure of abilities including attitudes which cannot be easily assessed otherwise.

Construction of MEQ

The examiner first selects possible fields (e.g. cardiovascular nursing, respiratory care, oncology nursing), a situation which is most relevant for their purpose. Suppose members of the class in oncology nursing were being assessed in relation to side effects of chemotherapeutic agents, it requires to not only thest the recall ability but also apply the facts while caring for the patients receiving such drugs.

Example: You are caring for Reena, a 54 year old female, diagnosed with carcinoma cervix. Until few days ago, her pain has been well controlled; you have reevaluated the pain control measures and reported to the physician concerned. He had ordered to initiate treatment with sustained release oral morphine. Her husband has expressed his concern that his wife will become addicted to the pain medication. What will you say to Reena's husband?

Short Answer Questions

Short-answer questions are open-ended questions that require students to create an answer. They are commonly used in examinations to assess the basic knowledge and understanding (Level 1) of a topic before more in-depth assessment questions are asked on the topic.

Structure of Short Answer Questions

Short answer questions do not have a generic structure. Questions may require answers of completion type like fill in the blanks, or supply a missing word, short descriptive or qualitative answers, diagrams with explanations etc. The answer is usually short, from one word to a few lines. Students may answer them as phrases or answer in bullet forms.

Examples

- List the 5 nursing diagnosis related to alterations in respiratory function
- Differentiate between sickle cell disease and sickle cell crisis
- A child suffering from acute exacerbation of rheumatic fever will have ------------ ESR.

Advantages

- Short answer questions are also relatively easy to set compared to many assessment methods
- Short answer questions are relatively easy to mark and can be marked by different assessors, as long as the questions are set in such a way that all alternative answers can be considered by the assessors.
- Short answer questions can be used as part of a formative and summative assessment.
- There is no guessing on answers; student must supply an answer.

Limitations

- Short answer questions are only suitable for questions that can be answered with short responses.
- They are open ended questions and students can answer freely as they prefer and this may make difficulty in scoring.
- Short answer questions are used only for testing knowledge thus promote memorizing and rote learning.
- Style and script of the examine may influence the assessor.
- There can be time management issue if the examinee is not careful to answer short answer questions according to the score/marks provided.

Designing a Good Short Answer Questions

- Write short answer questions based on learning objectives
- Make sure that the content of the short answer question measures knowledge appropriate to the desired learning goal
- Express questions with clear wordings
- Specify the short answer questions in such a way that the student understand the mode of answering (student should be able to answer it briefly in one or two sentences, or phrases)
- Provide clear instructions
- As far as possible provide direct questions
- While asking numerical answers, let the students know that they will get the full score if they mention the units
- Prepare a structured marking sheet
- Accept other possible answers too.

Rubric for Marking

Short answer questions are short and have more precise answers and hence, there is a possibility to list all the possible answers or points.

Questions	5	4	3	2	1	Total
Defining Answers/ points	Answer all points	75% of all the points answered	50% of all the points answered	25% of all the points answered	0% of all the points answered	

Multiple Choice Questions (MCQs)

Multiple choice questions (MCQs) have been shown to be more reliable in testing knowledge than the traditional essay questions. It represents one of the most important well-established examination tools widely used in assessment at the undergraduate and postgraduate levels of all professional examinations. The MCQ is an objective question for which there is prior agreement on what constitutes the correct answer. This widespread use may have led examiners to use the term MCQ as synonym to an objective question.

Guideline for Writing MCQ

Any examiner or teacher preparing MCQ should be aware of the stages of preparation that need to be taken care off. There are three stages in preparing a MCQ. These are: Planning stage, Writing stage and Testing stage.

Planning Stage

- Ensure question deals with an important and useful aspect of the subject.
- **Avoid trivia including:** common issues, serious conditions, important or frequent misunder-standings.
- Appropriate to expected level.
- Test knowledge around a central theme.
- Be clear about exactly what fact, concept or generalization is being tested.
- This central theme should be clearly defined in the stem.
- All options should refer to this theme.
- Decide on the ability you wish to test: Recall or recognition, Interpretation, Problem-solving.
- Consider how the information should be presented: Word description, Photograph, Radiograph, Tracing (e.g. ECG, visual field), Diagram (e.g. anatomical), Movie film,and Amplified sound (e.g. heart sounds).

Writing Stage

- Use simple and clear language.
- Avoid unfamiliar technical or unusual words.
- Check for ambiguity amongst fellow examiners or students.
- Anxious examinees imagine traps in questions.
- Write stem as a question or incomplete statement.
- If a question, each option must be a possible answer.
- If an incomplete statement, each response must follow grammatically and logically from the stem; i.e. stem + each option must be a complete statement .
- Avoid stems with just one or two words.
- Avoid clues to the correct answer.
- Avoid use of stereotyped or standard phraseology (e.g. "the pituitary gland is the master of the endocrine orchestra").
- Avoid unequal length of alternatives.

- No obvious inconsistencies between stem and a response.
- Avoid using opposite of the correct answer as a distractor.
- Avoid use of absolutes (e.g. "always", "only", "never").
- Avoid clues to the correct answer.
- Avoid use of synonyms or overlapping alternatives.

Distractors

- Avoid use of similar distractors, making the correct response more conspicuous.
- Use plausible and logical distractors.
- Obvious distractors increase chances of guessing.
- Derive distractors from common errors made by students.
- Derive distractors from common misconceptions held by students.
- If legitimate distractors cannot be found, recast question in a different format.
- Use eponyms, acronyms and abbreviations only if you expect students to know them
- Specify units.
- Particularly when using laboratory units, as they can vary from one laboratory to another.
- The normal range for a given laboratory may have to be quoted.
- Indicate opinion or authority if dealing with un-established facts.
- Indicate whose opinion or what authority the question is based on.
- Minimize negatively phrased questions.
- Avoid double negatives- They confuse examinees.
- If absolutely necessary, emphasize the word(s) conveying a negative aspect by using capitals or underlining.
- Avoid "all of the above" and beware of "none of the above".

Testing Stage

- Get agreement from fellow examiners that: the question is worth asking; it is clearly and unambiguously stated; distractors are reasonable and plausible.
- Test the question on students, if possible because it-
    - May represent a different interpretation of the question
    - May reveal what the question was actually testing
    - May have an opinion on importance and validity
    - Can indicate their answering strategy
    - May point out errors in the question.

Writing One Best Answer Questions

Basic Rules

Each question must focus on important concept as far as possible with a clinical problem. Each item should assess application of knowledge and not recall of isolated facts. Stem of each item should appear as a clear question and should be able to get an answer with the options covered. Distractors of each questions should be homogenous. Need to avoid technical errors while preparing each item so that there should not be undue benefit for the examinees. **Those questions should be avoided that ask which of the following statement is true or each of the following statement is correct except.** These questions are unfocussed and have heterogeneous options. Subject each question to these five rules, if the question passes all five your question is a good question

Item Template (Vignette)

To develop a good vignette it should include all or part of the following:
- **General information about the patient, Site of Care, Presenting Complaint** (e.g., complaining of abdominal pain), **Duration of symptoms** (e.g., that has continued for 2 days).
- **Patient health history and Physical Findings.**

Writing Options

- Most of the items should be in the stem.
- Stem should be relatively long.
- Options should be relatively short.
- Stem should have relevant facts.
- No additional data should be provided in the options.

There are different types of multiple choice questions namely type A, B, C, D, E, H, I, K, R and X labeled alphabetically according to the chronological introduction. These types are not included in this chapter as the book is meant for basic students.

Viva Voce or Oral Examination

This is an examination in which a face to face interview of the learner is taken by the examiner. It is an ancient method of evaluation of the learners and is usually termed as viva. Viva as a tool for evaluation tests all levels of knowledge, attitude, professional competence, interactive skills and ability to discuss and defend (example in a thesis defense).

Approaches Towards Viva Voce

Viva can be conducted in two ways. They are traditional approach and objective structured approach. In traditional approach, there is no prior planning and is conventional. The examiner may be asking questions according to situations and not based on any prior criteria. The student need to answer questions that the examiner asks from any part of the subject and no specific area of learning is concentrated. In this method there is no specific marking plan, no specific number of questions or type of questions. It lacks reliability, validity and objectivity. Difficulty levels of questions are not tested too.

Objective structured viva is a preplanned, objective via where the examiner uses tested questions, each student will get a specific number of questions and type of questions will be similar and the topic of viva is predetermined. It is considered as one of the most efficient method of viva voce.

Examiner's Role

In viva voce, the examiner has certain specific roles. These are:-

- The examiner should be courteous.
- Keep the student comfortable and offer a warm smile.
- Avoid careless attitude and show importance.
- Be time conscious.
- Show respect to student's individuality.
- Avoid arguments on difference in views.
- The examiner, should find what the students know rather than what he is expecting on a topic.

Examiner Should

- Make the student uncomfortable in anyway
- Not make fun on students
- Not disregard the student
- Not disrespect student views
- Not show impatience.

Viva should be conducted on must know areas and examiner should have a list of tasks and abilities to be tested and questioned. Inconsistency in scoring should be prevented using rating scales to score the learner.

Merits

- It gives opportunity to test the knowledge from all the 3 domains namely, cognitive, affective and psychomotor domains.
- Viva can be used for any type of assessment namely, formative or summative.
- It gives direct contact with the learner and provides opportunity to test interactive skills.
- It can be used to test personal attributes of learner such as attitude, approach, confidence, command over language.
- It provides flexibility in questioning for the assessor.
- Viva permits learner to express views and defend their views.
- Assessor can give good feedback and also can make judgement of teaching learning process.
- It has less chance for cheating or unfair practice.
- It provides facility for simultaneous evaluation by two or more evaluators.
- It is a way for quick assessment.

Demerits

- Subjectivity is an issue as it is influenced by the knowledge and experience of the examiner.
- Student may experience anxiety, fatigue, stress and difficulty to express due to language problems.
- It is time consuming.
- Judgment is influenced by many external factors and the view of examiners.
- It has less validity, reliability and objectivity.

- It is difficult to standardize
- It may test only recall ability
- Examiners may not be consistent
- There is and issue of probable cueing
- Personal contact with examiners may influence scoring
- Non availability of trained examiners to conduct viva can impact the result.

CLINICAL EVALUATION

It is a process by which judgments are made about learner's competence in nursing practice. Teacher arrives at a judgment regarding student's competency level in the clinical practice includes:

- Care of patients, families, communities
- Care of the environment of the patient
- Simulated experiences

Teacher should keep in mind that clinical evaluation is not an objective process. So the evaluator should implement fairness in clinical evaluation. Teacher's values, beliefs and biases influence the evaluation process in clinical practice. So it is imperative to develop awareness of these values and the evaluator should examine own attitudes so that he or she can avoid bias so that it cannot influence student's evaluations.

Self Report Technique

Interview

Interviews involve verbal communication between evaluator and evaluate, during which required information is collected. Interview may be structured, semi-structured or unstructured. In case of structured interview, evaluator use a preplanned format, which is designed by him/her self with a set of question and response. Each question that is asked in structured interview must have a definite answer. The order of the question is not altered at any time. On the other hand, unstructured interview is primarily used to identify level of attitude, assess in-depth knowledge on any subject. In unstructured interview set of question and answer is not planned before conducting the interview. Evaluator may ask describe your experience in emergency ward.

Questionnaire

Questionnaire is a printed self report form designed to elicit information that can be obtained through the written responses of the examine. Questionnaires can be designed to determine facts about an events or situation, or beliefs, attitude, opinion etc. Questionnaire may includes open ended or close ended item covering the subject matter which is already taught.

- **Open ended:** Allow person to respond in his own words.
- **Closed ended:** A person respond by selecting, ranking or creating one or more alternatives specified in the question.

For Example: Does negative reaction to a sick person have any bearing or caring for him as a patient?

   A   It makes no difference.

   B   It interfaces with patient care because one is unwilling to spend a lot of time with him.

   C   It interferes with patient care because one is likely to underestimate his needs.

Forced Choice Items

Forced choice items may also consist of words instead of statements. A list of stimulating words may be presented with respondents choosing those that best represent their attitudes towards selected objects or concepts.

Example

A list of role words and affect words – asked to choose 3 from each group that are descriptive of nurses

CLINICAL EVALUATION VS GRADING

Clinical evaluation is not the same thing as grading. In evaluation, observations and other data are collected and compared to a set of criteria to make judgments. From this, a quantitative symbol (grade) is given to reflect the data, and then a judgment is made about the performance. The clinical grade, such as Pass or Fail, A through F, is a quantitative symbol to represent evaluation. Clinical performance may be evaluated, but not graded, for example, in formative evaluations. Grades should not be assigned without sufficient evaluation data.

Formative Clinical Evaluation

Uses and Conditions

- Provide feedback
- Identify areas that need strengthening student's skill
- Extensive formative evaluations are requiring when there is still time to practice and learn
- It is not graded
- It allows immediate feedback on formative clinical evaluations and adapts the feedback to the learner's needs.

Summative Clinical Evaluation

- Summative clinical evaluation means at the end of instruction students will be evaluated to make judgment about the clinical performance.

Uses

- To give clinical grades
- To summarize the competencies.

Confirmative Evaluations

It refers to the evaluation that determines the learner's clinical competencies over time.

Clinical Evaluation Methods

Criteria for Selection

Select evaluation method that provides information on how well the student has achieved the clinical objectives/competencies. There are various clinical evaluation methods. One has to select the most realistic clinical evaluation methods. Teacher has to consider the nature of the clinical experience, resources available and the constraints while selecting the evaluation methods. It is also important to differentiate methods intended for formative vs summative evaluations and clarify these with the students. Teacher also needs to review the purpose and the number of required assignment completed by students in clinical practice. In deciding on clinical evaluation method, consider faculty time for completing the evaluation, providing feedback, and grading.

Types of Clinical Evaluation Methods

Observations

Observation methods are the most common method of collecting data on student performance. Observational methods are more subjective than other methods of evaluation but many times no other option is suitable. To assess student's clinical performance, it is widely used by teachers. Variety of tools like checklist, rating scale and anecdotal records is used for observation methods.

Threats to its validity and reliability are as follows:
- Teacher's values, biases and beliefs
- Over-reliance on first impression
- Different focus of attention by different teachers
- Teacher may arrive at incorrect judgment about the observation.
- Every observation session reflects only a small sampling of the behavior during the clinical experience.

Tools used for Recording Observations

- **Anecdotal record:** Narrative descriptions of observations
- **Check lists:** List of specific behaviors to be observed
- **Rating scales:** Recording of judgments about a student's performance on an objective, or behavior or competency.

Five Types of Rating Scales

- Letter: A, B, C, D, F
- Qualitative Labels: Excellent, Very good, Good, Fair, Poor
- Numbers: 1, 2, 3, 4, 5

- Frequency Labels: Always, Usually, Frequently, Sometimes, Never
- Other Labels: Independent, Supervised, Assisted, Marginal, Dependent
  N.B: Descriptors for each label/ letter or number improve objectivity and inter-observer reliability

Observation Checklist

Observation checklist is a measuring tool widely used in nursing by nurse educator, nurse researcher and nurse administrator for assessing particular set of behavior in a situation or performance in a specified area. Observation checklist is defined as a tool for data collection that allows evaluator to gather information based on predetermined criteria and make judgments.

It is also used to evaluate any object or event for presence of certain traits or characteristics. An observation checklist contains a set of items that describe the characteristics/traits/behavior of person and it is checked by the evaluator on the basis of presence or absence among those individuals, who are being evaluated.

Purposes

- To record observation systematically
- To assess the level of performance of students
- To diagnose unattained skill in a particular area
- To identify the instructional needs of students
- To find the effect of teaching in a particular area
- To provide feedback to the students.

Uses

- Observation checklist is used to evaluate classroom behavior of students.
- It is also used to assess clinical performance of students.
- Teacher or student can do self-evaluation by using checklist.

Types of Checklist

In teaching learning environment, based on purpose and user, observation checklist is categorized into two: a teacher evaluation checklist and a checklist for self-evaluation.

- **Teacher evaluation checklist**: It is a type of observation checklist, which is used by an individual who is observing the set of behavior of another person. The teacher evaluation checklist is used by the teacher for evaluating behavior or performance of students.
- **Checklist for self-evaluation**: This type of checklist is mainly used by the individual for self-evaluation, so that the evaluator and evaluatee is the same person. A teacher or student may use it to evaluate his/her own performance.

Ways to Increase the Quality of Observation

- **Comprehensiveness:** The observer should recognize all the desired learning outcomes for any particular nursing procedure or action. While a student nurse is performing a procedure, we need to observe students' resource management skill, time management skill, technical or operational skill, communication skill, risk management and prevention skill, etc. Any single learning area is never considered for comprehensiveness.

- **Connectedness**: Observation should be made within familiar learning contexts closely related to curriculum frameworks, learning experiences and pedagogical planning.
- **Contextualized**: Sensitive to the effects of context on performance and deriving assessment evidence from a variety of situations and occasions. If we want to assess student's skill in managing emergency situation, it is appropriate to observe during different occasions at the time of emergency ward posting/ intensive therapy unit/intensive care unit posting.
- **Authentic**: when observation is made, the topic or incident should be interesting, challenging, worthwhile and meaningful to students.
- **Holistic**: Emphasizing relatedness and connections in learning and involving performance on complex whole rather than separate components.

Advantages

- It facilitates data collection directly.
- Systematically data collection is possible.
- It helps in accurate data collection.
- It is easy to develop based on sample characteristics or specified subject matter.
- It is easy to use as it contains instruction or guidelines for user.
- It is useful to record verbal and nonverbal behavior of individual.
- It is more objective because observer does not need to justify like rating.
- It is easy to score and interprets.

Limitations

- Past behavior of a person cannot be identified through direct observation.
- It is time consuming because administration is on one to one basis.
- To obtain more authentic observation report, expensive audio-visual aids are required.
- Opinion or attitude is not possible to measure through observation checklist.
- A complete report of a problem or issue is not possible to be recorded using observation checklist.

Rating scale

Rating scale is a tool used for recording judgment of observation in a systematic process. It contains a set of items that describe some behaviors or characteristic and the function of the evaluator is to indicate to what extent these behaviors are observed among evaluatees.

Function of Rating Scale

- It directs observation towards specific set of behaviors that are predefined.
- It provides a common frame of reference for comparing same set of characteristics among evaluate.
- It provides most convenient method of recording on judgment of observation.
- It interprets the observation category through numerical values.

Types of Rating Scale

There are mainly three types of rating scale: Numerical rating scale, Graphic rating scale and Descriptive rating scale.

- **Numerical rating scale**: It is the simplest type of rating scale, in which numbers are assigned to indicate the degree of traits that are present among evaluatee. Commonly used rating scales are 3 point, 5 point or 7 point.
- **Graphic rating scale**: In this type of rating scale, a straight line is presented with pointed mark and each mark clearly indicates the specified characters or trait through descriptive phrases. The ratter is allowed to place a mark to indicate his/her opinion.
- **Rank order rating scale**: In rank order rating scale the ratter is required to indicate the peoples/objects in an orderly rank from high to low. The units of the scale are unequal.

Uses of Rating Scale

- **Characteristic/traits evaluation**: Rating scale is used to evaluate some specific traits, characteristics or behavior of person like, level of anxiety and feeling of happiness.
- **Process evaluation**: It includes the steps of performing any activity systematically. How a student nurse administers oral medication can be evaluated by a rating scale.
- **Product evaluation**: Any nursing activity or process is possible to evaluate in this and similarly, effect of nursing action or procedure can also be evaluated. Nursing is a service, therefore, in nursing; product refers to the effect of nursing activity, i.e., satisfaction, reduction of pain level and changes of skin temperature, etc.

Principles of Effective Rating

To rate effectively, an evaluator must follow some principles that guide to evaluate correctly by minimizing error.

- Measuring behavior/ traits /characteristics should be specific.
- Characteristics should be directly observable.
- Descriptive character and points on the scale should be clearly defined.
- Raters should be instructed to omit ratings, if they feel unqualified to judge.
- Rating from several observers should be combined, wherever possible.

Necessary Requirements to Develop Quality Rating Scale

- Rating scale should be developed based on purpose or objectives of measurement.
- Measuring characteristics or descriptions should be clear, specific and observable.
- Adequate number of item is necessary to measure a behavior or performance.
- Each level or category of particular traits should be distinguishable (i.e. severe pain, moderate pain, mild pain and no pain).
- Each rating scale must have an instruction towards raters regarding rules of uses.
- Rating scale must have a scoring key, which helps to interpret the results.

Advantages

- It is useful for measuring those behaviors that are not easily measured by others means.
- It is easy to administer because less training is required.
- Rating scale can be completed quickly.

Limitations

- It is highly subjective in nature. Rater's errors and bias is a common problem.
- If ambiguous terms are used to describe character, then rater can become confused and actual rating is not obtained.

Likert's scale

Likert's scale is a ordinal psychometric measurement device developed by Rensis Likert, from University of Michigan, in 1932. Likert's scale is generally used for assessing attitudes, opinions, beliefs and values of person.

Definition

Likert's scale refers to a measuring device containing a number of declarative statement and response category with assigned numerical values that measures one's attitude, opinions or values in relation to any event, concept or practice.

The Likert's scale is a series of questions or items that ask respondent to select rating ranges from one extreme to another.

Description of Likert's scale

The original version of Likert's scale includes five response categories and each response category was assigned with numerical value from 1 to 5. The scoring value is increased from negative to positive response. Commonly used response categories are agreement, evaluation and frequency. The options for agreement is strongly agree, agree, uncertain, disagree and strongly disagree. A Likert's scale may contain 10–20 items and each item is an element of whole concept that is being measured. To avoid bias, half of the items are quoted positively and another half is quoted negatively. After administering the scale, the respondents are instructed to rate each statement. The values obtained from all item are summated and total score obtained from each individual respondent. According to predefined category, total score is interpreted.

Example 1

- **Tool:** Assessing opinion on mental illness
- **Instruction:** The respondents are instructed to read each statement carefully and place a tick mark in the response column that best suitable to them.

	Strongly Disagree	Disagree	Uncertain	Agree	Strongly Agree
People with mental illness are not treated at home					
Mental illness is not manageable					
Mental illness always occur in adulthood					

Example 2

How satisfied are you with nursing services?	ES	MS	SS	Neutral	SDS	MDS	EDS

ES = extremely satisfied,   **MS** = moderately satisfied,   **SS** = Slightly satisfied,
SDS = Slightly dissatisfied,   **MDS** = Moderately dissatisfied,   **EDS** = Extremely dissatisfied

Advantages

- It gives a deeper insight regarding respondent's thoughts and feeling
- It is easily understood, therefore, it is a universally accepted tool for data collection.
- It allows respondents to select their degree of agreement within a range of choice
- It is a quick, efficient and inexpensive method for data collection.
- The method of construction of Likert's scale is less cumbersome

Limitations

- It may fail to measure the true attitudes of respondents.
- Individual's response may be influenced by previous statement.
- Some individuals may avoid extreme category.
- Total score may be same for two persons but attitudes or opinions in all dimensions of the concept may vary.

Thurstone Scale

Thurstone scale was the first formal tool developed by psychologist, Robert Louis Leon Thurstone, in 1928, to measure attitudes towards religion. He developed three methods for constructing the unidimensional scale: the **method of equal-appearing intervals**; the **method of successive intervals**; and the **method of paired comparisons.** Although the methods of construction were different for three scales, the resulting scale was rated the same way by respondents.

Method of Equal-Appearing Intervals

- **Step 1**: At the beginning of scale construction, a large number of statements are developed on the topic of interest. The topic may be people's attitude towards 'early marriage' or 'alcohol consumption'. Positively and negatively quoted items are constructed on the selected topic. If the selected topic is attitude towards alcohol consumption, the items may be:
  - Alcohol consumption is injurious for health
  - People gain extra energy after consuming alcohol.
  - Alcohol consumption decreases activity level.
- **Step 2**: The list is given to a panel of judges to rate each item on a scale of 1 to 11. Panelists are instructed to indicate, to what extent each item is favorable or unfavorable. The panelist should not respond in terms of their own agreement or disagreement with the statements; rather, respond in terms of the judged degree of favorableness or unfavorableness. The lowest score (1) indicates extremely unfavorable item and the highest score (11) indicates an extremely favorable item.
- **Step 3**: In third step, the median value and interquartile range (IQR) is calculated for each item. If the total items are 50, then 50 median scores and 50 IQRs is obtained.
- **Step 4**: Each item's median value is tabulated in ascending order (smallest to largest). In other words, the 1s should be at the top of the table and the 11s should be at the bottom.
- **Step 5**: For each set of medians (i.e. 1s. 2s, 3s), IQRs is tabulated in descending order (largest to smallest) (Table 2).

TABLE 2: Partial table with the data sorted according to ascending medians with their respective, descending IQRs.

Item number	Median	IQR
45	1	1.5
33	1	1
12	1	1
40	1	1
17	1	1
7	1	0
6	2	4
44	2	3
31	2	3

- **Step 6**: In this stage, items are finally selected for the scale based on the results of 4th and 5th step. The item that is considered as best has the highest median value but lowest IQR value.

Methods of administration

The prepared tool is administered to all participants and they are instructed to read each item and indicate their response in terms of agreement or disagreement.

Item No	List of Items	Response	
		Agree	Disagree
1.	Alcohol consumption is injurious for health		
2.	People gain extra energy after consuming alcohol.		
3.	Alcohol consumption decreases activity level.		

Scoring

Each person's score is calculated from the scale value of item. For example, a person selected 3 items as agree and scale value of those items was 2.2, 1.6 and 4.9, respectively. He/she would have an attitude score of 2.2 + 1.6 + 4.9 = 8.7/3 = 2.9, indicates unfavorable to alcohol consumption.

Advantages

- Easy to administer
- Easy to score
- Facilitates higher level of statistical calculation, as data is ratio level.
- Item representativeness is achieved.

Limitations

- Development process is complex
- Development cost is higher

Common Errors Committed with Rating Scales Adversely Affecting the Validity of the Scale are:

- **Leniency Error:** It occurs when teachers rate all students on the higher end of the scale.
- **Severity Error:** It occurs when teachers rate all students on the lower end of the scale.
- **Central Tendency Error:** This occurs when teachers are hesitant to rate the students on either end of the scale. They use the middle part only.
- **Halo Effect:** It is a judgment based on a general impression of the student.
- **Personal Bias:** This occurs when the teacher's personal bias influences ratings.
- **Logical Error:** It occurs when the teacher gives similar ratings for items that seem logically related.

Strategies to Prevent Errors in Ratings of Observations

- Be alert to the possible influences of one's own values, attitudes, beliefs in observing and in drawing conclusions.
- Collect sufficient data before drawing conclusions.
- Do not rate items when you do not have the data on it.
- Use clinical objectives to focus observations, and give feedback to student about what you have observed.
- Rate each objective separately. Avoid making the common rating errors
- Make a series of observations in varied settings over a period of time.
- Do not rely on first impression. They may not be correct.
- Discuss observation with student and be willing to change rating if new data are presented.

- Review the clinical experiences and ask if they provide sufficient data for completing the rating. Other clinical competencies may be needed.
- Avoid using rating as the only source of data. Use multiple evaluation sources.
- If the rating from is ineffective for judging student performance, then revise and re-evaluate. Make sure that the rating scale is valid and reliable.

Simulation

Simulation is the second type of clinical evaluation method. It creates an experience that represents reality without the constraints of real-life situations. It presents situations that require problem solving, decision making, critical thinking, fostering development of cognitive skills. It can take the form of paper-and pencil format, videos, models, and case scenarios. It is appropriate for formative evaluations

Disadvantages of Simulation

- Very expensive
- Requires space to house and large labs
- Requires the faculty to learn the technology.

Conferences

Ability to present ideas orally is an important outcome of clinical practice. This is possible in a conference. Sharing information about a patient, leading others in a discussion about clinical practice, presenting ideas in a group format, are important skills to be developed. Conferences provide a method for developing oral communication skills, problem solving, decision making skills, and how to conduct discussions that stimulate higher order learning.

Types of Conferences Appropriate for Clinical Evaluation

- **Clinical Conferences:** Discussion about a specific patient
- **Post Conferences:** At the conclusion of a clinical day
- **Issue Conference:** Involves group discussion of issues associated with clinical practice, professional, cultural, ethical, etc
- **Critical Incident conference**: In which details of significant incident in practice are explored by the group.

Criteria to Evaluate Conferences

- Present ideas clearly and logically
- Participate actively in group discussion
- Offer ideas relevant to the topic discussed
- Demonstrate knowledge of the topic
- Assume leadership role
- Lead the group
- Contribute multiple perspectives to the discussion.

Clinical Examination

For any clinical examinations, the examiner should identify the objectives and the dimensions to be evaluated in the clinical examinations. Clinical examinations are set up outside of the clinical setting to test clinical performance for summative evaluation. Clinical examinations provide greater control over the environment in which practice occurs, limiting the effect of distractions on performance.

Clinical examinations should include observation of actual patient care situation to evaluate student's ability to assess and transfer learning to a reality situation. Clinical examinations should evaluate multiple objectives. They includes several different evaluation methods including a viva voce with models, videos, simulations etc. Students may be given scenarios and they are asked to complete several activities, such as, complete assessment through evaluation of interventions. Questions related to critical thinking can be integrated into these questions.

Games

Games are contests played with rules, goals, and certain activities to perform for the purpose of learning. Examples of games of medical trivia, puzzles and board games. They may be used for clinical evaluations, but they are primarily for formative evaluations to give immediate feedback

Media Clips

Media clips are short segments of a videotape, a film, an interactive video or other forms of media. These are viewed by students and discussed in a clinical conference, written assignments or group activities. They are appropriate for assessing students' abilities to apply concepts to patient situations depicted in the film, identify problems, discuss multiple approaches, possible explore their consequences, engage in critical thinking. It may be graded and valuable as formative evaluations.

Portfolios

A student portfolio documents meaningful projects that take place in the clinical setting over a period of time. Nitko (1996) differentiates 2 types of portfolios:

- **Best Work Portfolio:** They include evidence of students' demonstration of competence and achievements in clinical settings. These are appropriate for summative evaluations.
- **Growth and Learning Progress Portfolios:** Designed to monitor students' progress and self-reflection of learning outcomes at several points in time.

Steps in Setting up Portfolios

- Identify the purpose of the portfolio. Is it best practices or growth portfolio?
- Identify the type of content to be included in the portfolio. E.g. number of papers, projects.
- Decide on the criteria for evaluation of the portfolio

Self-Evaluation

Developing the ability to evaluate own learning and competency is an important outcome of a nursing program. Self-evaluation begins with the first nursing course. Self-evaluations are appropriate for formative evaluations.

Purpose of Self-Evaluation

- To discuss student's clinical performance and obtain their perception of their competency.
- To identify strengths and areas for future learning
- To provide feedback
- To enhance communication.

Objective Structured Clinical Evaluation (OSCE)

When used correctly, the Objective Structured Clinical Evaluation (OSCE) can be highly successful as an instrument to assess competence in medicine (Ronald Harden).

Traditional clinical examination appears to have validity but reliability of the same is suspected as candidates are tested on different cases and judged by different examiners. In order to overcome the same, objective clinical examinations are developed in 1970s. The prototype of this is the objective structured clinical evaluation. In OSCE, the candidates rotate through a series of stations at which they are asked to carry out a (usually clinical) task. In each station they are observed and scored as they carry out the task. Other situations, they may interact with clinical materials, writes notes, answers questions. All candidates are given the same clinical and other challenges and assessed by same judges.

Background about OSCE

OSCE started in 1972 Dundee, Scotland by R. Harden and F. Glesson. First literature about OSCE was published in the year 1975, in British Medical Journal (BMJ). It is used in undergraduate as well as postgraduate courses and for formative and summative evaluations and in many disciplines.

Modification of OSCE

- OSLER: Objective structured long examination record
- OSPE: Objective structured practical examination
- OSVE: Objective structured video examination
- OSTE: Objective structured teaching evaluation
- OSPRE: Objective structured performance-related examination
- OSSE: Objective structured selection exam.

Characteristics of the OSCE

- It is used to measure clinical competence with predetermined criteria
- It follows an examination format or framework
- There will be one or more examiner's in each station to monitor the examinee
- The examiners score the students as and when they complete a task
- Different types of tests can be incorporated into OSCE making it more comprehensive.

Harden's 12 Tips for Organizing an OSCE

- What is to be assessed?
- Duration of station

- Number of stations
- Use of examiners
- Range of approaches
- New stations
- Organization of the examination
- Assigning priority
- Resource requirements
- Plan of the examination
- Change signal
- Records.

Advantages of the OSCE

- It is considered as a very valid examination and can be used along with other types of examination.
- Examiner can use it for large number of students and can control the process of examination and its complexities.
- It can be used for both formative and summative evaluations.
- It promotes team work among faculty of the department.

Disadvantages of the OSCE

- It tests knowledge in compartments
- It is tiring and demanding for both examiners and examinees
- Need many faculties
- Requires the whole department cooperation and is time consuming
- Sometimes distressing to students.

Written Assignments

Written assignments after a clinical experience are valuable and effective in evaluating students' problem solving, decision making, and critical thinking, understanding of content relevant to clinical practice, and ability to express ideas in writing.

Types of Written Clinical Assignments

- **Journaling:** Journaling provides a way of reflecting on feelings and attitudes and documenting the cognitive development of the student throughout the duration of the course. It helps the student to "think loud".
- **Short Papers:** They are problem-oriented papers to assess student's critical thinking and other cognitive skills. For example, Take a position about an issue in clinical practice and present an argument to support their position.
- **Term Papers**: Term papers may be completed about clinical practice, providing an opportunity for students to critique relevant literature, summarize their ideas and demonstrate the use of theories and concepts for analyzing clinical problems. One can evaluate students' writing abilities.

CLINICAL TEACHING METHOD

- **Nursing Care Plans:** Nursing care plan is framework developed by nurses to analyze patient's health status, identify health problems, plan for required care, implement care and ultimately evaluate the effects of nursing care. It helps the student nurse to provide more complete, unified and need-based care.

- **Nursing Case Study:** Nursing case study is one of the common and a useful clinical method of teaching. The patient is selected by the student with the help of clinical instructor and ward sister. Then the student is allowed to take care for the same patient at regular basis. Student performs in-depth assessment of the patient, recognize actual and potential health problem, prepare a plan to solve patient problem, provide care based on identified problem and evaluate changes of health status. While planning cares to solve patient problems nursing student refers book, journal and consult with supervisor for necessary guidance. Nursing students also compare actual patient's health status with theoretical information.

- **Importance of case study**
  - Regular patient care through student's concentrated effort improves patient care.
  - Student gains a greater understanding about patient's health problem and response to the care.
  - Student acquires information about systematic organization of relevant information.
  - Student develops a sense of responsibility in providing health education at right time.
  - It helps to learn the application of problem solving approach.
  - It helps to develops a sense of observation.
  - Students learn effective uses of resources.
  - It helps to improve communication of student nurses.
  - It gives the opportunity to become familiar with professional literature.

- **Process Recording**: It is the recording of the conversation during the interaction between nurse and patient in the psychiatric set up. Used to analyze student's interaction and communications skills with patients/ families.

ATTITUDE ASSESSMENT

For nurse educators, one of their most important instructional goals is student's acquisition of desirable interests, attitude, appreciations, values and commitments. But most often, educators are worried about achievement of cognitive or intellectual goals and acquisition of specific nursing skills. The reasons attributed to non-compliance to attitude measurement are:

- Evaluating attitudes are so often vague or ill defined
- Believe that attitudes can neither be precisely defined nor objectively measured.

Definition

An attitude has been defined as a relatively enduring organization of beliefs, around an object, subject or concept that predisposes one to respond in some preferential manner (Rokeah,1968)

All attitudes are learned and unlike purely rational ideas, they are linked to emotions. It has three components namely, a cognitive or knowledge element, an affective or feeling element and a tendency to action. Affective domain gives five levels of behaviors that signal positive attitudes of different intensity (Krathwohl et. al, 1956).This behavior illustrate the kind of specification that must occur before attitudinal objectives can be measured. These behviors are receiving, responding, valuing, organization and characterization by a value complex. Most of the nurse educators agree that one of the most important attitudes that nurse ought to exhibit in the willingness to adapt care to individual patient needs. This statement lacks the specificity needed for evaluation.

Specification

Willingness to adapt care to patient needs may be demonstrated by one or more of the following action:
- Makes special efforts to contact family when patient is in distress.
- Allows family to bring home made food for a renal patient
- Changes standing orders and or usual procedures to facilitate physical comfort or safety.
- Changes standing orders and or usual procedures to reduce psychological stress.
- Requests a change in medication and / or treatment procedures to increase the effectiveness of the treatment.

These actions can be observed and recorded by clinical teachers if the task is to evaluate willingness to adapt care to individual patient needs. So now it is measurable and can assign a grade for these attitudinal changes.

Measurement of Attitudes

Methods to assess attitudes may be considered in four dimensions.
- Who is the respondent, self or others?
- How is the response obtained in a direct or indirect way?
- What is the form of the question – fixed or free answer?
- For which purpose the method of assessment is useful for individual or group evaluation?

Attitude Scales

Most commonly used scale is Likert type which consists of a series of statements representing attitudes toward a given object or concept.
Example: The most important nursing function is making professional judgments.

Semantic Differential

A kind of graphic rating scale developed by Osgood, 1964. The respondent is asked to describe a person, an experience, an idea or an object on several bipolar scales.
Example: Forced choice methods- variation in response style is reduced when all persons are required to select from the same responses. It can be presented in different formats. One format requires selection of one of the two statements in a pair.

Example: Are you more attracted?
- To a person with a quick and brilliant mind.
- To a person with understanding and sensitivity.

Q Sort (Third Choice Method)

Q-sort consists of a set of independent verbal statements, single words, phrases or pictures.

Example: On each card, a statement describing a teaching practice may be typed and nurses may be asked to sort the cards according to whether they approve or disapprove of each student

Indirect Methods

- This camouflage the purpose of test,
- The person taking the test cannot anticipate the correct response and thus has no use to the socially desirable answer.

Example: Social interaction inventory (SII). To assess verbal responses that nurses tend to make to patient in emotion – laden situations.

Example: Free answer vignette, description of the picture etc. It has long been recognized that what is perceived and remembered is influenced by one's attitudes.

TOOL USED FOR OBSERVATION OF COVERT BEHAVIOR

Traditionally nurse educators use this method- Rating scales and check lists are used for observations

Anecdotal Records

Here the observer is free to note any behavior that appears significant. Observer describes observations exactly, avoiding mixing facts and interpretation. Record is made soon after the action to eliminate errors of recall. Cumulated over a period of time the description of incidents provides a rich picture of behavior.

Responsibilities of the Observer

To report only the facts of incidents this must be objective. Two types of incidents mainly recorded: characteristics of a person; exceptional conduct of the person. As anecdotes accumulate, search through records regarding manifestations of particular attitudes that show up repeatedly. A summary on these recurring patterns, gives useful information about individual's objectivity of observation can be increased by defining carefully what is to be noted and providing checklist or recording form for uniform data collection. Two forms used for directed observation that includes Clinical rating scales and Clinical performance records

Clinical Rating Scales

Most common and least helpful scales are clinical rating scales. The rater checks how often a given behavior occurred or how completely an attitude was exhibited.

Clinical Performance Records

The categorization and classification of many critical incidents in nursing into major areas of cognitive and non-cognitive behaviors led to the development of the performance record. (Flanagan, Gosnellt Fivars, 1963)

Critical Incident

Critical incident is a sample of clinical performance record, where intention of a person or act is clear to the observer. Critical incident technology resembles a structures version of the anecdotal record. It is a set of procedure or collection of behavioral observations intended to assist in solving practical problems or developing principles.

Incident is a behavioral description of a complete activity and it follows ABC rule in describing a behavior

- A— Antecedents to the behavior.
- B— Behavior itself
- C— Consequences of behavior

It use only facts, not opinions or interpretation is recommended. Critical implies to activities that makes a significant positive or negative contribution to whatever variable is being studied. Uses are similar to anecdotal records.

It also provides free standing instrument or in conjunction with other structured instruments like checklists and rating scales. Use of critical incident in summative evaluation is limited. Formative evaluation it can be used when either structured methods are not applicable. It is not used for grading.

Needs of Educational Assessment in Nursing

The need of educational assessment is not only realized by teacher, students or parents, but it is required to fulfill the expectation of society and nation.

- **Teaching function:** Educational assessment is one of the important functions of nursing teacher. A teacher is able to plan, organize, conduct and evaluate teaching learning activity with the use of educational assessment.
- **Learning function**: Teacher as well as the students, both assess their skills and abilities, thereby learning their strengths and weaknesses in teaching learning process.
- **Development of professional nurse**: In every field of nursing, education, administration, practice and research, require professional nurse. Nurse becomes as a professional by providing excellent services with their updated knowledge, skills and competency and it is the result of continuous assessment.
- **Providing standard nursing service:** To maintain or maximize the standard of nursing service, employer not only looks at the quality of nursing personnel but they continuously monitor the process: how nursing service is delivered and output: the effect of nursing care.
- **Human resource management**: Nurses are large segment of population in healthcare services. In the development of a student nurse to a professional nurse, his/her learning outcomes and competencies are evaluated a number of times and at various stages of career with the use of educational assessment.

- **Meeting societal expectations**: As a professional, every nurse has the responsibility and accountability towards society that they will provide safe care and optimize health status of society's people. It would not be possible if health needs are not assessed; standard of nursing education is not maintained; standard of nursing service is not maintained.

Importance of Educational Assessment in Nursing

At the end of the day, we assess ourselves to know how productive was the day? To what extent a planned task was completed? If not completed, then what was the probable reason? How to overcome those problems in relation to task accomplishment? We may get all answers, if assessment is proper. The way we assess ourselves, we may be assessed by others also and our present and future actions are based on this assessment. Assessment is important in every person's life and every day more or less we engage in assessment either formally or informally.

Nursing is a professional discipline where educational assessment has an important role. Educational assessment is important in nursing in every aspect, such as:

- It is important to recognize learning needs of nursing students, nursing staff, and any other nursing professional.
- It is required to organize teaching and learning experience for different groups of learners in various teaching programs of nursing.
- It is essential for determining the learning outcome of a lesson, unit or program.
- It helps to find the effect of teaching methods and teaching aids of nursing students.
- Nursing students are awarded after completion of nursing course successfully.
- Throughout an educational program in nursing, assessment is important for diagnosing student's problem
- It is also important to maintain the education standard in nursing.
- It is essential in monitoring the quality of educational program in various organizations.
- It is essential in maintaining the standard of nursing service.

SUMMARY

Evaluation, assessment and measurements are interrelated and each has a significant role in teaching learning process. Evaluation is a process that includes measurement and value judgment whereas measurement is concerned to the quantitative description of learner's behaviors. Educational assessment indicates a systematic process of data collection, organization, analysis and interpreting meaningfully for the purpose of educational goal attainment. Educational assessment serves many purposes for the teachers, students, institution and for the society. The scope of evaluation is expanded in nursing education, nursing management, nursing practice and nursing research. With increasing scope of evaluation, it is also necessary to control the process of evaluation.

Evaluation becomes more valid and reliable with the use of principles, which guide the evaluator to minimize errors. There are mainly two types of evaluation: formative and summative and both are used according to the purpose of evaluation. Each type of evaluation has some merits and demerits and both are quite different in terms of purpose, frequency, time of feedback, etc. In adopting any type of evaluation certain general steps are followed by the evaluator and he/she need to select the appropriate measuring instrument.

The important qualities of a measuring instrument include validity, reliability, objectivity and practicability. A number of evaluation test are used in different time of program that mainly involve written test or viva test. Written tests include Essay Questions, Modified Essay Questions, Short Answer Questions, and Multiple Choice Questions. Each type of written test has specific characteristics, merits and demerits.

In viva or oral tests, some other skills are assessed that are not possible to be assessed in written test. Other than theoretical evaluation, clinical evaluation is also an important aspect of assessment. As a method of clinical evaluation, observation is very popular and commonly used tools are Checklist, Rating scale and Anecdotal record. To develop clinical skills among nursing students, commonly used teaching methods are Nursing Care Plans, Nursing Case Studies, Case Presentation, Nursing Rounds, Bedside clinics, Process Recordings, Nursing care conferences, Demonstration, Field trips etc. With the use of different clinical teaching methods, it is possible to close the gap between theoretical and practical learning experience.

ASSESS YOURSELF

LONG ANSWER QUESTIONS

1. What are the principles involved in the construction of essay test?
2. Write five essay items in area of your subject specialization.
3. Discuss the principles guiding the construction of objective tests.
4. Explain the principles to be considered in writing short answer form of test.
5. Explain the importance of OSCE
6. What is simulation? How will you use simulation in nursing education?
7. What are the purposes of student assessments?
8. How will you use rating scales in clinical evaluation?
9. How will you test attitudes?
10. How will you use observation as a method of testing?
11. What are the advantages and disadvantages of viva/ oral examination?

SHORT ANSWER QUESTIONS

Differentiate Between
  (i) Formative and summative evaluation
  (ii) Validity and reliability
  (iii) Short notes and modified essay questions
  (iv) Test analysis and item analysis

SHORT NOTES

1. Easy scoring
2. Summative assessment
3. Guessing on answer
4. Assessing in-depth knowledge

Contd...

MULTIPLE CHOICE QUESTIONS

1. **Tests that show how well a student performed in relation to other students is known as-**
   A. Norm-referenced
   B. Criterion-referenced
   C. Function referenced
   D. Teacher-student referenced

2. **In contrast to summative evaluation, formative evaluation-**
   A. places greater demands on issues of validity and reliability
   B. is used more in decision making
   C. is used more for final judgments
   D. is used more to monitor learning progress

3. **Self evaluations are appropriate for:**
   A. Formative evaluation
   B. Summative evaluation
   C. Summative and formative evaluation
   D. Confirmative evaluation

4. **Check list is a tool, that mainly used to record-**
   A. narrative description of performance
   B. list of specific behavior of student
   C. judgments of student's performance
   D. students behavior that are rare

5. **Advantage of essay test is indicated by all of the statement, except:**
   A. it can tap complex level of thinking
   B. It is relatively easy to construct
   C. It allow coverage of more topic
   D. It is free from grading bias

6. **A test that measures the intended learning outcome also satisfy:**
   A. Reliability
   B. Validity
   C. Justifiability
   D. objectivity

7. **Miller's pyramid helps a teacher to:**
   A. prepare tests for professional competence
   B. construct questions for cognitive domain
   C. test attitude
   D. prepare tests on psychomotor domain

Contd...

8. **To prepare MCQ one should be aware of the 3 stages that includes-**
   A. Planning, writing and testing
   B. Testing, composing, Evaluating
   C. Preparing, Analyzing, Evaluating
   D. Preparing, writing, Responding

9. **Short answer questions has the advantage of-**
   A. summative evaluation
   B. guessing on answer
   C. assessing in-depth knowledge
   D. easy scoring

10. **In a method of evaluation, students are instructed to rotate through a series of stations for performing clinical task. The method is known as-**
   A. Objective Structured Clinical Evaluation
   B. Objective Unstructured Clinical Evaluation
   C. Definite Structured Clinical Evaluation
   D. Direct Structured Clinical Evaluation

ANSWERS TO MCQS

1. (A)	2. (D)	3. (A)	4. (B)	5. (D)	6. (B)	7. (A)
8. (A)	9. (D)					

BIBLIOGRAPHY

1. Kleehammer, K., Hart, AL, Keck, JF. (1990). Nursing students perception of anxiety-producing situations in the clinical setting. Jr. of Nursing Education, 29, 183-187.
2. Krathwohl, D.R., Bloom, B.S. and Masia, B. B. (Eds.). (1964). Taxonomy of educational objectives: Handbook II: The affective domain. New York: McKay.
3. Oermann, MH. (1996). Research of teaching in the clinical setting.In K.R. Stevens (Ed.), Review of Research in Nursing Education (Vol. VII, pp.91-1246). New York: National League for Nursing.
4. Oermann, MH. (in press). Differences in the clinical experiences of ADN and BSN students. Journal of Nursing Education.
5. Oermann, MH, and Gaberson, KB. (1998). Evaluation and testing in nursing education, New York, NY: Springer Publishing Co.
6. Osgood C.E (1964). "Semantic Differential Technique in the Comparative Study of Cultures"American Anthropologist. Vol 66, Issue 3 June 1964Pp 171–200
7. Pagana, K.D. (1988). Stresses and threats reported by baccalaureate students in relation to an initial clinical experience. Journal of Nursing Education, 27, 418-424.
8. R. M. HARDEN AND F. A. GLEESON (1979) Assessment of clinical competence using an objective structured clinical examination (0s CE). Medical Education 13, 41-52
9. Reilly, J.A. and Oermann, M.H. (1992). Clinical Teaching in Nursing Education. New York: National League for Nursing.
10. Rokeah. M (1968) A Theory of Organization and Change Within Value-Attitude Systems" Journal of Social Issues Vol. 24, Issue 1
11. Shon, D.A. (1990). Educating the reflective practitioner. San Francisco, CA: Jossey-Bass.

⊙⊙⊙

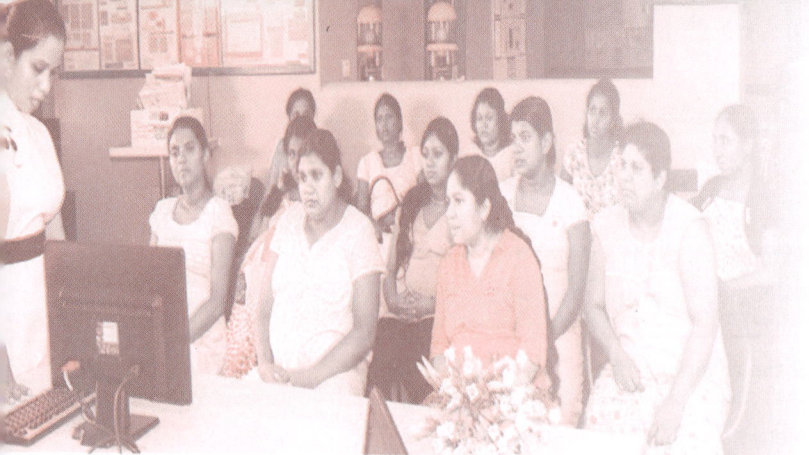

Information, Education and Communications for Health (IEC)

— Gitumoni Kanwar

CHAPTER OUTLINE

Health Behavior and Health Education

- Definition of Health behavior
- Concept of Health Behavior
- Process of Behavior Change
  - Awareness
  - Neutrality
  - Action
  - Environment
  - Retention

Planning for Health Education

- Definition of Health Education
- Aims and Objectives of Health Education
- Importance of Health Education
- Principle of Health Education
  - Interest
  - Participation
  - Comprehension
  - Reinforcement
  - Motivation
  - Learning by Doing
  - Known to Unknown
- Characteristics of Effective Health Education

Health Education with Individuals, Groups and Communities

- Individual Approach
- Family Approach
- Group Approach
- Community Approach
- Mass Approach

Communicating Health Messages

Methods and Media for Communicating Health Messages

- Media
  - Television
  - Radio
  - Internet
  - News Papers
  - Printed Material
  - Direct Mailing
  - Posters Billboards and Signs
  - Health Measures and Exhibitions
  - Flock Methods

📖 LEARNING OBJECTIVES

After completing this unit the learner will be able to

- Describe the concpet of health behavior and helath education
- Explain different aspects of planning health education

- Construct health education with individuals, groups and communities
- Discuss the factors influencing communicating health messages
- Use mass media for transmitting health information where ever necessary

INTRODUCTION

Today the focus of healthcare is on promotive and preventive aspects of health. The Ministry of Health and Family Welfare Government of India has emphasized on holistic approach to health. The emphasis has been given on promotion and protection of health with behavior change of the people in the community. The behavior modification can be achieved through well planned health education. The quality of life of the individuals has been influenced by their health behavior. Incorporating healthy behaviors such as regular exercise, balanced diet, meditation, quit smoking, stop alcohol can delay the onset of chronic disease. This chapter pays attention to the role of health education, communication and information (ICE) in health promotion and prevention to ensure optimum health. Therefore, health education generates awareness through dissemination of information by accurate planning as well as the appropriate implementation. This chapter also discusses different approaches to health education with individuals, groups and communities and methods and media necessary for communicating health messages.

INFORMATION, EDUCATION AND COMMUNICATION

The utmost aim to achieve a healthy life of the people in every community can be facilitated by enhancing their knowledge on preventive and promotive aspects of health. Provision has to be made available to provide adequate information even to the rural individuals, families, groups and community. Planning and implementation of health education with communication strategies helps us to achieve this goal. Hence, information, education and communication (ICE) has been combined to accomplish the desired behavior change among the people of the society.

Information

It is described as one or more facts that are received by a human, which have some form of worth to him. The facts and figures that are received by humans have to be true and factual to be labelled as information. In other words, information is intangible news and facts, which an individual uses to bridge discontinuities and gaps that are prevalent in his mind.

Education

It serves as an essential means to assist deliberate behavior change to promote health and prevent disease, which in turn helps the people to lead a functional productive life. Education is the process by which behavioral change takes place in an individual as a result of experience, which he has undergone.

Communication

It is the exchange of ideas, facts, feelings, thoughts, opinions and information, which are vital in facilitating human interaction through words, symbols or actions. Communication enables involvement between two or more individuals in sharing information and messages. It is a two-way process.

While the "information", "education", and "communication" have separate entity and significances, when grouped together collectively as "Information, Education, Communication (IEC)", they are well-known to the people associated with healthcare agency. The development of worldwide web in this century and swift progress in information technology has imperative implications in enhancement of quality of life.

Definition of "IEC" refers to a public health approach aiming at changing or reinforcing health-related behaviors in a target audience, concerning a specific problem and within a pre-defined period of time, through communication methods and principles.

HEALTH BEHAVIOR AND HEALTH EDUCATION

Health behavior is expressed as the action adopted by the individuals to protect, to maintain and to promote their health status. Our lifestyle is closely interrelated with health behavior. The epidemiological studies have established the relationship between onset of illness and regular exercise, taking adequate amount of fruit and vegetable, consumption of more green leafy vegetables, drinking milk, low fat, low caloric intake, proper sleeping habit, socialization etc.

Definition of Health Behavior

- Health behavior is defined as "combination of knowledge, practices and attitudes that together contribute to motivate the actions we take regarding health". (Farlex Partner Medical Dictionary)
- Health behavior is: "An action taken by any person to maintain, attain or regain good health and to prevent illness. Health behavior reflects a person's health beliefs. Some common health behaviors are exercising regularly, eating balanced diet, obtaining necessary inoculations" (Mosby's Medical Dictionary).

Concept of Health Behavior

The behavior of the people develops from his family, ethnicity culture and social tradition of the community he belongs to. It is possible to predict risks to inhabitants' health by observing their health behaviors for a longer period of time. Public health policies are developed for the population most in need. It is observed that the health activities, which have increased chance of developing morbidity and mortality are physical inactivity, sleep deprivation, unprotected sex, lack of recreation, low consumption of fruit and vegetables, inadequate rehydration, tobacco use, alcohol use, drug misuse and inadequate emotional expression. These health behaviors are called risk factors and these are modifiable. The lifestyle modifications with healthy behavior have considerable impact on onset of chronic diseases, disability and mortality. Our attitude, belief and behavior contribute to the prevention of illness. The current leading causes of death are cardiovascular diseases, hypertension, cancer, and acquired immune deficiency syndrome (AIDS) are closely associated with the person's lifestyle. Our attitude, belief and behavior contribute to the prevention of illness. The root cause of development of these illnesses can be prevented by modification of behavior or changing behavior of the people.

Process of Behavior Change

The behavior of an individual get shaped from his childhood throughout the different developmental stages. The progress of behavior modification takes place with the likes, beliefs, values, attitude, knowledge and the life experiences of a person. The modification of behavior is only possible with the conscious, deliberate and deeply committed effort of a person. It requires strong will power and firm decision to modify/change or adopt a new behavior. The decision of change of behavior sustains with constant feedback with positive reinforcement and motivation. People undergo different stages of activities during transformation of behavior. These activities are called the ***process of behavior change***.

Awareness (Fig. 1)

The first step of behavior modification or change is awareness. It is imperative to create awareness among people about the need of a particular behavior modification. Emphasizing about the causes, consequences, and cures for particular problem behavior increases awareness of the people. Once insight is developed on the problem, their attitude, belief and values are shaken.

Neutrality (Fig. 1)

They strive during this step to change their attitude. People search for more information about that change and outcome benefits of the change. Information education materials help to build knowledge base. Interventions like feedback, interpretations, and examples from the community and media campaigns that can amplify responsiveness of the people. The change of negative attitude brings individuals to the zone of neutrality. The healthcare provider becomes successful when the community accepts the message.

Action (Fig. 1)

The attitude of these persons gets changed from zone of neutrality to the positive attitude in this stage. The positive attitude is reinforced with their knowledge gain and personal experiences. They then take strong decision to change their behavior. Committed will of the people helps them to take action for modification in behavior. Simulated exercise reinforces the correct action, as for example: role playing, demonstration, and role model from real life situations. Positive feedback encourages people to enhance the action.

Environment (Fig. 1)

Maintenance of the environment motivates the person to continue the modified action. The family, community and healthcare provider support health behavior change by caring and maintaining trusting relationships. Evaluation of the desired outcome is essential. Achievement of desired benefit in visual forms or with objective data provides positive energy. The health benefits add force to the action. The risk behavior modification such as alcoholism needs maintenance of the

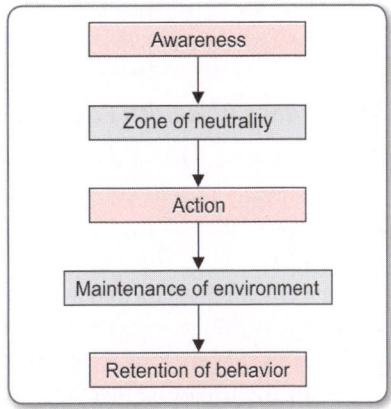

Fig. 1: Different methods and media for communicating health messages

environment. It is better to keep him away from the partners of drinking, excess money and free time. Sometimes, other stimulants may be necessary to remove these behaviors, for example, smoking.

Retention (Fig. 1)

Retention is the stage when the changed behavior remains same for longer period. Successful behavior changes the people and helps them re-energize with repeated information at intervals. The person comes to know how much improvement has taken place due to his effort in changing behavior. So, he is boosted to continue the same. This is then converted into habit and inculcated with the other health behaviors. Thus, the process of behavior change takes place.

Definition of Health Education

Health education has been defined as:
- "The sum of all experiences in school and elsewhere that favourably influence habits, attitudes and knowledge, related to individual, community and racial health."
- "Any combination of learning opportunities and teaching activities designed to facilitate voluntary adaptations of behavior that are conducive to health." (Green LW)
- Health education has been defined in many ways by different authors and experts. **Lawrence Green** defined it as "a combination of learning experiences designed to facilitate voluntary actions conducive to health."

Aims and Objectives of Health Education

The primary aim of health education is the deliberate behavior change of the community. The aim and objectives of health education can be listed as follows:
- To assist people in modification of health behavior to maintain healthy lifestyle
- To create awareness among people of their health needs
- To ensure that people realize the right to health
- To alter the attitude of people towards health
- To make the people understand that health is an asset of the community
- To provide the people the latest knowledge and skill
- To promote the utilization of health services available.

Importance of Health Education

The health education always emphasizes on the need-based desired behavior changes or lifestyle modification among the people of the community. The importance of health education is as follows. It:
- Enhances the quality of life and the health status of the people
- Increases activity of daily living of the people with chronic illness
- Makes people aware and increase the utilization of health services
- Creates healthy environment to improve hygiene and sanitation
- Ensures safe drinking water and appropriate nutrition
- Reduces the costs of healthcare for individuals by encouraging preventive practices
- Strengthens the community with reproductive and child health program
- Helps in successful implementation of all health programs.

Principles of Health Education

There is internal learning by which a man grows in to an adult individual. It's possible to extract certain principles of learning and use them in health education.

Interest

According to the psychological principle, people give importance to the things of their interests. Therefore, it is essential that the topic of the health education must relate to the interests of the program and the people. That will ensure active participation from the people. The health educator should be able to determine the health needs of the society. The education of healthcare providers must address the priority health needs of the people and problem within the society.

Participation

The individual and community health are closely interwoven and dependent. Hence, health education is commonly given to the adult learners. Hence, active learning methods are the better choice. The various active participatory methods are group discussion, panel discussion, work shop, symposium, role play etc.

Comprehension

The health educator must detect the level of understanding of the community people to whom the teaching is directed. During communication of the health messages, the health educator should keep in mind the use of simple words, which can be comprehended.

The change of behavior among the children is effective with practice of health habits instead of abstract. The health educator emphasizes on practicing the skill, while the aim is to change habit of the children.

Reinforcement

Health education programs can be successful to change the people mind set with repeated information at intervals. Repetition is useful to assist comprehension and understanding. Reinforcement is a process whereby behavior with desirable consequences is repeated. The positive reinforcement helps the people to adapt themselves and develop their knowledge and skill.

Motivation

Motivation is the internal process that activate, guide, and maintain behavior over time. It is a force, which results in persistent behavior directed towards a particular goal. People can be motivated by the outside forces or incentive like praise, love, rivalry, rewards, punishment and recognition. The people will be deeply committed, when they receive feedback on their progress toward meeting the goals. The motivation is an essential factor for health education to be successful. Learning is best when the people are well motivated and they are actively involved in the process. The health educator must respect the self esteem of the individuals.

Learning by Doing

An effective health education is based on the principles of learning by doing. Active learning is best to achieve the desired outcome and provide persistent change for longer period. The importance of learning is well described by the proverb "'If I hear-I forget, if I see- I remember, if I do-I know". The healthcare provider needs to demonstrate the expected behavior modification or change. The individuals are appealed to carry out the task as demonstrated to them. Health habits should be cultured through self determination practice.

Known to Unknown

The health educators should proceed from, the known to the unknown while communicating health messages. The education should be based on the previous knowledge of the group and then continue with new knowledge. The existing knowledge of the individual serves as base for better understanding. Hence, interest on the topic can be stimulated and insight into the problem can be build up.

Characteristics of Effective Health Education

- Based on previous knowledge of the individuals
- Emphasizes benefits of action by using clear, simple language
- Promotes feasible actions with available resources within the community
- Encourages discussion and learner participation for active learning
- Attracts the attention of the community with entertainments
- Uses different methods such as songs, dance, drama, role play, role model, puppet show, kirtan-katha and story-telling, etc.
- Uses demonstrations and simulations to develop correct practice
- Repeats feedback for reinforcement of action periodically.

Planning for Health Education

A good planning is pre-requisite for an effective health education. While planning health education we must develop strategies for desired behavior change. It is important to find out local traditional and sociocultural methods for communication. The healthcare provider plans health education for success of the heath program of the state.

Steps of Planning Health Education

- Assess the need or problems persistent in the community
- Identify the problem according to the priority need
- Collect information on cultural background and socioeconomic status
- Assemble data on available resources and strength of that community
- Assess previous knowledge of the target audience
- Determine objectives according to the topic
- Prepare of the teaching material and audiovisual aids
- Involves the community leaders for better acceptance and support
- Design monitoring and evaluation tools to assess the outcome.

Health Education With Individuals, Groups and Communities

The target of the health education is behavior change. The success of the information and education is evaluated as the prevalence or incidence of the specific problem. Selection of appropriate approach is necessary to achieve the targeted behavior change. The different approaches are individual approach, family approach, group approach and community approach.

Individual Approach

Individual approach is a personal contact and face to face discussion. The individual approach can be adopted by the health educator through the different life span of an individual i.e. infant, toddler, school age, adolescent, adults and old age. This ways health education can be provided according the needs at different stage of life. Topics for the health counselling may be selected as per prevalence of the problem. The individual approach provides more stress on a particular behavior change of an individual, such as, heavy alcohol consumption. Use of individual approach promotes verbalization due to maintenance of confidentiality.

Family Approach

Family approach is also a personal contact and face to face discussion with couples and family. The community health nurse use home visit as family approach. The health education topic is selected according to the need of the family. This approach helps the couples and the family to deal with the health problems effectively. The educator should create trustworthy and friendly environment, which allows them to talk deeply about a particular problem. The family approach provides better understanding because it promotes discussion.

Group Approach

Group approach is an effective way of teaching a group of people such as pregnant women, post-menopausal women, etc. on a common topic of their interest. The members of the group are helped to think, discuss, decide and then follow up their decisions by action. This ways it enhances the acceptance of ideas, makes the people responsible about their health and lets them adopt preventive and curative measures themselves to restore health and save time.

Community Approach

The most important step in community approach is to encourage the community to distinguish their needs. This approach encourages better community participation on a particular health need. The advantage of community approach is that a large number of target people at a time can be covered. The various methods used in this approach are dance, drama, flock songs, flock drama etc.

Mass Approach

Mass approach is used when the message or information is to be given to a large number of persons. When the target population is large, mass media is used to reach the population without much difficulty. There are various methods and media used in mass communication, for example, exhibitions, campaigns, radio, news papers, etc. Mass communication is the method used by communication industries that creates a relationship between the media and their viewers.

COMMUNICATING HEALTH MESSAGES

Communicating health messages is the sharing of information, exchange of ideas and transmission of messages between two or more persons about preventive and promotive measures of health. The available resources, customs and cultural background, traditional practices, socio-economic level and the environmental situations are considered while developing strategies for communicating health messages. Information, education and communication combine strategies are used to assist people to care for their health actively. The activities involved during communication of health messages empowers the individuals to take decision for behavior modification or change. The accomplishment of the public health initiative depends on the effective communication of the health messages. One should keep in mind the process of communication, channels of communication, and facilitators of communication, while communicating health messages. Different methods and media were used for communicating health messages.

Methods and Media for Communicating Health Messages

The foundation of every successful public health program mostly depends on information, communication and education. There are different methods and media used to deliver health education to the community. The various methods and media of communicating health messages may be grouped as given in Fig. 2.

These are the several **methods** by which health education is imparted. Any one or combinations of these methods can be used to communicate health messages as per the objective to be achieved. The different methods used in the teaching learning process have been already discussed in Chapter 6, Methods of Teaching, of this book.

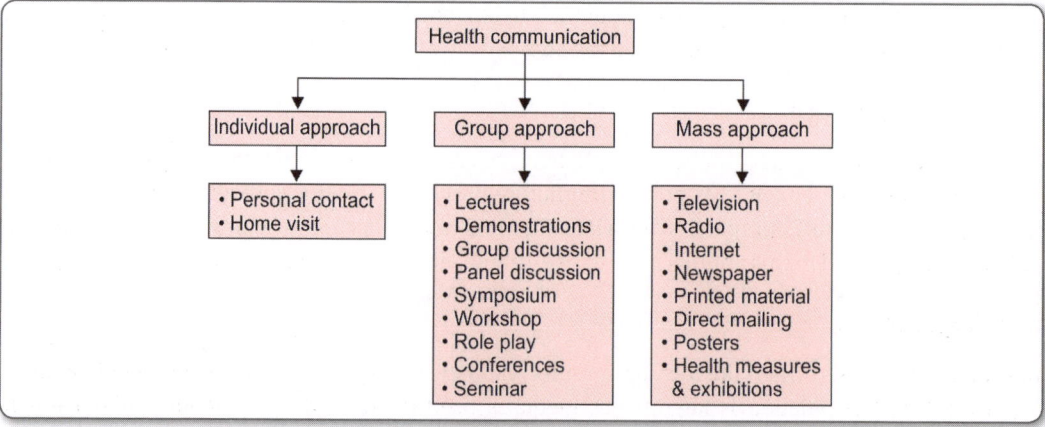

Fig. 2: Different methods and media for communicating health messages

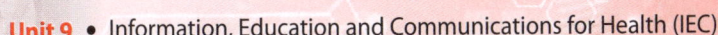

Media is an agency through which communication takes place and media are needed to deliver the message to the target audience. The various media for communicating health messages are discussed below:

Television

The most popular media is television with variety of shows. Television is useful as an aid in creating awareness and persuades public opinion. It is very much effective in introducing people with new ideas, things and increase understanding level by the help of visual presentation. The disadvantage of the television is; it is a one way communication channel. The television is utilized as a prospective media for communicating health messages. However, television is not self sufficient to cover all the areas of desired behavior change.

Radio

Radio is almost available in everyone's house. A large number of people love listening to radio programs. It is a social favorite media and found nearly every home. In many developing countries, the radio has a broader audience than television. Radio is helpful for the people, who cannot read and write. It can reach to the remotest people because it is cheaper than television. Radio is a mass communication approach. A large number of populations are covered with health information and news. Radio serves as a strong medium of communication of voice messages in local languages.

Internet

The invention of the World Wide Web or worldwide computer network has changed the earth to a global village. The communication became very faster and easy with the help of internet. This service can be used for knowledge transfer, gather information, e-mail and chat. On the website, there are huge amount of health-related information available from different agencies like World Health Organization and the ministry of health and family welfare Govt. of India.

Newspapers

Newspapers are the oldest method of mass communication. It is very popular among the literate group. Newspapers provide latest detailed news on local and national matters. Political news and law and order situation of the society are center of attention of the newspapers. Unfortunately, health issues have little focus on newspapers.

Printed Material

Most widely used printed materials in health communication are magazines, newsletters, pamphlets, booklets, leaflets and hand-outs. These materials can only facilitate the literate group of the society. Printed materials are versatile to create awareness and provide knowledge. These materials reinforce the health education and information in detail. These materials can be created in low cost for a large amount, for example, pamphlets on breast self examination, family planning, weaning of baby, etc.

Direct Mailing

Direct mailing is one among the cheapest media of communication. These are sent to the village leaders such as, Sarpanch of the panchayat, gaon burha and ward member, etc. Direct mailing is a means of personal communication. It is a powerful media to generate public awareness.

Posters, Billboards and Signs

Posters and sign boards are very much helpful to generate awareness among all the group of people. These are projected to draw attention of the public in a simple and artistic way. Posters are effective media to create awareness on different topics of health, such as safe drinking water, immunization etc. This display is best at hospitals, bus stops and railway stations where a person has to wait some time. The posters should be relevant with the community, as it is viewed by the large number of individuals. A poster is less effective to change the behavior of people.

Health Measures and Exhibitions

A systematically organized health mela or exhibitions attract large number of people. At the same time many topics were presented in visual from with the help of photographs, models and printed materials. Through exhibition, depth and consequences of a particular health behavior is represented beautifully. It is a powerful medium to increase knowledge, generate awareness and change attitude of all people of a community. The exhibited items were explained by a healthcare provider.

Flock Media

Every community have their traditional flock forum. The flock media, which are originated from different culture such as kirtan, katha, flock songs, ghazals, kawalis, dances, dance drama, dramas, street plays and puppet shows are efficient media for communication. These methods transmit health messages through entertainment. This media acquires more acceptance from the people as it is rooted in their culture.

Using Mass Media

- The mass communication media has prospective means to cover a large number of people word wide.
- It is a public communication, which reaches mechanically or electronically to the people.
- The different mass media used to spread health messages are television, radio, newspaper, wide range of printed media and flock mediums as discussed before.
- The health information is delivered to millions of people at the same time.
- It empowers the public to change their attitude towards health behavior. Still it is not sufficient to change human behavior.
- These media is used as an aid along with other methods of communication. For effective communication, they should be used in combination with other methods.

COMMUNICATION FOR HEALTH CARE AND NURSING PRACTICE

The essential nursing functions are preventive, restorative, promotive, curative and rehabilitative. In all these the 'Effective Communication Skill' is the most important determinant of the nursing care outcome. While following the steps of Nursing Process, whether in hospital set-up, community health fields or home-nursing, communication skill is vital right from health assessment till the end of nurse-client interactions.

Deciding about the appropriate matters, methods and supportive aids for communication require a nurse to learn and have hands-on training in all aspects of successful nurse-client communication.

SUMMARY

We have discussed various aspects of information, education and communication in this unit. The activities undertaken by an individual to keep himself healthy are health behaviors. Information, education and communication combines approaches are utilized to empower the individuals, families and communities to play active roles in achieving, their own health. The aim of health education is to promote specific desired behavior to maintain health and prevent illness. There are various methods and media used for the successful communication of this information. The lecture, demonstrations, group discussions, panel discussions, workshops, role plays, radio, television, internet, posters, and printed materials are some example of methods and media of communication. The success of the health program undertaken by the ministry of health and family welfare depend on the transmission of information with effective communication.

ASSESS YOURSELF

LONG ANSWER QUESTIONS

1. Explain the principles of health education.
2. Why do nursing students need to plan for health education for community?
3. How are health messages communicated to the mass?
4. Plan a health education for mothers regarding immunization/personal hygiene.
5. Discuss in details mass media communication.
6. Enumerate the different types of Media. Write down the advantages and limitations of use of print media as a medium of communication.
7. Explain the utility of television as an effective mass media of providing education.
8. Discuss the characteristics of effective health education.
9. Explain demonstration method with its advantages and disadvantages.
10. Explain health education with individual, groups and communities.

SHORT ANSWER QUESTIONS

1. List any four principles of health education.
2. Enumerate the media for communicating the health messages.

Contd...

3. Name any two types of mass media.
4. Any four advantages of Lecture method.
5. Enlist four types of mass media.
6. Mention two differences between seminar and symposium.
7. Define the health education.
8. List down the different Flock methods.
9. Enumerate the two properties of Seminar.
10. Essentials of information, education and communications.

SHORT NOTES

1. Health measures and exhibitions
2. Symposium
3. Role play
4. Internet
5. Use of mass media in health education
6. Role of mass media in health care industry
7. Use of television and radio as media for ICE
8. Explain the objectives of health education
9. Process of behavior change
10. Importance of health education

MULTIPLE CHOICE QUESTIONS

1. **The meaning of ICE is:**
   A. Information Control Education
   B. Initiative Control Education
   C. Information Communication Education
   D. Information Communication Entertainment

2. **The different group approach of communication are:**
   A. News paper, discussion, demonstration   B. Lecture, symposium, direct mailing
   C. Conferences, exhibition, role-play   D. Group discussion, symposium, seminar

3. **In which year the Alma Ata declaration of Primary Health Care was conducted:**
   A. 1978   B. 1938
   C. 1956   D. 1925

4. **Principles of health education:**
   A. Interest, participation, involvement
   B. Comprehension, reinforcement, motivation
   C. Learning by doing, participation, simulation
   D. Known to unknown, comprehension, accomplishment

Contd...

5. The process of behavior change through health education usually involves appropriate approach except:
   A. Personal approach
   B. Individual approach
   C. Family approach
   D. Community approach

6. Which of the following is a mass approach of media?
   A. Group discussion
   B. Internet
   C. Panel discussion
   D. Symposium

7. Which statement is true for mass media?
   A. Mass media transmit messages to few people
   B. Mass media does not use flock method
   C. Mass media falls under group approach
   D. Mass media are one way communication

8. Advantages of demonstrations:
   A. Persuades the onlookers to adopt recommended practices
   B. Upholds the principles of learning by doing
   C. Bring desirable changes in behavior
   D. All of the above

ANSWERS TO MCQS

1. (C)	2. (D)	3. (A)	4. (B)	5. (A)	6. (B)	7. (D)
8. (D)						

BIBLIOGRAPHY

1. Albert Bandura. Health Promotion by Social Cognitive Means. Health Educ Behav. 2004; 31:143-64
2. Bartholomew LK, Parcel GS, Kok G. Intervention Mapping: A Process for Developing Theory and Evidence-Based Health Education Programs. Health Educ Behav. 1998;25: 545-63. http://www.ncbi.nlm.nih.gov/pubmed/9768376
3. Basavanthapa BT. Communication and Education Technology for nurses. 1st ed. New Delhi: Jaypee Brothers Medical Publishers (P) Ltd; 2011. p.351-69
4. WHO EMRO. Child health and development: Information, education and communication. http://www.emro.who.int/child/community-information/
5. Conner M. Health Behaviors. Available from: http://userpage.fu-berlin.de/~schuez/folien/conner2002.pdf
6. Farlex Partner Medical Dictionary, Farlex 2012. Definition:Health behavior. Available from: http://medical-dictionary.thefreedictionary.com/health+behavior
7. Green LW. Int J of health education. 1979;22:161-8

8. Green LW; Kreuter MW; Deeds SG; Partridge KB; Bartlett E. Public Health education planning: a diagnostic approach. Available from: http://www.popline.org/node/499039

9. Mosby's Medical Dictionary, 9th ed. 2009, Elsevier. Definition:Health behavior. Available from:http://medical-dictionary.thefreedictionary.com/health+behavior

10. Neeraja KP. Textbook of Communication and Education Technology for Nurses. 1st ed. New Delhi: Jaypee Brothers Medical Publishers (P) Ltd;2011. p. 514-25

11. Nutbeam D. Health Literacy as public Health goal, a challenge for contemporary health education and communication strategies into 21st century. Health promotion International 2000;15:259-267. Available from: http://heapro. oxford journals.org/content/15/3/259. full pdf + html

12. K Park. Park Textbook of Preventive and Social Medicine. 23rd ed. Jabalpur: Banarasidas Bhanot Publishers; 2015. p.854-67

13. Roy NR. Maharajan and Gupta Text Book of preventive and Social Medicine. 4thed. New Delhi:Jaypee Brothers Medical Publishers (P) Ltd; 2013.p.555-75

14. Schroeder S. We can do better-Improving the health of the American people. New England J of Med. 2007;357:1221-8.

15. Sudha R. Nursing Education Principles and Concepts. 1st ed. New Delhi: Jaypee Brothers Medical Publishers (P) Ltd; 2013. p.78-92

16. US Department of Health and Human Services 1990 Health People 2000: National Health Promotion and Disease Prevention Objectives. US Department of Health and Human Services, Public Health Service, Washington, DC.

17. WHO: Education for Health: A manual for Health Education. Primary Health Care. Geneva. WHO 1998. Available from: http://www.who.int/healthpromotion/about/HPR%20Glossary%201998.pdf

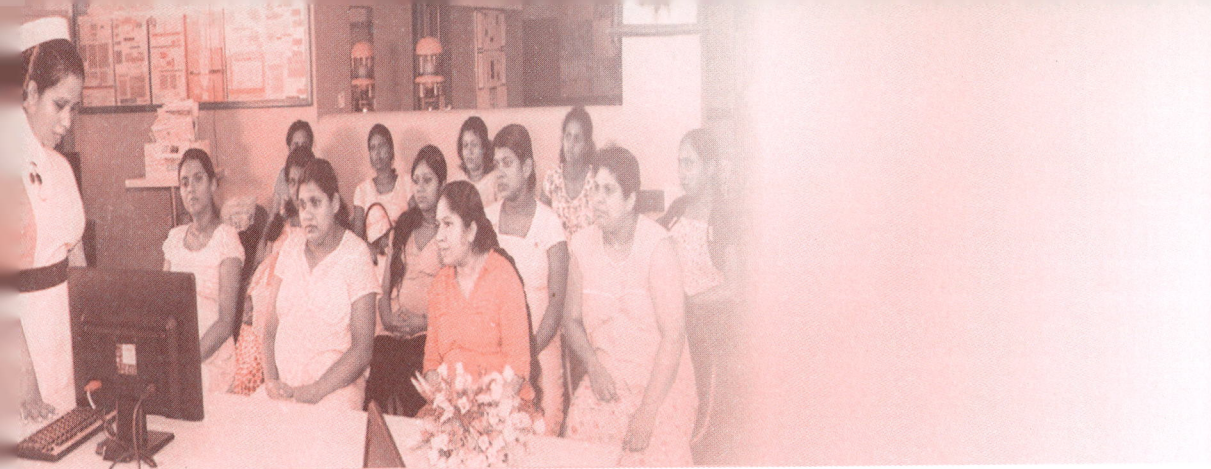

Index

Refer 't' for table and 'f' for figure, respectively.

Nursing Knowledge Tree

An Initiative by CBS Nursing Division

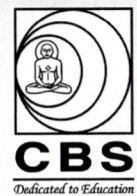

C B S
Dedicated to Education

Nursing Books Catalogue 2021-22

Books for All

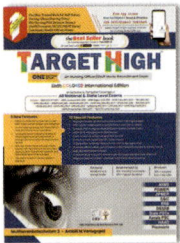

Target High
Muthuvenkatachalam S et al.
978-93-90619-55-9
6/e, 2022
MRP: ₹1499/-

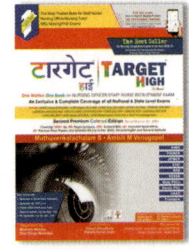

Target High (In Hindi)
Muthuvenkatachalam S et al.
978-81-94025-65-8
2/e, 2020
MRP: ₹1299/-

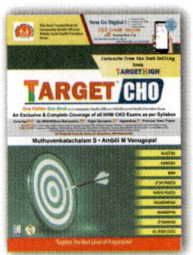

Target CHO
Muthuvenkatachalam S et al.
978-81-940256-0-3
1/e, 2020
MRP: ₹495/-

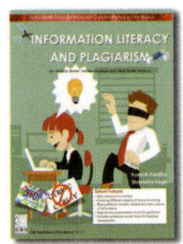

Information Literacy and Plagiarism
for Medical, Dental, Nursing Graduates
and Allied Health Sciences
Ramesh Pandita et al.
978-93-86827-13-5
1/e, 2018
MRP: ₹370/-

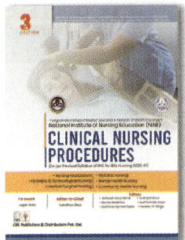

PGI NINE
Clinical Nursing Procedures
Sandhya Ghai
978-93-90619-56-6
3/e, 2022
MRP: ₹1295/-

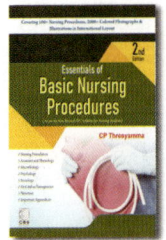

Essentials of
Basic Nursing Procedures
CP Thresyamma
978-81-94523-47-5
2/e, 2020
MRP: ₹795/-

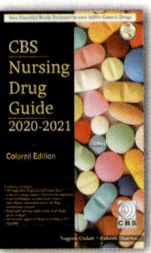

CBS Nursing Drug Guide
2020-2021
Yogesh Gulati et al.
978-93-88178-53-2
1/e, 2020
MRP: ₹1050/-

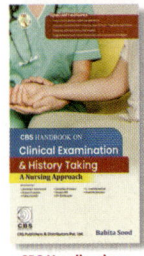

CBS Handbook on
Clinical Examination & History Taking
A Nursing Approach
Babita Sood
978-81-948693-9-9
1/e, 2021
MRP: ₹350/-

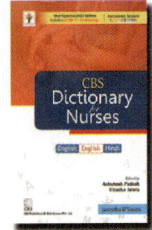

CBS Dictionary for Nurses
Jacintha D'Souza
978-93-90619-06-1
1/e, 2021
MRP: ₹595/-

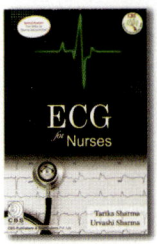

ECG for Nurses
Tarika Sharma et al.
978-93-89261-88-2
1/e, 2019
MRP: ₹350/-

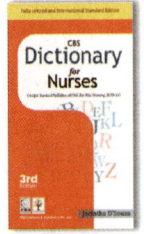

CBS Dictionary for Nurses
Jacintha D'Souza
978-93-90619-29-0
3/e, 2022
MRP: ₹450/-

Read, Review & Buy

Now, buying CBS Nursing Books is extra convenient with 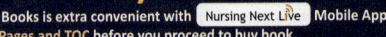 Mobile App.
Get a Glimpse of Sample Pages and TOC before you proceed to buy book.

Download the App from
Google Playstore or scan
here to download

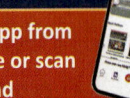

Community Health Nursing

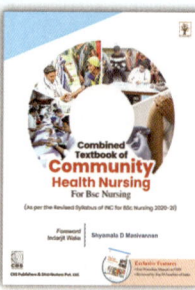

**Combined Textbook of
Community Health Nursing**
For BSc Nursing
Shyamala D Manivannan
978-93-90619-37-5
1/e, 2022

TBA

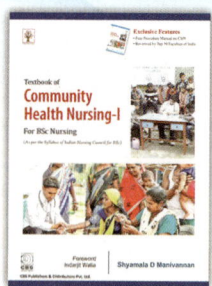

**Textbook of
Community Health Nursing-I**
For BSc Nursing
Shyamala D Manivannan
978-81-23927-01-5
1/e, 2018

MRP: ₹750/-

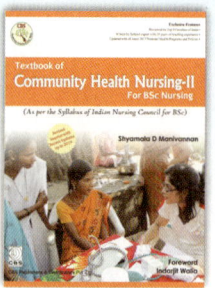

**Textbook of
Community Health Nursing-II**
For BSc Nursing
Shyamala D Manivannan
978-93-86827-22-7
1/e, 2018

MRP: ₹450/-

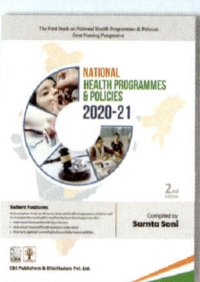

**National Health Programmes &
Policies 2020-21**
Samta Soni
978-93-90619-13-9
2/e, 2022

MRP: ₹695/-

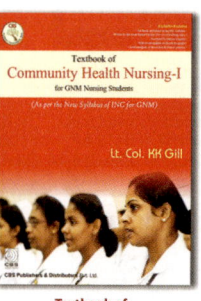

**Textbook of
Community Health Nursing-I**
For GNM Nursing Students
Lt. Col. KK Gill
978-93-86827-17-3
1/e, 2018

MRP: ₹550/-

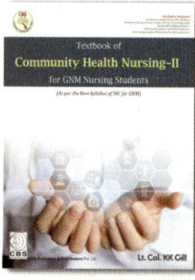

**Textbook of
Community Health Nursing-II**
for GNM Nursing Students
Lt. Col. KK Gill
978-93-88178-57-0
1/e, 2019

MRP: ₹525/-

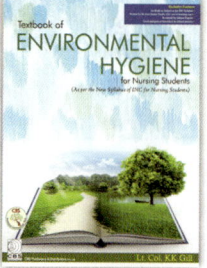

**Textbook of
Environmental Hygiene**
for Nursing Students
Lt. Col. KK Gill
978-93-88178-56-3
1/e, 2018-19

MRP: ₹225/-

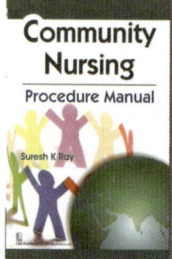

**Community Nursing
Procedure Manual**
Suresh K Ray
978-81-23929-35-4
1/e, 2017

MRP: ₹265/-

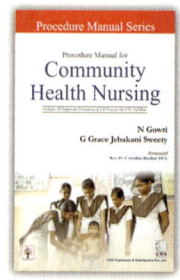

**Procedure Manual for
Community Health Nursing**
N Gowri et al.
978-81-948693-6-8
1/e, 2021

MRP: ₹195/-

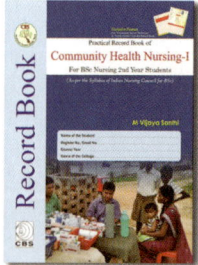

**Practical Record Book of
Community Health Nursing-I**
for BSc Nursing 2nd Year Students
M Vijaya Santhi
978-81-23926-84-1
1/e, 2016

MRP: ₹450/-

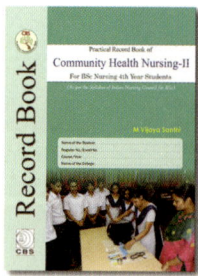

**Practical Record Book of
Community Health Nursing-II**
for BSc Nursing 4th Year Students
M Vijaya Santhi
978-93-88108-77-5
1/e, 2018-19

MRP: ₹575/-

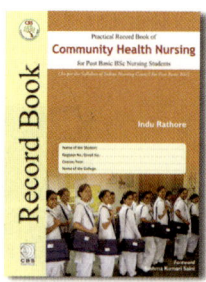

**Practical Record Book of
Community Health Nursing**
for Post Basic BSc Nursing Students
Indu Rathore
978-93-86827-06-7
1/e, 2017

MRP: ₹475/-

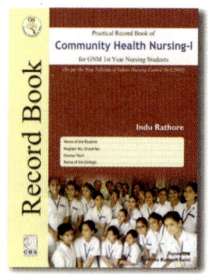

**Practical Record Book of
Community Health Nursing-I**
for GNM 1st Year Nursing Students
Indu Rathore
978-93-86827-07-4
1/e, 2018-19

MRP: ₹350/-

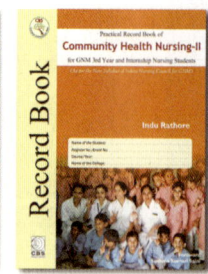

**Practical Record Book of
Community Health Nursing-II**
**for GNM 3rd Year and
Internship Nursing Students**
Indu Rathore
978-93-86827-30-2
1/e, 2018-19

MRP: ₹395/-

Buy online :
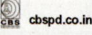   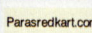 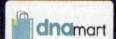 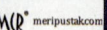

Nursing Foundation

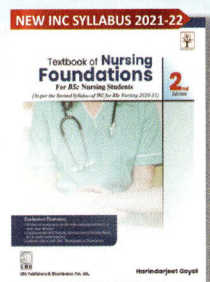

**Textbook of
Nursing Foundations
for BSc Nursing Students**
Harindarjeet Goyal
978-93-90619-12-2
2/e, 2022
MRP: ₹950/-

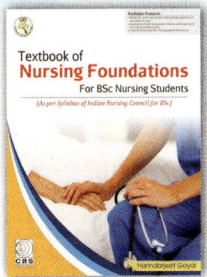

**Textbook of
Nursing Foundations
for BSc Nursing Students**
Harindarjeet Goyal
978-93-88108-94-2
1/e, 2020
MRP: ₹950/-

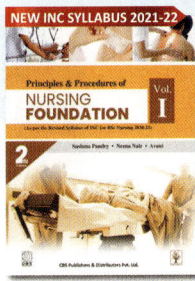

**Principles & Procedures of
Nursing Foundation Vol-I
for BSc Nursing**
Sushma Pandey et al.
978-93-90619-57-3
2/e, 2022
TBA

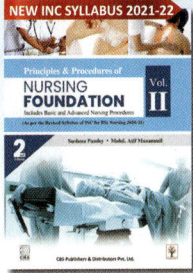

**Principles & Procedures of
Nursing Foundation Vol-II
for BSc Nursing**
Sushma Pandey et al.
978-93-90619-19-1
2/e, 2022
TBA

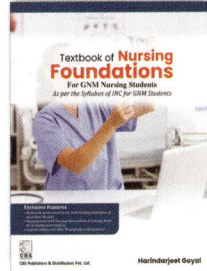

**Textbook of
Nursing Foundations
for GNM Nursing Students**
Harindarjeet Goyal
978-93-90619-70-2
1/e, 2022
MRP: ₹850/-

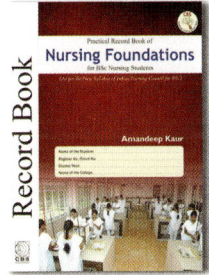

**Practical Record Book of
Nursing Foundations
for BSc Nursing Students**
Amandeep Kaur
978-93-88108-96-6
1/e, 2018-19
MRP: ₹425/-

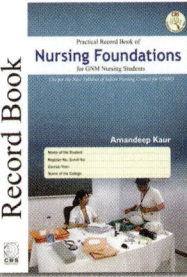

**Practical Record Book of
Nursing Foundations
for GNM Nursing Students**
Amandeep Kaur
978-93-88178-50-1
1/e, 2018-19
MRP: ₹350/-

Medical Surgical Nursing

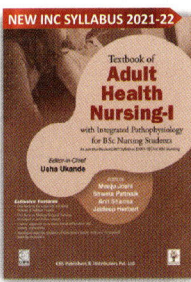

**Textbook of
Adult Health Nursing-I
with Integrated Pathophysiology
for BSc Nursing Students**
Usha Ukande
978-93-90619-20-7
1/e, 2022
TBA

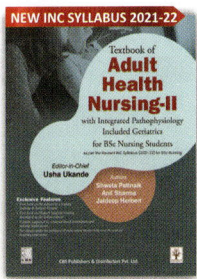

**Textbook of
Adult Health Nursing-II
with Integrated Pathophysiology
Included Geriatrics for BSc Nursing Students**
Usha Ukande
978-93-90619-86-3
1/e, 2022
TBA

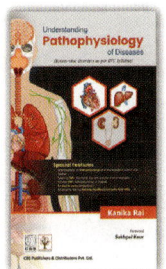

**Understanding
Pathophysiology of Diseases**
Kanika Rai
978-93-90619-11-5
1/e, 2022
MRP: ₹395/-

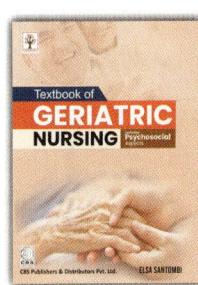

**Textbook of
Geriatric Nursing
Including Psychosocial Aspects**
Elsa Santombi
978-93-90619-79-5
1/e, 2022
TBA

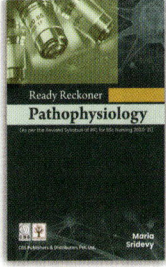

**Ready Reckoner
Pathophysiology
for Nurses**
Maria et al.
978-93-90619-05-4
1/e, 2022
TBA

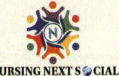

MSN/Pharmacology/Pathology

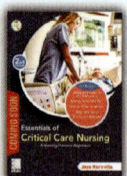

Essentials of Critical Care Nursing
A Nursing Process Approach
Jaya Kuruvilla
978-93-90619-61-0
2/e, 2022
TBA

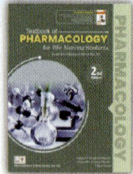

Textbook of Pharmacology
For BSc Nursing Students
Joginder Singh Pathania et al.
978-93-90619-27-6
2/e, 2022
MRP: ₹650/-

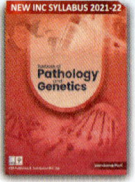

Textbook of Pathology and Genetics
Vandana Puri
978-93-90619-87-0
1/e, 2022
TBA

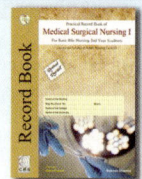

Practical Record Book of Medical Surgical Nursing I
for Basic BSc Nursing 2nd Year Students
Rakesh Sharma
978-81-23928-00-5
1/e, 2018-19
MRP: ₹550/-

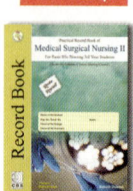

Practical Record Book of Medical Surgical Nursing II
for Basic BSc Nursing 3nd Year Students
Rakesh Sharma
978-81-23928-01-2
1/e, 2018-19
MRP: ₹475/-

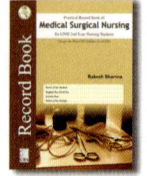

Practical Record Book of Medical Surgical Nursing
for GNM 2nd Year Nursing Students
Rakesh Sharma
978-93-86827-04-3
1/e, 2017
MRP: ₹475/-

Child Health Nursing & Pediatric Nursing

Exclusive Marketing & Distribution Rights

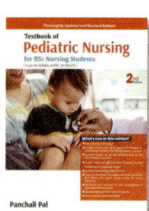

Textbook of Pediatric Nursing
for BSc Nursing Students
Panchali Pal
978-81-948693-2-0
2/e, 2021
MRP: ₹795/-

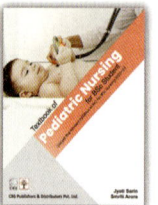

Textbook of Pediatric Nursing
for BSc Nursing Students
Jyoti Sarin et al.
978-93-90619-78-8
1/e, 2022
TBA

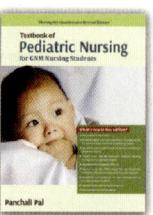

Textbook of Pediatric Nursing
for GNM Nursing Students
Panchali Pal
978-93-90619-71-9
1/e, 2022
TBA

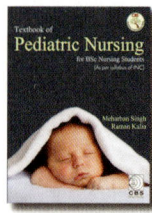

Textbook of Pediatric Nursing
for BSc Nursing Students
Meharban Singh et al.
978-93-88108-72-0
1/e, 2018
MRP: ₹725/-

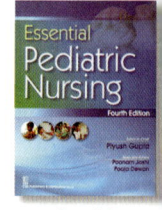

Essential Pediatric Nursing
Piyush Gupta
978-93-86217-87-5
4/e, 2017
MRP: ₹750/-

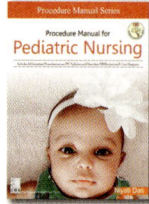

Procedure Manual for Pediatric Nursing
Niyati Das
978-93-88108-86-7
1/e, 2018
MRP: ₹325/-

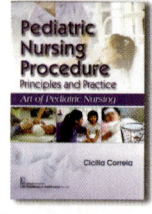

Pediatric Nursing Procedure Principles and Practice
Cicilia Correia
978-93-86310-74-3
1/e, 2017
MRP: ₹450/-

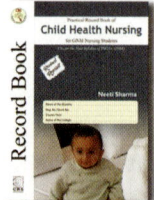

Practial Record Book of Child Health Nursing
for GNM Nursing Students
Neeti Sharma
978-93-86827-53-1
1/e, 2017
MRP: ₹325/-

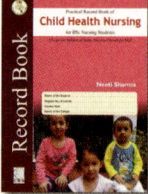

Practial Record Book of Child Health Nursing
for BSc Nursing Students
Neeti Sharma
978-93-86827-05-0
1/e, 2017
MRP: ₹310/-

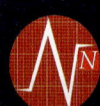
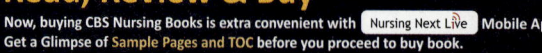

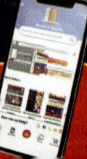

Mental Health Nursing & Psychiatric Nursing

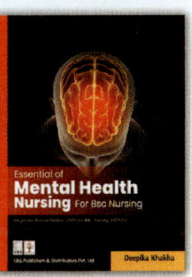

Essential of Mental Health Nursing
for BSc Nursing
Deepika Khakha
978-93-90619-73-3
1/e, 2022

TBA

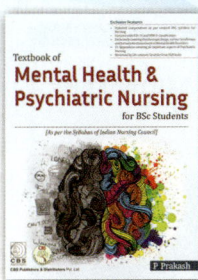

Textbook of Mental Health & Psychiatric Nursing
P Prakash
978-93-89261-91-2
1/e, 2019

MRP: ₹625/-

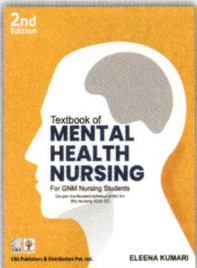

Textbook of Mental Health Nursing
for GNM Nursing Students
Eleena Kumari
978-93-90619-72-6
2/e, 2022

MRP: ₹395/-

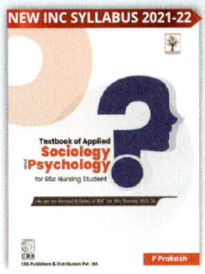

Textbook of Applied Sociology and Psychology
for BSc Nursing Students
P Prakash
978-93-90619-54-2
1/e, 2022

MRP: ₹395/-

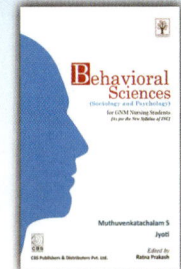

Behavioral Sciences
(Sociology and Psychology)
Muthuvenkatachalam S et al.
978-93-90619-04-7
1/e , 2021

MRP: ₹350/-

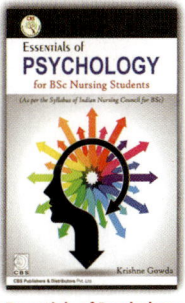

Essentials of Psychology
for BSc Nursing Students
Krishne Gowda
978-81-23927-11-4
1/e, 2017

MRP: ₹340/-

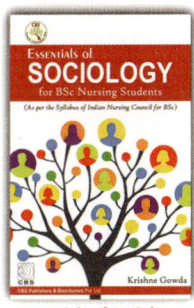

Essentials of Sociology
for BSc Nursing Students
Krishne Gowda
978-93-86217-51-6
1/e, 2017

MRP: ₹395/-

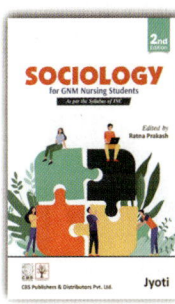

Sociology
for GNM Nursing Students
Jyoti
978-81-948693-1-3
2/e, 2022

MRP: ₹210/-

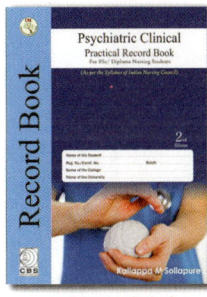

Psychiatric Clinical Practical Record Book
for BSc/Diploma Nursing Students
Kallappa M Sollapure
978-93-88108-81-2
2/e, 2018-19

MRP: ₹395/-

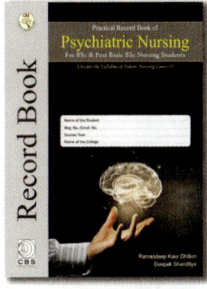

Practial Record Book of Psychiatric Nursing
for BSc & Post Basic BSc Nursing Students
Ramandeep Kaur Dhillon
978-93-88108-80-5
1/e, 2019

MRP: ₹415/-

Midwifery, Obstetrical & Gynecological Nursing

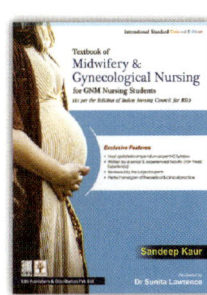

Textbook of Midwifery and Obstetrical Nursing
for BSc Nursing Students
Sandeep Kaur
978-93-89261-90-5
1/e, 2020

MRP: ₹995/-

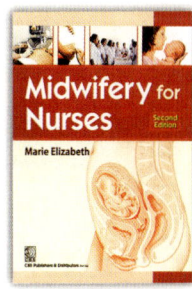

Textbook of Midwifery & Gynecological Nursing
for GNM Nursing Students
Sandeep Kaur
978-93-90619-18-4
2/e, 2022

MRP: ₹895/-

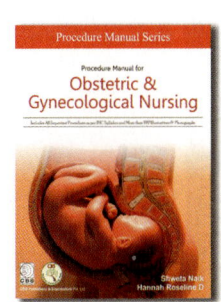

Textbook of Midwifery for Nurses
Marie Elizabeth
978-81-23922-14-0
2/e, 2018

MRP: ₹650/-

Procedure Manual for Obstetric & Gynecological Nursing
Sheweta Naik et al.
978-93-88178-60-0
1/e, 2018-19

MRP: ₹235/-

Midwifery, Obstetrical & Gynecological Nursing

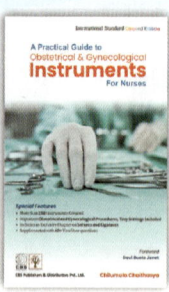

A Practical Guide to Obstetric & Gynecological Instruments for Nurses
Chilumula Chaithanya
978-93-90619-03-0
1/e, 2022
MRP: ₹250/-

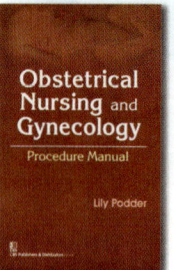

Obstetrical Nursing and Gynecology Procedure Manual
Lily Podder
978-81-23925-81-3
1/e, 2017
MRP: ₹265/-

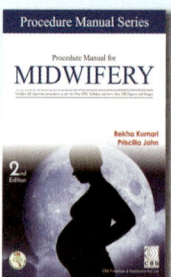

Procedure Manual for Midwifery
Rekha Kumari et al.
978-93-89261-94-3
2/e, 2019
MRP: ₹225/-

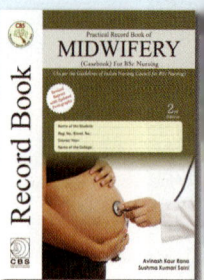

Practical Record Book of Midwifery (Casebook) for BSc Nursing
Avinash Kaur Rana et al.
978-93-88178-65-5
2/e (R/R), 2018-19
MRP: ₹675/-

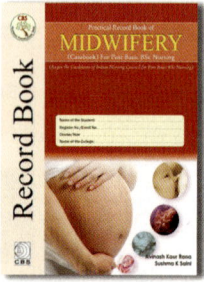

Practical Record Book of Midwifery (Casebook) for Post Basic BSc Nursing
Avinash Kaur Rana et al.
978-81-23927-07-7
1/e, 2016
MRP: ₹375/-

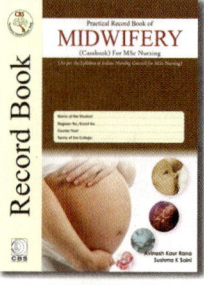

Practical Record Book of Midwifery (Casebook) for MSc Nursing
Avinash Kaur Rana et al.
978-93-86217-97-4
1/e, 2017
MRP: ₹625/-

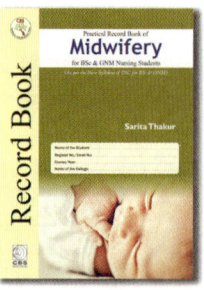

Practical Record Book of Midwifery for BSc & GNM Nursing Students
Sarita Thakur
978-93-86827-33-3
1/e, 2017
MRP: ₹415/-

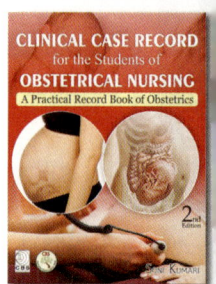

Clinical Case Record for the Students of Obstetrical Nursing
A Practical Record Book of Obstetrics
Soni Kumari
978-93-88178-51-8
2/e, 2018
MRP: ₹475/-

Nursing Research/Biostatistics

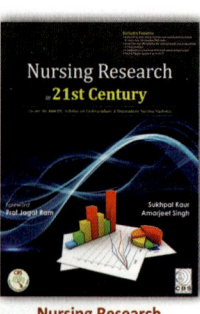

Nursing Research in 21st Century
Sukhpal Kaur et al.
978-93-89261-89-9
1/e, 2020
MRP: ₹725/-

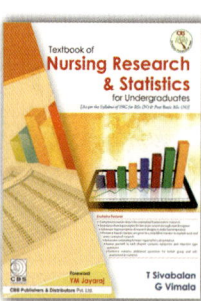

Textbook of Nursing Research & Statistics for Undergraduates
T Sivabalan et al.
978-93-88178-61-7
1/e, 2018
MRP: ₹525/-

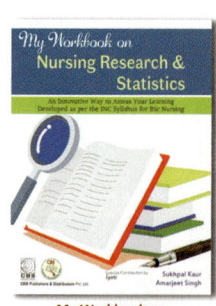

My Workbook on Nursing Research & Statistics
Sukhpal Kaur et al.
978-93-88108-75-1
1/e, 2019
MRP: ₹150/-

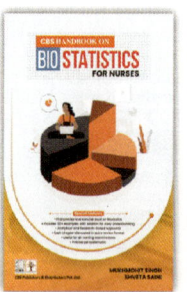

CBS Handbook on Biostatistics for Nurses
Mukhmohit Singh et al.
978-93-90619-10-8
1/e, 2022
MRP: ₹195/-

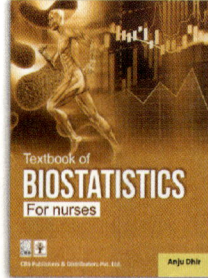

Textbook of Biostatistics for Nurses
Anju Dhir
978-93-90619-47-4
1/e, 2022
TBA

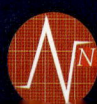

Read, Review & Buy
Now, buying CBS Nursing Books is extra convenient with Nursing Next Live Mobile App.
Get a Glimpse of Sample Pages and TOC before you proceed to buy book.

Download the App from Google Playstore or scan here to download

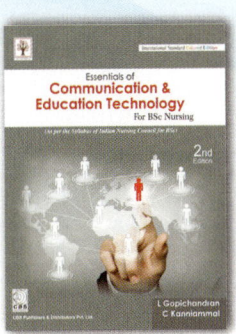

**Essentials of
Communication & Education Technology
for BSc Nursing**
L Gopichandran et al.
978-93-88178-58-7
2/e, 2019

MRP: ₹495/-

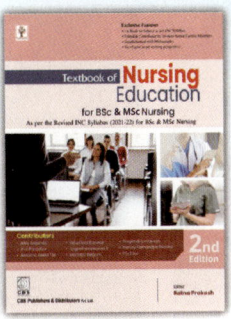

**Textbook of
Nursing Education
for BSc & MSc Nursing**
Ratna Prakash
978-93-90619-53-5
2/e, 2022

TBA

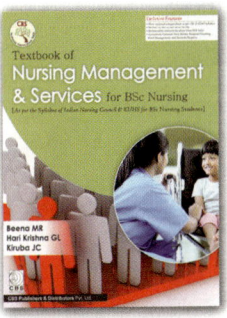

**Textbook of
Nursing Management & Services
for BSc Nursing**
Beena MR et al.
978-93-88178-62-4
1/e, 2019

MRP: ₹625/-

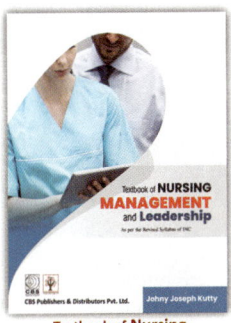

**Textbook of Nursing
Management & Leadership**
Johny Joseph Kutty
978-93-90619-40-5
1/e, 2022

MRP: ₹695/-

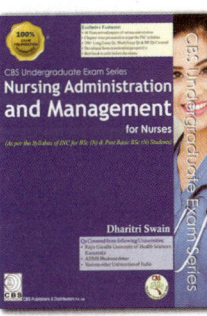

**CBS Undergraduate Exam Series
Nursing Administration
and Management for Nurses**
Dharitri Swain
978-93-86827-42-5
1/e, 2018

MRP: ₹350/-

Read, Review & Buy

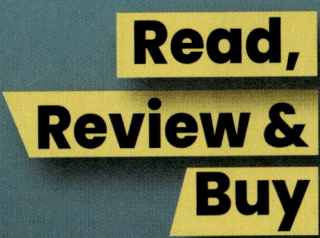

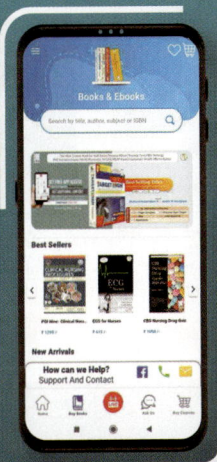

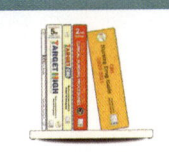

Books & Ebooks

Section is **Live** Now

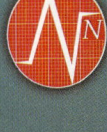

Now, buying CBS Nursing Books is extra convenient with **Nursing Next Live** Mobile App.

Get a Glimpse of **Sample Pages and TOC** before you proceed to buy books.

Best Discounts & Special Offers on all the Books.

Microbiology

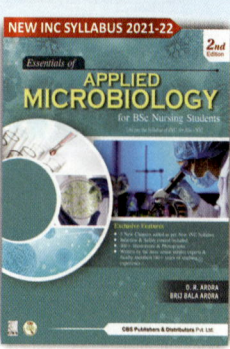

Essentials of Applied Microbiology
for BSc Nursing Students
D.R. Arora et al.
978-81-945234-4-4
2/e, 2020

MRP: ₹575/-

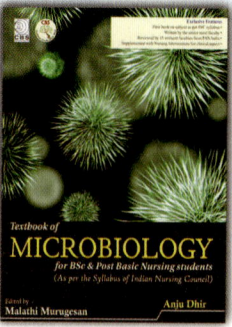

Textbook of Microbiology
for BSc & Post Basic Nursing Students
Anju Dhir
978-93-88108-82-9
1/e, 2018

MRP: ₹725/-

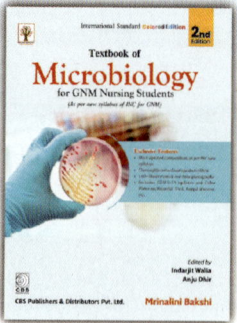

Textbook of Microbiology
for GNM Nursing Students
Mrinalini Bakshi
978-93-90619-12-2
2/e, 2021

MRP: ₹225/-

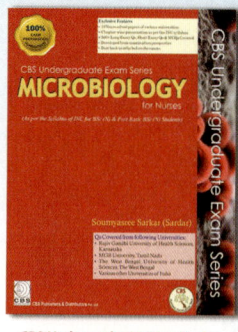

CBS Undergraduate Exam Series Microbiology for Nurses
Soumyasree Sarkar
978-93-86310-49-1
1/e, 2017

MRP: ₹275/-

English/First Aid/Computer

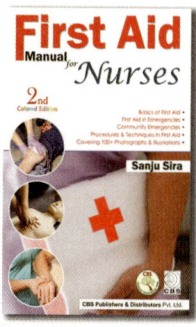

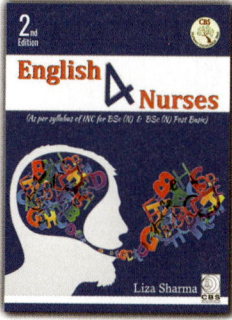

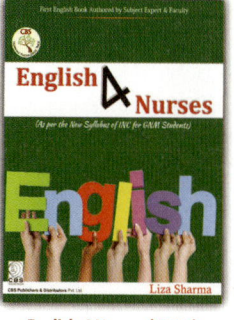

Communicative English 4 Nurses
for BSc Nursing Students
Liza Sharma
978-93-90619-26-9
1/e, 2022

TBA

English 4 Nurses (BSc)
Liza Sharma
978-93-89261-95-0
2/e, 2019

MRP: ₹415/-

English 4 Nurses (GNM)
Liza Sharma
978-93-86827-09-8
1/e, 2017

MRP: ₹350/-

First Aid Manual for Nurses
Sanju Sira
978-93-88178-55-6
2/e, 2019

MRP: ₹310/-

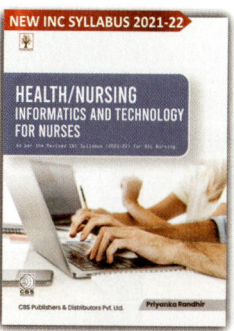

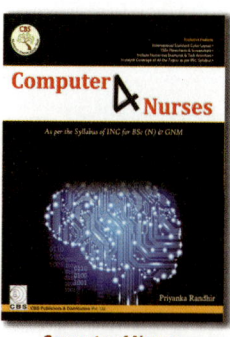

Health/Nursing Informatics and Technology for Nurses
Priyanka Randhir
978-93-90619-21-4
1/e, 2022

TBA

Computer 4 Nurses
Priyanka Randhir
978-93-86310-48-4
1/e, 2017

MRP: ₹370/-

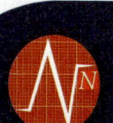

Read, Review & Buy
Now, buying CBS Nursing Books is extra convenient with Nursing Next Live Mobile App.
Get a Glimpse of Sample Pages and TOC before you proceed to buy book.

Download the App from Google Playstore or scan here to download

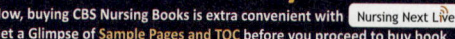

Anatomy & Physiology/Biochemistry & Nutrition

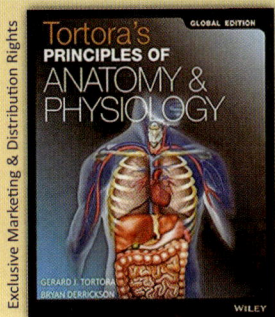

**Tortora's Principles of
Anatomy & Physiology**
Gerard J. Tortora
978-81-26567-61-4
GLOBAL Edition, 2017

MRP: ₹3495/-

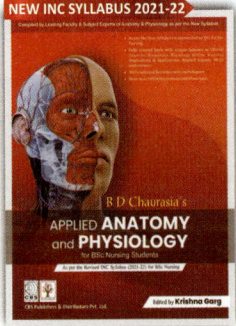

**BD Chaurasia's
Applied Anatomy and Physiology
for BSc Nursing Students**
Krishna Garg
978-93-90619-65-8
1/e, 2022

TBA

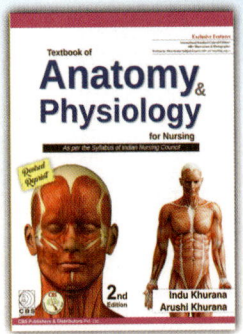

**Textbook of
Anatomy & Physiology for Nursing**
Indu Khurana et al.
978-93-86827-12-8
2/e, 2018

MRP: ₹995/-

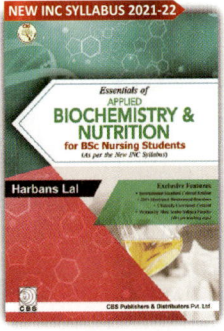

**Essentials of APPLIED
Biochemistry & Nutrition
for BSc Nursing Students**
Harbans Lal
978-93-90619-41-2
1/e, 2022

MRP: ₹450/-

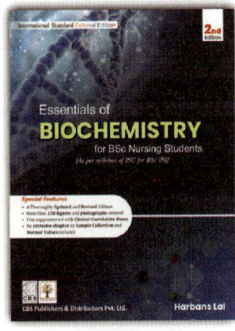

**Essentials of
Biochemistry
for BSc Nursing Students**
Harbans Lal
978-81-948693-3-7
2/e, 2022

MRP: ₹450/-

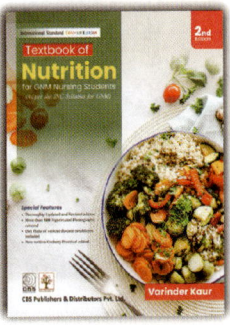

**Textbook of
Nutrition
for GNM Nursing Students**
Varinder Kaur
978-93-90619-02-3
2/e, 2022

MRP: ₹295/-

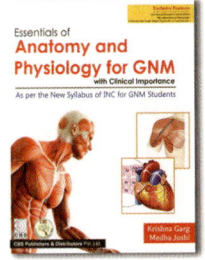

**Essentials of
Anatomy & Physiology for GNM
with Clinical Importance**
Krishna Garg et al.
978-93-86827-11-1
1/e, 2018

MRP: ₹475/-

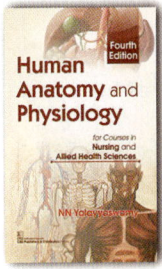

**Human Anatomy and Physiology
for Nurses**
N.N. Yalayyaswamy
978-93-87085-16-9
4/e, 2018

MRP: ₹395/-

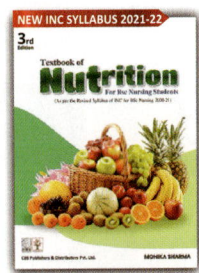

**Textbook of
Nutrition
for BSc Nursing Students**
Monika Sharma
978-93-90619-02-3
3/e, 2022

MRP: ₹370/-

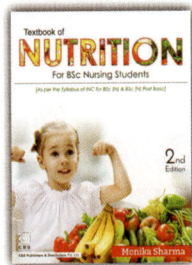

**Textbook of Nutrition
for BSc Nursing Students**
Monika Sharma
978-93-89261-92-9
2/e, 2019

MRP: ₹370/-

Nursing Knowledge Tree

NURSING NEXT SOCIAL

Nursing Next Live

Others

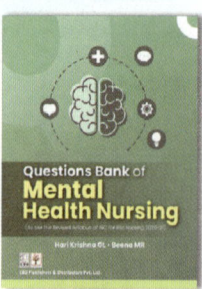

**Questions Bank of
Mental Health Nursing**
Hari Krishna GL et al.
978-93-90619-46-7
1/e, 2022

TBA

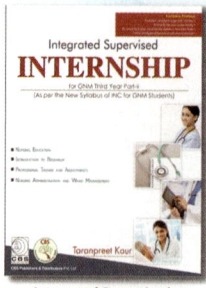

**Integrated Supervised
Internship**
for GNM Third Year Part-II
Taranpreet Kaur
978-93-88108-89-8
1/e, 2018

MRP: ₹415/-

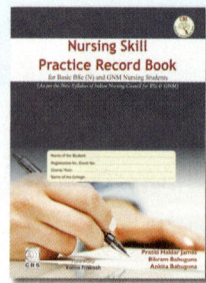

**Nursing Skill
Practice Record Book**
for Basic BSc (N) and GNM Nursing Students
Pratiti Haldar James et al.
978-93-86827-38-8
1/e, 2018-19

MRP: ₹310/-

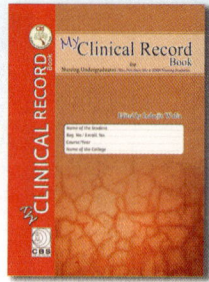

**My Clinical Record Book
for Nursing Undergraduates**
(BSc, Post Basic BSc & GNM Nursing Studen
Indarjit Walia
978-81-23927-04-6
1/e, 2017-18

MRP: ₹325/-

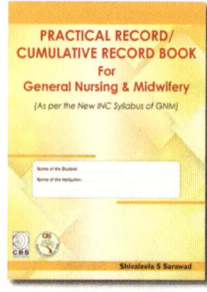

**Practical Record/
Cumulative Record Book
for General Nursing & Midwifery**
Shivaleela S Sarawad
978-93-86827-03-6
1/e, 2018

MRP: ₹225/-

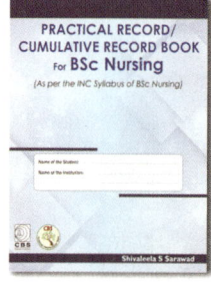

**Practical Record/
Cumulative Record Book
for BSc Nursing**
Shivaleela S Sarawad
978-93-86827-01-2
1/e, 2017

MRP: ₹210/-

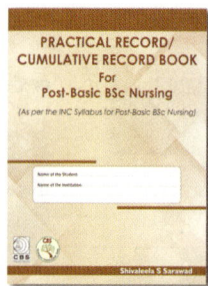

**Practical Record/
Cumulative Record Book
for Post-Basic BSc Nursing**
Shivaleela S Sarawad
978-93-86827-02-9
1/e, 2018

MRP: ₹225/-

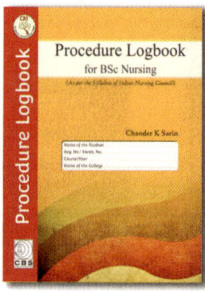

**Procedure Logbook
for BSc Nursing**
Chander K Sarin
978-93-86310-46-0
1/e, 2017

MRP: ₹210/-

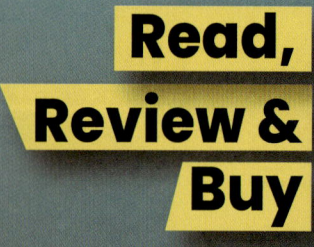
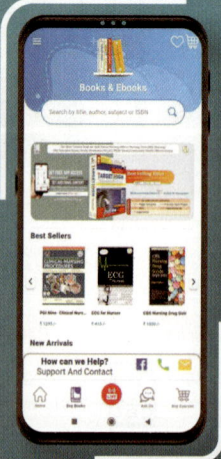
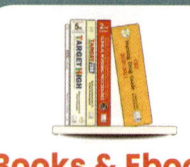
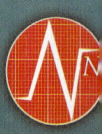

KUHS Series (Kerala University of Health Sciences)

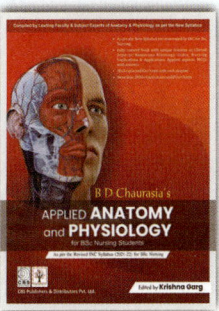

BD Chaurasia's
Applied Anatomy and Physiology
for BSc Nursing Students
Krishna Garg
978-93-90619-65-8
1/e, 2022

TBA

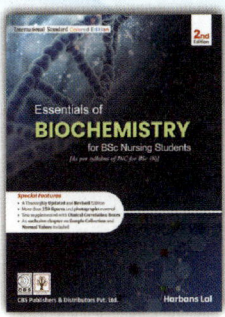

Essentials of Biochemistry
for BSc Nursing Students (As per KUHS)
Harbans Lal
978-81-948693-3-7
2/e, 2022

MRP: ₹450/-

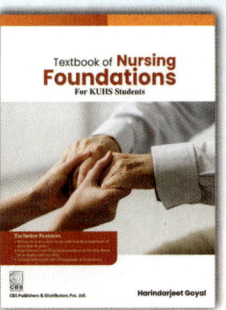

Textbook of
Nursing Foundations
for BSc Nursing (As per KUHS)
Harindarjeet Goyal
978-93-90619-38-2
1/e, 2022

MRP: ₹950/-

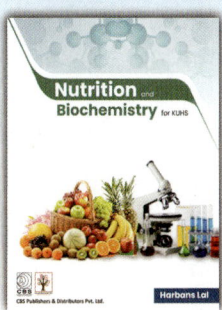

Textbook of
Nutrition & Biochemistry
for BSc Nursing (As per KUHS)
Harbans Lal
978-93-90619-32-0
1/e, 2022

MRP: ₹450/-

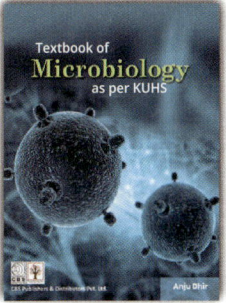

Textbook of
Microbiology
for BSc Nursing (As per KUHS)
Anju Dhir
978-93-90619-49-8
1/e, 2022

MRP: ₹725/-

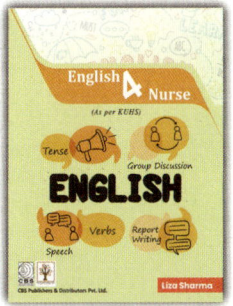

English 4 Nurses
for BSc Nursing (As per KUHS)
Liza Sharma
978-93-90619-33-7
1/e, 2022

MRP: ₹495/-

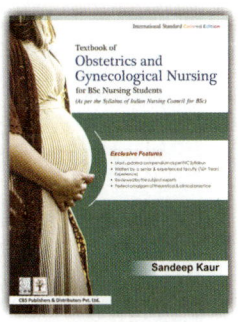

Textbook of
Obstetrics & Gynecological Nursing
for BSc Nursing (As per KUHS)
Sandeep Kaur
978-93-90619-48-1
1/e, 2022

MRP: ₹895/-

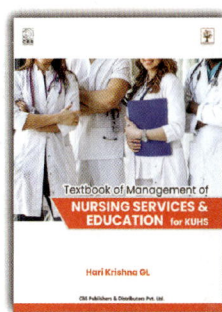

Textbook of
Nursing Management
for BSc Nursing (As per KUHS)
Hari Krishna GL et al.
978-93-90619-39-9
1/e, 2022

MRP: ₹695/-

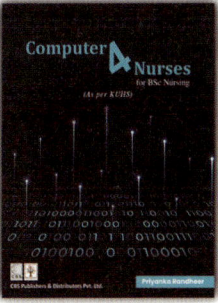

Computer 4 Nurses
for BSc Nursing (As per KUHS)
Priyanka Randheer
978-93-90619-62-7
1/e, 2022

MRP: ₹370/-

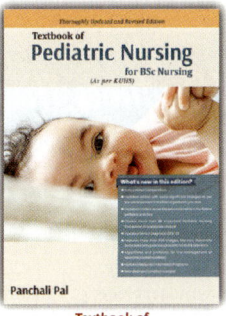

Textbook of
Pediatric Nursing
for BSc Nursing (As per KUHS)
Panchali Pal
978-93-90619-80-1
1/e, 2022

MRP: ₹795/-

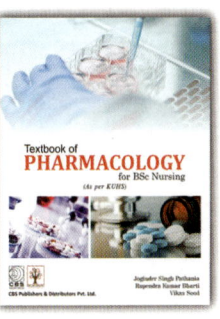

Textbook of
Pharmacology
for BSc Nursing (As per KUHS)
Joginder Singh Pathania et al.
978-93-90619-28-3
1/e, 2022

MRP: ₹650/-

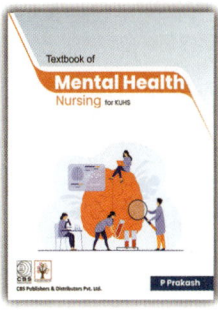

Textbook of
Mental Health Nursing
for BSc Nursing (As per KUHS)
P Prakash
978-93-90619-81-8
1/e, 2022

MRP: ₹625/-

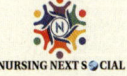

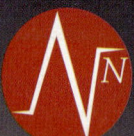
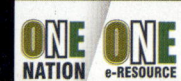
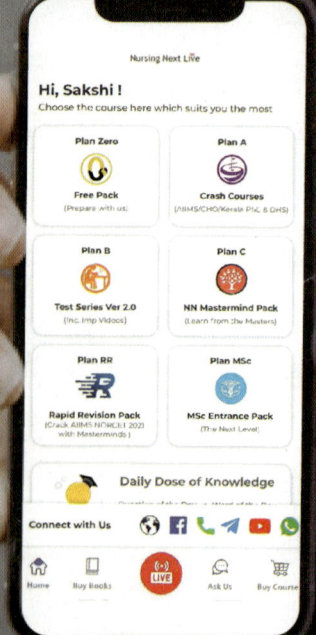
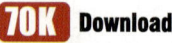
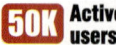

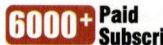

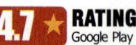

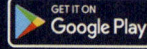
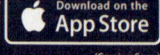
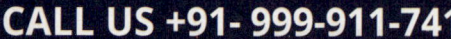